MANAGING CARE IN PRACTICE

Managing Care in Practice

This book forms part of the core text for the Open University course K303 *Managing Care* and is related to other materials available to students, including two more texts also published by Routledge:

- *Managing Care in Context* (Book 1)
- *The Managing Care Reader* (Course Reader).

If you are interested in studying this course, or related courses, please write to the Information Officer, School of Health and Social Welfare, The Open University, Walton Hall, Milton Keynes MK7 6AA, UK.

Details are also given on our web page at www.open.ac.uk

> The management of social care has never posed as many challenges as now, as practitioners navigate their way through the complexities of social care delivery against a background of constant change and the incentives for integration and the breakdown of traditional barriers.
>
> *Managing Care in Practice* offers a rich and diverse source of material for social care managers that illuminates the complexity and provides potential models with a proven track record, as well as introducing us to the model of practice-led management. It has been built on the direct experiences of frontline managers and is a credible tool for busy managers, since it is evidently based on reality.
>
> (Peter Kemp, Director of Social Services, Durham)

> This fine new course was prepared with extensive input from health and social care users. It gives comprehensive guidance to all the management themes needed by first line managers and succeeds in situating them firmly within a framework where the service user is at the centre of the care picture. As such it is well situated to deliver the much more service user-focused aims of modern health care policy.
>
> (Jude Wildwood, User Involvement Worker)

> For those of us who became managers by accident or by being in the right place at the right time and therefore received little initial training or preparation for becoming a manager, it is good to know that books such as this are around. This book will prove an invaluable guide to the new manager. It might also benefit the more experienced manager and challenge their thinking.
>
> (Martin Armitage, Project Manager Mental Health and Learning Disabilities, Easington Primary Care Trust)

Managing Care in Practice

Edited by

Janet Seden and Jill Reynolds
The Open University

A maze ... is a kind of machine with people as its moving parts.
(Carol Shields, 1997, *Larry's Party*, London, Fourth Estate, p. 218)

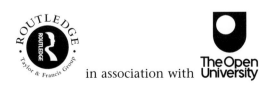

in association with **TheOpen University**

This book forms part of an Open University course K303 *Managing Care*. Details of this and other Open University courses can be obtained from the Course Information and Advice Centre, PO Box 724, The Open University, Milton Keynes MK7 6ZS, United Kingdom: tel. +44 (0)1908 653231; e-mail ces-gen@open.ac.uk

Alternatively, you may visit the Open University website at www.open.ac.uk where you can learn more about the wide range of courses and packs offered at all levels by The Open University.

To purchase this publication or other components of Open University courses, contact Open University Worldwide Ltd, The Open University, Walton Hall, Milton Keynes MK7 6AA, United Kingdom: tel. +44 (0)1908 858785; fax +44 (0)1908 858787; e-mail ouwenq@open.ac.uk; website www.ouw.co.uk

First published 2003 by Routledge
11 New Fetter Lane, London EC4P 4EE

Simultaneously published in the USA and Canada by Routledge
29 West 35th Street, New York, NY 10001

Routledge is an imprint of the Taylor & Francis Group

Copyright © 2003 The Open University

Edited, designed and typeset by The Open University.

Printed and bound in the United Kingdom by the Cromwell Press Limited.

ISBN 0-415-29864-4 (hbk)

ISBN 0-415-29865-2 (pbk)

1.1

30543B/k303b2prelimsi1.1

Contents

Contributors

Hilary Brown is Professor of Social Care at Canterbury Christ Church University College and a consultant in adult protection issues.

John Burton is an independent consultant who has worked in children's and adults' social care services, mostly residential care, since the 1960s. He has been a care worker, a manager, an inspector, a tutor, a researcher, an advocate, and a writer and consultant. John remains close to service users and frontline workers, and is directly involved with several social care innovations and projects.

Julie Charlesworth is a Lecturer in Management in The Open University Business School. Her research interests include inter-agency working, local governance, public management, and the role of volunteers in health and social care services. Her publications focus on partnership in health and social care, health improvement, local politics, and qualitative research methods.

Les Gallop has a background in social work, social work management and social services training and staff development. He now works part-time at Leicester University School of Social Work and at the Centre for Social Care Studies, De Montfort University. He also works independently in social care-related fields and for District Audit.

Roger Gomm is a lecturer in the School of Health and Social Welfare at The Open University. He has considerable experience of writing open learning courses relevant to adult services. He has practice knowledge and experience of financial management in the voluntary social care sector.

Martin Ousley has experience of working in and managing children's services units in social services. He has also developed management reporting from databases and he managed the data migration team at Anite Public Sector.

Mark Peel is Director of Social Work studies at The Open University. He has experience as an academic and a social work manager of supporting, appraising and supervising staff at different stages of their professional development. Through the National Open Learning Diploma in Social Work Programme, he is involved in the training of more than one in ten social workers in the UK.

Jill Reynolds is a Senior Lecturer in the School of Health and Social Welfare at The Open University. She has experience as a manager, training adviser and supervisor in the voluntary sector in the UK and Australia. Her work at the OU has involved writing on mental health and social work. Her research interests and publications include education, training and practice issues, feminist practice, identity and singleness, and meanings of care and support. She co-edited *The Managing Care Reader* (2003, Routledge).

Anita Rogers is Lecturer in Human Resource Development in the School of Health and Social Welfare at The Open University. She has been in the UK for four years, coming from southern California where she was involved in human resource development in education and health care. At the same time she was head of employee development at a San Diego university. The focus of her research is on the formation of scholarly communities of care in health and education, and the development of post-industrial leadership processes.

John Rowlands is a Social Services Inspector working on children's social care policy for the Department of Health. His current interests are information requirements, costs, service planning and children's outcomes indicators. He previously worked as a social worker and manager in local authorities and the voluntary sector.

Jeanne Samson Katz is a Senior Lecturer in the School of Health and Social Welfare at The Open University. Her primary teaching and research interests relate to caring for dying and bereaved people in different settings. Most recently she has undertaken two Department of Health-funded research projects exploring the terminal care needs of older people in residential and nursing homes and the related training needs for carers.

Janet Seden is a Lecturer in the School of Health and Social Welfare at The Open University. She worked as a probation officer and social worker and lectured at Leicester University before taking up her present post in 1999 as Lecturer in the School of Health and Social Welfare at The Open University. She is the author of *Counselling Skills in Social Work Practice* (1999, Open University Press), and has published on the assessment and provision of services for children and their families; social work processes; children and spirituality; and practice teaching. She is also a counselling tutor and supervisor.

David Shemmings is a Senior Lecturer in social work at the University of East Anglia. He is the author of numerous publications on empowerment and participation. Currently he is researching adult attachment theory in later life filial relationships. Before moving to UEA in 1988, David was a senior manager in Essex Social Services Department, which included responsibility for children's services and community care. He is the co-ordinator of Making Research Count in the Eastern Region.

Yvonne Shemmings had 13 years' experience as a qualified social worker, supervisor and manager in children's services and community care before her current role as an independent consultant. She has written and researched extensively on child protection and adult care. Her book *Death, Dying and Residential Care* was published by Avebury in 1996. To help promote research-mindedness in practice, Yvonne has developed an online service offering support to practitioners and managers seeking evidence-based information.

Gary Spolander is Head of Performance Management for Wolverhampton City Primary Care Trust. He is a tutor for The Open University, and previously was a visiting lecturer for Birmingham University. He has operational experience in the NHS and Social Services, including experience as an approved mental health social worker.

Adrian Ward is Senior Lecturer in Social Work at the University of East Anglia. He has written extensively about group care, and is an experienced practitioner, manager and groupworker. He has managed a therapeutic children's home, and established the MA in Therapeutic Child Care at the University of Reading.

Editors' acknowledgements

This Open University book has been written in collaboration with several people. The editors would like to thank the various contributors.

First, thanks go to the authors who wrote or collaborated with the course team in writing the chapters: their details are given in full on pages vii–ix. The editors also want to thank Giles Darvill, John R. Hudson, Patricia Kearney, Steve Onyett, Richard Poxton, Eileen Shearer and Ganga Westwood for their ideas and suggestions during the early stage of the production process, and Fran Orford for providing the cartoons.

We greatly appreciate the help of a large number of people across the UK who generously gave time to work with us. They include the managers, practitioners and service users who attended the many workshops and interviews that we set up in Belfast, Bristol, Leeds, Leicester, Edinburgh, Newcastle, Durham, Oxford, Stoke, Witney, York and Carlisle during 2000 and 2001. Thanks also to the workers and members at Redcar and Cleveland Mind and Coram Family. In Leicester, thanks to City Social Services Family Centre and Children's Homes Managers (Child Care Resources), Family Service Unit, Homestart, the Rathbone Project, Compass Children's Services, and the Centre for Deaf People. Thanks are also due to Milton Keynes Homestart, Broxtowe Family Centre, Surestart Mansfield and Penny Hajek for their help with interviews. Special thanks to the service users and managers at all these places whose comments, ideas and examples appear throughout this book, and to the managers who wrote or recorded their diaries for us, whose work we have quoted extensively.

This book has gone through a rigorous developmental testing process. Our thanks to Ganga Westwood and her equal opportunities group of Rohhss Chapman, Amerjeet Rebolo, Louise Townson, Judith Ward and Jude Wildwood, plus the critical readers group of Martin Armitage, John Burton, Kate Doyle, Robin Jackson, Ann Marsden, Lorraine Morgan, Christine Vigars and Jill Walker, and the course testers group of Tim Clement, Sue Robson, Joan Green, Caroline Picking and Diane Savage. We welcomed the advice given by our external assessor, Professor Richard Whipp of Cardiff Business School and Pro-Vice Chancellor of Cardiff University, whose encouragement helped shape the whole project.

The editors would also like to express gratitude to their colleagues in the K303 *Managing Care* course team: Dorothy Atkinson, Brian Dimmock, Jeanette Henderson, Ingrid Jefferys, Wendy Rose and Anne Bullman (the course manager); editors Jenny Monk and Amanda Smith, graphic designer Siân Lewis and graphic artist Sara Hack; and the course team assistant Kathy McPhee. Also our thanks to other academic colleagues in The Open University, in particular Mike Aiken, Jane Aldgate, Celia Davies,

Ronny Flynn, Roger Gomm, Julie Johnson, Vivien Martin, Linda Miller and Jenny Spouse for their academic input, comments and support.

Finally, we want to convey our thanks to the staff of The Open University who processed the text and to everyone at Routledge who was involved in its printing and distribution.

Janet Seden and Jill Reynolds, The Open University, October 2002

Acknowledgements

Grateful acknowledgement is made to the following sources for permission to reproduce material in this book.

Text

Chapter 4

Figure 4.1: Hackman, J. (1983) *Perspectives of Behaviour*, with permission of McGraw-Hill Companies.

Tables

Chapter 7

Table 7.1: York City Council, 2001.

Figures

Chapter 3

Figure 3.1: Blanchard *et al.* (1986) 'Leadership and the one minute manager', *Developing Competence and Commitment*, p. 74, © Blanchard Management Corporation, 1985.

Chapter 8

Figure 8.1: screenshot, Copyright © Data Analysis Network for Children's Services.

Illustrations

Chapter 1

p. 21: Copyright © Fran Orford Cartoons.

Chapter 2

p. 35 and p. 47: Copyright © Fran Orford Cartoons.

Chapter 3

p. 76: Copyright © Fran Orford Cartoons.

Chapter 4

Chapter 5

Chapter 6

Chapter 7

Chapter 8

Chapter 10

Chapter 11

Chapter 12

Introduction

This book provides a new look at management in action in care settings. The authors write about the day-to-day realities of managing care and apply the knowledge that fits with the purposes, values and concerns of users and practitioners in care settings. The book forms part of the course materials for the Open University course *Managing Care*. It includes ideas from the established management literature and introduces the key theme of *practice-led management*, by which we mean an active engagement with the interface between the best of practice and management issues.

The companion volume, *Managing Care in Context*, looks at the pace of change in social care services and how that shapes the contexts in which managers work. *Managing Care in Practice* is also embedded in the contemporary frameworks within which managers work, such as legal requirements, competing values, user involvement, performance measurement and initiatives such as Best Value. However, our focus here is on exploring and developing the practice issues and tasks that such contextual elements create for managers.

The contributing authors represent a wide range of academics, researchers, managers and practitioners drawn from educational institutions, health and social care advisory bodies, and government departments as well as The Open University academic team. Therefore, there is a variety of written styles and a diversity of approaches reflecting the different writers' interests, experience or specialist knowledge. All the contributions aim to offer knowledge that will enable managers in care settings to develop and enhance their own practice in the context of the fast-changing environments in which they work.

Managing Care in Practice selectively draws on theories for practice for their relevance to the social care field, and works through them in relation to real examples from different care settings. Readers are helped to discriminate between different theories and models and encouraged to think about their applicability to their own practice or interests. There are no 'quick fixes' or simple guides to action. Managing in social care requires a responsive, active engagement with the dilemmas, constraints and opportunities of daily practice.

What is a practice-led manager? We argue that a practice-led manager keeps to the fore service users and the best outcomes for them when managing services. They are managers whose management practice is informed by the values and ethics of social care, while at the same time meeting the requirements of government, employers and policy makers. This balancing act is not easy: it requires innovative thinking and creativity. It is also a management style informed by user involvement and practitioner experience and knowledge for making decisions about services. Above all, it is a model of managing where the leadership offered is active and not passive, although sometimes the decision to 'wait' or 'monitor' is a positive choice.

The practice-led manager engages with the problems, acts on the concerns and keeps in touch with the issues of service users and workers. This means they do not have neat and easy solutions at their fingertips. Policies and practice are worked out at the interfaces of public policy directives, workers' experience and service users' voices. Practice-led managers are not management gurus, whose magic wand makes all well. Far from it – managing in care means accepting human frailty, including your own, and the inevitability of making mistakes at times. These mistakes are then used to find learning points for the future, while still trying to improve matters in the present.

Practice-led management means tolerating uncertainty and anxiety while seeking the best possible solutions in the circumstances. It means facing dilemmas and conflicts of interest and trying to find a way through. This includes the challenge of working in partnership with a range of people and organisations. While this theme of practice-led management is developed and articulated more fully in some chapters than others, it underpins the approach throughout this book.

Managing Care in Practice is informed by the experiences of frontline managers as they engage with their tasks. Appendix 1 gives a full description of the process of consultations with managers, practitioners and service users (for the purposes of preparing this book and the other course materials). Managers' voices are heard throughout the book: expressing their dilemmas, concerns, solutions, joys and frustrations. Despite the pressures, demands and stresses of the work, many managers we spoke to asserted they would not change their job.

For many frontline managers there is considerable job satisfaction when services are improved for individuals or a particular group. There is the satisfaction of a service user's quality of life being changed for the better, or of enabling a worker to obtain a qualification. Managing a team can be a very positive experience. The practice wisdom of these contributors is there to illustrate theoretical ideas and to ground discussions in the realities of life in care agencies. There is a balance between managers sharing their struggles and difficulties as well as their good times and achievements. Management is rarely one or the other: it is more of a mixed experience.

Managers can be blamed when things go wrong in care services. Yet at the same time they are expected to learn 'on the job', with little opportunity for management training. More recently there has been a growing awareness that better management is the key to improving services and that attention to managers' training needs is essential to achieve this. The application of management theory to care in an integrated way is still in its infancy. There continues to be some scepticism when management theories are applied to the daily realities of care work.

This is healthy and this book seeks to encourage a dialogue about how managers of care might apply well-established management ideas and acquire the confidence to compare and evaluate different approaches to managing.

Therefore, this book will be useful if you already have a management post, or if you are planning to become a manager as your next career step, or if you are simply interested in how care services are organised and managed. Whether you are a care co-ordinator, or a social work team manager, or a manager of a children's home, a day centre for disabled people, an early years education/care centre, or a nursing or care home for older people, there is something of interest to you here. If you are involved in educating other people this book will be a key resource to help you keep up with demands for improved education and training in social care management or to mentor workers through Scottish and National Vocational Qualifications (S/NVQs). As new awards based on occupational standards are introduced, this relevant and accessible textbook can support such curricula and help candidates preparing for vocational assessment at levels 4 and 5. It can also support the development of a post-qualifying portfolio on 'enabling others'.

Structure of the book

This book is written in an accessible style, with helpful summaries of key points at the end of each section of a chapter. There is a logical progression that makes it worthwhile to read the chapters sequentially. However, the contributions are also written to make sense as independent chapters, so you may prefer to dip into different parts of the book. Each part has an introduction, which gives more detailed guidance on the chapter themes. The index can be used as a guide to key terms and discussions.

Part 1 Managing with Knowledge and a Vision sets the agenda for practice-led managing. What makes a good leader? What kind of vision for change and what kind of knowledge and values do managers need? Some leaders use their personality and strong ideas to abuse and harm. Conveying your vision to other people and leading from the evidence about good outcomes in care is one way of being ethical and providing strong leadership based on professional wisdom and knowledge rather than personal power. An approach that draws on evidence-based practice can underpin and ground management decisions in what is thought to work best. What skills and qualities for building a team work together well? Some people think it is easier to choose their own team from the outset. However, few managers have this luxury, so we consider how to draw out the best from the group they have inherited. Change is pervasive in care, so we look at how it is best managed and what kind of initiative managers may want to take. These are all important issues for managers to get to grips with.

Part 2 Managing Services for People is the hub of what managing care is about and some key issues predominate. Services are rarely the responsibility of a single agency nowadays. What is it like for people when they fall through the net because no one takes responsibility for co-ordinating a response to their needs? The issues of working in partnership and achieving effective collaboration are not simply administrative concerns. It is essential to manage co-ordination well; to make sure that people receive a service that meets their needs; and to ensure that each agency plays its part in doing that effectively. Money is also a people issue. Services need to be paid for and service users worry about whether they can afford what they need. In inter-agency meetings to co-ordinate services, managers must be clear about what resources their agency can commit. Understanding budgets and Best Value is a crucial part of managers working together at a local level. Likewise, issues of sharing information are key. Who needs to know? What for? What are people's concerns about the ways confidential information is shared in practice? Decisions about money and information are changed by the requirement to work across agency boundaries. The final chapter in this part, 'Managing to protect', brings the multi-agency working agenda full circle, as responsibilities to protect adults and children are explored at societal, agency and individual levels. Too often people have been neglected or suffered harm because no one managed their situation in a way which ensured they were safe and their rights to dignity, choice, respect and privacy were protected.

Part 3 Managing Learning and Development in the Team develops a theme begun in Part 1. Here we focus on the need for managers to learn all the time, through the situations they are called on to manage. We begin by considering how mistakes happen and suggesting that mistakes in care settings are an inevitable part of the complexity of the issues service users bring to agencies. Managers learn through the mistakes and challenges they experience, and this learning should lead to improved services. Managers also learn from the users of their services, as well as from the workers they manage, as they respond to the significant events in their lives, such as moving home, changing job or coping with loss. This kind of learning from experience is embedded in the very nature of the job. Taking account of significant feelings and crises in people's lives is an essential part of managing care. We argue that managing with humanity is also an essential part of a manager's role. The final chapter takes a holistic view of managers' responsibilities for the professional and career development of their staff. We explore how, from the moment a worker joins the team, the manager is involved in their career development. This responsibility for development continues through induction, supervision and appraisal up to the time a member of staff moves on.

Part 1 Managing with Knowledge and a Vision

Introduction

Managers of care services need knowledge and a vision. They need knowledge about 'what works' in their field, knowledge about the impact of services on service users and carers, and a vision that can encourage and unite people to work together and cope with unrelenting change. This may sound like a tall order, so in Part 1 we seek to unravel the practicalities of managing and the skills required, through real-life examples from different care settings.

The central theme running throughout this book – *practice-led management* – is introduced and developed in Part 1. Newly appointed managers moving on from a role as practitioner bring a wealth of practice expertise and judgement, providing a solid foundation for acquiring management skills. If their background is not in practice, or it is in a very different area of expertise from the people they manage, they need to inform themselves and develop their understanding of key practice issues. Managers generally move from being responsible for their own practice to taking on responsibility for other people's practice. They are no longer judged solely on what they do, but on the efforts of the whole team or unit. Therefore, managers have a key role in developing the practice of other people and ensuring they work competently. This involves managers in developing the ability to appreciate the different ways other workers might approach key tasks, and the validity of their expertise as practitioners. Managers also pass on information and their own practice knowledge. When managing a multidisciplinary team, there is the challenge of managing and supporting people with different training, professional expertise and contributions to make to the work.

There are connections between managers who are practice-led and those who aspire to develop an organisation that learns from and improves its practices. The notion of a 'learning organisation' is highlighted for consideration in Chapter 1. The need for managers to learn and encourage other people in learning – from the team, through skill development, through shared and distributed leadership, in responding to and initiating change, and in using evidence from research and practice – relates to the discussion throughout Part 1. The theme of learning and development in the team is taken further in Part 3. The conscious use of learning from practice, so that an organisation is transformed at all levels to provide more satisfaction to its service users and a better working environment for its staff, is rare but increasingly seen as central to effective organisations. Frontline managers can contribute to efforts to learn from practice and participate in a feedback loop that brings improvements. Indeed, they hold critical information that their organisation needs.

In Chapter 1 'Becoming a manager: acting or reacting?', Reynolds looks at issues for people who are managing for the first time, and points to some key areas of development. The twin facets of managerial work are explored: *acting* – planning and shaping practice and services towards good outcomes for service users; and *reacting* –

dealing with unexpected events and responding to new directives. How can managers find a balance, so that they feel in control of their job rather than controlled by it? The suggestions include keeping a focus on the organisation's primary task, extending the areas of choice available, and turning intentions into obligations, all of which are considered in turn. Good time management also helps managers to cope, although sometimes there may simply be too much to do.

In Chapter 2 'Managing the team', Ward emphasises the crucial contribution of teamwork. The team is the way in which managers get things done. Careful nurturing and developing of teamwork skills can mean the whole is greater than the sum of its parts. Using examples drawn from residential care, Ward demonstrates the interdependence of team members and the importance of good communication between them. The team leader can be seen as requiring some of the skills of an orchestral conductor: bringing out the best in people to enhance the performance of the whole group. In practice, this means focusing on the interpersonal dynamics of leadership, and thinking about how to inspire people and help them to inspire each other. 'Leadership and vision' is the subject of Chapter 3, in which Rogers and Reynolds consider how managers can encourage leadership from other people, whether in their team, in the organisation or in collaborative work with different agencies. They explore leadership style, and the extent to which managers can and should adapt their personal style to the different needs of situations and people. Frontline managers may not always feel they have much opportunity to influence the grander vision and strategy of their organisation. Rogers and Reynolds argue that, none the less, they play a role in the vision sequence, even at the level of putting it into practice and looking for better ways of doing things. Practice-led managers relay their experience from the front line back to more senior management so that they can contribute to strategic planning.

In Chapter 4 'Managing change', Rogers and Reynolds consider the context of change in care services. They argue that managing *is* managing change and describe it as a continuous process, rather than a neat and tidy event with clear start and finish points. Different models are used and applied to an example of a major change process in a service for adults with learning disabilities. Here again, the vision of what might be, and how to do things better, acts as a major incentive to everyone concerned to take part in change that is inevitably disruptive for individuals.

In the final chapter in this part, 'Supporting evidence-based practice and research-mindedness', David and Yvonne Shemmings consider the manager's role in encouraging team members to inform their practice through the conscious and judicious use of evidence. This means developing critical skills in appraising research studies and becoming aware of the scope and limitations of the different research methods. More widely, it includes consulting service users and carers about their experience, using theoretical frameworks and drawing on a range of sources of practice experience and wisdom. These different sources of knowledge inform the kind of managing called for in the title of Part 3. The levels of awareness of current research findings among workers and managers in social care do not appear to be generally high. Shemmings and Shemmings suggest that the changes needed would involve a transformation of practice. None the less, they argue there are things managers can do to change attitudes and stimulate enquiry and they outline some practical steps.

Chapter 1
Becoming a manager: acting or reacting?

Jill Reynolds

1.1   Introduction

In this chapter I look at some of the key issues for new managers in getting to grips with the role. For people who are managing care services for the first time there is often a big transition to be made from being 'a practitioner' to being 'a manager'. What are the overlaps and distinctions between these two roles? Managers in the front line are still likely to be near to the delivery of a service, and they are responsible for the quality of that service and the practice that goes into it. A theme here is what it means for managers to be 'practice-led'.

Care services are going through major change: the government's vision is that they should be 'proactive' (Neate, 2000). This implies creativity and taking initiatives. So, active managers are needed who can take hold of the work, sometimes in new kinds of organisations or with unfamiliar groups of staff working together, and shape their own roles and the kind of service being offered. As well as *acting* with confidence, there is a place for *reacting*. Managers are the channel for a great deal of information and communication, and they need to be responsive to all of it. This chapter explores how managers can balance the different demands on them; how they can be clear about the objectives of their organisation and their role in achieving them; how they can manage their time in unpredictable environments; and how they need to use their judgement in problem solving and decision making. There are no easy formulae to resolve these matters. Many managers were consulted in the development of this book and this chapter draws on their experience and ideas (see Appendix 1 for a description of the consultation process).

The aims of this chapter are to:

- review what is involved in moving from practice in care services to management
- argue the importance of a continued focus on practice and a practice-led approach to managing
- consider the manager's role in working towards a 'learning organisation'
- discuss the potential for managers to extend their ability to make choices over how they spend their time
- review the manager's different roles in making decisions.

1.2   From practising to managing

> But being a manager is not something you set out to do is it?
>
> Are you sure?
>
> I think it's much more that you sort of just become a manager, don't you? You know, you start off doing a real – I mean a – you know, an actual job and then you end up getting promoted. And then you're the manager.
>
> (Watson, 1994, p. 29)

It is not unusual for new managers in all fields to feel that they are searching for their identity. If you are a new frontline manager, the personal change of moving into a management position will often concern self-concept (Who am I?) as you begin to develop your new sets of relationships at work. Some managers in our consultations referred to 'loss' as an aspect of taking on a management role:

> There's also an issue of loss in there, isn't there? About the loss of the previous role as well as the new exciting management role. So often people would be promoted within the team, or at least within an area where you know your colleagues quite well, and it's about being able to leave that role behind and adopt another role.
>
> (Community manager, manager consultations)

The move is often experienced as an organisational move from being 'one of us' to being 'one of them': for example, those people who sit in an office or who allocate work. Somehow, through this move, people seem to treat you differently. Conversations appear to end abruptly when you arrive on the scene, and you do not get included so readily in those small but interesting discussions that are non-work-related. Much of this hinges on the notion of 'in-groups', 'out-groups' and group identity, and some of the edges are smoothed out as relationships are re-established, especially in terms of trust (Gallop, 2001).

How big is the change from practitioner to manager? Links can be made between the different roles. The kinds of work that make up the world of practice span a wide range, much of which involves an ability to manage yourself. Practice is a meeting place between the needs of service users and the responses and initiatives that an agency offers. Practice is both *what* is done and *how* it is done.

While the activities of practitioners in social care are not easily defined, as they will vary by context, some common skills are needed. Making and maintaining relationships with service users, undertaking assessments, planning appropriate responses, evaluating risk and potential for harm, and developing arrangements for joint working are all central to the care task (NVQ Level 4 New Care Awards, 1998). Most of these revolve around working with people, which gives an immediate connection with much managerial work.

Rosen points out that good practice and good management both involve working with people to achieve tasks; working to solve complex problems, or to manage those that are insoluble; and working to achieve change in social situations and relationships (Rosen, 2000, p. 16). The core difference is probably that the manager's focus is on managing the practice of other people.

The people aspects of the frontline manager role were emphasised by many of those interviewed during the research for this book (see Appendix 1):

> Giving people the ability to do the job that's in front of them.
> (Project manager, mental health services, manager consultations)

> First line management means to me the staff in the project, first and foremost. I give supervision very high priority in my work, because unless the staff in the team remain focused, motivated, clear about their roles, supported, I don't believe this project could function.
> (Team manager, voluntary sector project, manager consultations)

> Somebody who really values you as a person and values the skills and experience that you bring, and a person who can really harness that and develop that and listen to your ideas in a team, and take your ideas forward, but also give you ownership of what you've contributed. I feel very strongly that management is a role to get the best out of your workers.
> (Project worker, voluntary sector project, manager consultations)

Most people's idea of a manager is someone who is *responsible for the work of others* (Stewart, 1991). However, to limit a definition to being in charge of people would exclude those who have a more strategic role, for instance in a newly developing area, or those who liaise across departments or divisions in relation to a specialist aspect such as fostering and adoption. Watson suggests that *organising* is a key feature of managing:

> Managing is organising: pulling things together and along in a general direction to bring about long-term organisational survival.
> (Watson, 1994, p. 33)

If the job shapes the activities of the organisation as a whole in some way, and helps it to keep going, this makes it managerial in Watson's view. Practitioners and managers in social care might question his stress on *organisational* survival. This is perhaps a limited aim in comparison with striving for better standards and provision. Indeed, the boundaries of many organisations may change or disappear as new forms of partnership develop to make services more accessible and logical from the service user's point of view. On the other hand, if the organisation is not there to argue for the continued existence of services, these too may disappear. Is it the *organisation* that is important or the *services* that it provides, and can one be had without the other?

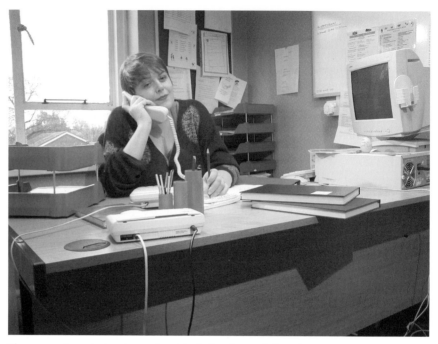

The move from being 'one of us' to being 'one of them'

Practice-led management

The focus of this book is on frontline managers in care services. The major change at this level of managing is from engagement in direct practice with service users and their families to *managing the practice of others*. Depending on the context, however, this does not always mean leaving involvement in practice completely: it may be a matter of different balances between managing and practising in different contexts.

Managers in residential and other forms of group care, for instance, may be crucially involved in direct work themselves, while needing to keep an organisational overview that 'pulls things together and along'. In many areas there are 'senior practitioners' who have their own caseload and supervise colleagues on practice issues; some will have line management responsibilities in this role. Of course, many practitioners also have some management responsibilities, perhaps involving responsibility for their budgets, or liaison with others on behalf of the organisation. Causer and Exworthy (1999) remark that, for these reasons, making a hard-and-fast distinction between managers and practitioners is difficult. From this point of view perhaps practising and managing can be seen as a continuum, and identifying the managing aspects in particular jobs may be more important than seeking to define some jobs as managerial and others as not.

These links between practice and management are very important in considering the role of the frontline manager. Whatever the layers and length of lines of accountability and management in an organisation, the frontline manager is the closest person in the managerial hierarchy to the delivery of the service or the practice. This is sometimes called *operational* management. It gives the frontline manager a unique perspective on the needs of service users, the responses they receive and the extent to which responses meet needs. The main business of agencies concerned with social care is to ensure the best possible quality of life for those who use their services. While *strategic* decisions by senior managers about the shape and kind of service will set the overall parameters, the frontline manager is in touch with the action 'at the sharp end', and this carries particular responsibilities. In small organisations the frontline manager may also be the chief executive, in which case they will be involved at both these levels. According to Rosen (2000, p. 14), the frontline manager in care services also has a key *professional* role to see that:

- practice standards are set and maintained
- practitioners are supported in complex and personally demanding practice
- practitioners are developed in knowledge- and evidence-based practice.

The frontline manager effectively models practice for the people being managed.

Because practice is so important in forming the interface between the agency and those who need its services, we have developed the term *practice-led management*. We argue that frontline managers (and their agencies) need to be practice-led, keeping in focus the demands of practice situations. This involves being responsive to what service users want. As well as direct consultation with users of the service, managers make judgements based on what they learn from practitioners. Practice-led managers do not put up a professional screen or hide behind agency policy. They promote to their senior managers the issues and challenges that emerge in the practice context, and take what opportunities they can to influence the policies and decisions surrounding these. The reason for the strong focus on practice is that packages of care and other kinds of support are not just items to be taken off the shelf and handed to people. Social care requires relationships, and the overall term for what happens in the spectrum of different relationships is *practice*.

Managing a transition

While it can reassure new managers to recognise the links between practice and management, the move from practitioner to manager is none the less experienced as a transition. Getting used to the different role and focus can involve an initial shock and some stress. Like all transitions, this needs recognition and time to practise skills in a new context, acquire new skills and generally build up confidence. Stewart (1991, pp. 7–8) cites a study of new sales managers by Hill (1991), who argues that new managers have four immediate tasks:

1   learn what it means to be a manager
2   develop their ability to judge others
3   learn more about themselves
4   learn to cope with stress and emotion.

The first one is the only task that is strictly for managers: the others may be present in any job, and in social care they are likely to be major elements in all areas of work. The difference is probably one of degree. While you are likely to be judging others in most practice decisions, the difference as a manager is the level of responsibility that you hold. Much of the time the buck stops with you, and you will want to feel confident in your judgement of other people, and indeed in how you judge *their* judgement of service users and their needs.

New managers have to come to terms with letting others do the work that they perhaps used to do, which is not always as easy as it sounds (Gallop, 2001). According to Josefowitz (1987) there are several possible delegation barriers:

- You did it well yourself, and someone else might not do it as well.
- Someone else might do it better, and you fear being replaced.
- If someone else does it, what is there for you to do?
- You might not have time to show someone else.
- There is no one to delegate to – which might really mean that there is no one you trust or who seems to have time.

One experienced manager recalls:

> When I first became a manager, I tried to do everything myself, because I had standards, and there were some people on the team who weren't meeting them, and I was very tempted to do it all. Now you can't work like that because it's not possible for one person to do everything.
>
> (Project Manager, Mental Health Services, Primary Care Group, manager consultations)

Not only is it impossible for one person to do everything, but also it is part of a manager's role to develop the competence of others so that their work meets the required standards; this includes allowing them to make mistakes and learn from them.

There may be some tensions here between being a practice-led manager and managing the work of other people. New managers may wonder how much they need to maintain their own practice base. How much is 'enough' and where does this tip over into clinging on to tasks that someone else should be doing? It is common to feel particularly uneasy when managing people from different practice backgrounds. Can social workers manage nurses and vice versa? Is it necessary to develop practice skills that were not part of an initial training? Credibility is often gained from having some practice experience (see, for instance, Kitchener *et al.*, 2003), but it might be argued that this does not have to be in precisely the same field as those being managed. Perhaps what is important is that the people who are managed feel understood in what they are trying to do. This might involve spending time with them as they do their work.

Becoming a manager is a gradual process: not every aspect of the new role can be in place right from the start. New managers need to be mindful of what kind of induction they need for their work and to plan a feasible programme for their development in consultation with more senior managers.

Key points

- Practising and managing have many common features.

- The frontline manager has a key role in managing the practice of other people.

- Becoming a manager can be a stressful transition.

- Managers need to learn to delegate and help others develop rather than try to do everything themselves.

1.3   Learning and developing

The transition to a new managerial role involves new learning, such as learning to give up some of the familiar work. Managers also learn to take on new responsibilities of organising that require more of an overview of where the work of the unit is going. ('Unit' is used here as a general term to cover a team, a project, or even the whole organisation.) Managing the interfaces of practice and the processes of consultation with service users and carers may be other areas for learning and development. The manager will probably be managing resources on a grander scale than before and learning how to use (or ration) them appropriately.

In managing other people, managers also have to think about their learning. As noted earlier, people need to be supported in personally demanding practice, and to be developed in practice informed by knowledge. The manager's role in professional development is considered in more detail in Chapter 12. Here the discussion turns to the manager's responsibility for the learning of others, and the relevance of this for a practice-led approach. The frontline manager is the person to whom practitioners look for support and guidance in their work. The manager's response to this affects the experiences and opportunities for others to learn and develop. Managers often have the opportunity to help people make links in their learning from practice. Learning from practice also holds implications for organisational change, and managers can use this kind of knowledge to help their organisations to learn and develop.

The phrase 'the learning organisation' originated in the USA in relation to business and getting a competitive edge in the market (see, for instance, Argyris and Schön, 1996; Pedler *et al.*, 1991; Senge, 1990). It builds on a sociological tradition of theorising the relationship between organisational structure and behaviour. The emphasis is on the organisation as a system which has to adapt, through learning, to the changing demands created by its environment (Gould, 2003). The concept has become of interest in health and social care services, with a focus on the 'competent workplace' as a necessary environment to foster competent staff.

The precise meaning of a learning organisation is hard to define. It may be more important at the level of a vision to be worked towards rather than as something actually accomplished. The process is continuous: it is hard, after all, to imagine an organisation that has no need to learn. Pearn and his colleagues quote Dixon's (1994) conceptualisation that learning organisations make:

> intentional use of learning processes at individual, group and system level to transform the organization in ways that are increasingly satisfying to [all] its stakeholders.
>
> (Pearn *et al.*, 1997, p. 18)

What kinds of action can managers take to help individuals learn, and how can they contribute to the learning of the organisation as a whole? They are in a strong position to promote learning from practice and enthuse others through a practice-led approach. Encouraging work towards qualifications is one way of doing this; another is to look routinely for learning in practice situations, and to share what has been learned with others. Example 1.1 describes a manager who was supported by his organisation in his vision of learning for continuous improvement.

EXAMPLE 1.1 Learning for continuous improvement

1   A manager of a group of nine residential and day care centres for adults with learning difficulties within a social services department encourages staff to take up a programme of National Vocational Qualification (NVQ) training. He becomes the first manager countywide to receive an NVQ in management.

2   Two heads of establishments join in as driving forces for the programme, and 20 people start on their care NVQs; others prepare their management portfolios or for training and development in assessment and verification. Contracts are drawn up between managers and candidates

concerning available time and other resources for learning. National occupational standards are used for the supervision of managers and frontline staff, so that staff become familiar with the standards used in NVQs. Service users regularly provide witness statements on staff performance.

3   National occupational standards are used for defining requirements – for internal and external commissioning and for reviews. The drop-out rate from NVQ activity is negligible. There are many more in-house training groups. Users are involved in applying the standards to their personal plans and in reviews of establishments: for instance, some do college-based training in kitchen hygiene. Almost everyone in the centres is engaged in the use of standards or the preparation and assessment for NVQs. Staff recruitment, absence due to sickness and staff turnover all improve. Some say this is attributable to the use of occupational standards.

Through this process staff learned to:
- define a vision of a quality service
- develop a pattern of teamwork
- improve the competence of individuals
- involve service users in their own development and in service and staff development
- develop learning skills such as analysis, written recording and verbal presentation.

(Source: adapted from Darvill, 2001)

It seems that the opportunity for workers to study and prepare together for vocational qualifications, and the way in which service users became involved as a matter of course, produced a major cultural shift in the group of centres discussed by Darvill. Example 1.2 shows how ordinary processes of intervention can lead to learning.

EXAMPLE 1.2 Enquiry, learning and knowledge creation

A team in a voluntary child care agency explores the need for work with homeless young people. Initial contacts suggest a complex set of circumstances leads some young people to choose travelling as a response. The team initiates a research project to enquire into the needs of young travellers. The findings become the basis for a report, and a series of presentations to politicians and officials convey the analysis of the problem and proposals for action.

The team adopts this process for each of its initiatives:
- investigation of need
- action

- evaluation
- enquiry.

When analysis suggests that another agency should be involved, partnerships are negotiated appropriately.

(Source: adapted from Gould, 2003)

The work in this example goes beyond organisational learning, as it involves sharing findings with other community agencies and individuals.

Sadly, it is all too easy to find examples of the problems that are created when an organisation does not encourage learning, and when feedback about improvements is not acted on. Of course, learning does go on in all organisations, whether it is encouraged or not, but learning can be negative as well as positive. According to Darvill (2001), people can learn to:

- keep out of trouble, avoid responsibility and minimise risk to themselves or their organisation
- find excuses and cover up
- put obstacles in the way of other people's progress.

However, while there are always obstacles, all managers have scope to act positively. Even if the manager and the unit are working within an overall organisational culture that is negative, the manager can still influence the attitudes of others around them. Chapters 4 and 5 discuss different strategies for introducing change and new ideas. Few people work in organisations that can claim to be fully learning organisations. It can be frustrating if your perceptions and attitudes are further along this path than those of your leaders or managers, but such a situation may just be part of the process of ongoing learning.

Key points

- Managers are involved in learning and development for themselves as well as those for whom they are responsible.

- There are ways of building in learning from practice in the workplace.

- The organisational culture affects how much scope there is for transformation at the level of the organisation, but managers do have opportunities to influence this culture.

1.4   The manager's job

We have noted connections between practice and managing, and the skills transferable between them. We turn now to the scope of the manager's job. What are the key features of the job of managing care and what qualities does it require? Core tasks are often described as managing:

- *people*
- *activities*
- *resources*
- *information*

and doing this through *managing yourself* (Martin and Henderson, 2001, p. 22). We shall use this as a framework for discussion.

Box 1.1 lists 11 qualities (or skills) of successful managers identified from research and experience by Pedler *et al.* (1994).

BOX 1.1 The qualities of successful managers

1   Command of basic facts

2   Relevant professional knowledge

3   Continuing sensitivity to events

4   Analytical, problem-solving, decision/judgement-making skills

5   Social skills and abilities

6   Emotional resilience

7   Proactivity – inclination to respond purposefully to events

8   Creativity

9   Mental agility

10   Balanced learning habits and skills

11   Self-knowledge

(Source: Pedler *et al.*, 1994, pp. 23–4)

Decision- and judgement-making skills

We shall apply the qualities listed in Box 1.1 to the work of managers of care services, starting with decision- and judgement-making skills.

Managers are responsible for the maintenance of good services, for moving events forward and for making sure that what is supposed to happen *does* happen. While many decisions may be made, or shaped up, by practitioners in the front line, the manager needs to be sure that planned action is in line with agency policy, legal requirements and available resources. Consultation and feedback from users and carers, practitioners' assessments, agency procedures, the provision and input of other agencies, local information, research findings, law and government policies are all elements that may play a part in helping managers to make decisions.

What *is* a decision? Most people make many small decisions during a day, the majority of which pass without great consideration. There are also more formal decisions that are generally acknowledged as such: the matters that are recorded in day books, on case files, through case conferences or at policy meetings. The kind of decisions to pay attention to here include the formal ones but we shall extend the net to *any* decision that affects the quality of practice and therefore the quality of the service that users receive. It is not always easy to recognise these as such and, unfortunately, it is often only when it becomes clear that something is not right that with hindsight a wrong decision can be spotted. It may be the accumulation of quite small decisions that leads to problems and complaints. Using the lens of decision making in particular, but also referring to other key qualities listed in Box 1.1, we return to the framework of the manager's core tasks.

Managing people

This is likely to involve some input into the recruitment, selection and appointment of staff (and perhaps volunteers) – plenty of decisions there. There are also decisions about what style of induction, support and supervision people need in order to be able to do their jobs. What levels of responsibility can or should they be carrying? How will they be encouraged to develop their knowledge and skills and move on in their careers? How will the ethos of the unit be developed? Qualities listed in Box 1.1 that are useful in the decisions involved in managing people are *relevant professional knowledge, social skills* and *emotional resilience* as well as *self-knowledge.*

Managing activities

Here there are decisions about who gets what services – rationing decisions as well as assessments of need and its resolution. Then there is workload allocation. There are professional judgements to be made over appropriate actions to take – routine ones as well as those relating to perceived risks or in response to a crisis. There are decisions about the end or completion of a service, perhaps because the work required has been concluded, or because the problem is deemed intractable. How will the effectiveness of activities be evaluated? The qualities of *analytical skills, sensitivity to events, professional knowledge* and *creativity* are important here.

Managing resources

Rationing again comes into play but there may also be scope for innovation. What new resources should be developed? Budgets need to be argued for, allocated and accounted for: one way of spending money needs to be weighed against alternative options. Which resources will give best value? Who needs to be involved in their evaluation? *Proactivity, creativity* and *mental agility*, as well as a good *command of basic facts*, all have a part to play.

Managing information

What is important and enduring among the deluge of information a manager receives, and where else does it need to go? Where is information stored? If mainly in the manager's head, how can it be got out of there and sent to others who need it? What new kinds of information should be sought – perhaps from users, potential users and carers – and how will that process be managed? What are the boundaries for confidentiality for such information? Again *proactivity, creativity* and *mental agility* are important and well-established *learning habits* are also needed.

Managing yourself

How do you manage your day and end it feeling that you have done enough of what needs to be done? What are the priorities? What kind of a manager do you perceive yourself to be, and how does that match others' perceptions and expectations? How do you look after yourself? *Self-knowledge* and *emotional resilience* are key here.

All of these features of a manager's work are considered in more detail in other chapters in this book. The final section of this chapter looks further at the problem-solving and decision-making aspects of the manager's role. The following sections look in particular at managing yourself: how do you achieve an acceptable balance between acting and reacting?

Key points

- Decision- and judgement-making skills are required in all aspects of managing care.

- The qualities found in successful managers generally are also relevant to managers of care services.

1.5   Acting or reacting?

John Hutton, when he was health minister, emphasised the need for an *active* and a *proactive* welfare state: 'a really proactive service making its contribution in communities felt, up and down the country' (Neate, 2000, p. 11).

Proactive managers respond purposefully to events; they also take the initiative before events overtake them. It is hard to be proactive when you are finding your way in a new role, and the title of this chapter highlights the sense that many new managers experience of either *acting* or *reacting*. Finding a balance can involve some discomfort. Acting can mean 'playing a part'. This language of the theatre is well suited to taking on a new role. The notion of the different roles of a manager is explored well in the management literature (see, for example, Handy, 1999; Mintzberg, 1975).

Sometimes you have to play the part of a manager before you feel as if you really *are* a manager. There may be aspects of control that are uncongenial – imposing deadlines, confronting people about their work – and acting the role can be a way of coping with this. Acting also means 'taking action', which is an important antidote to the feeling that many new – and not so new – managers have of being at everyone's beck and call, without the time to see a piece of work through to its completion. There can be a strong sense that the job simply involves reacting to other people's demands and, if this is so, it will be rather unsatisfying.

Reacting has its place, too, however. People need to know that they have been listened to and responded to. The frontline manager is an important channel of communication between practitioners, service users and senior managers and often needs to be in reacting mode. This requires them to face in more than one direction. Of course, managers may be in other modes at different times: just being, perhaps, or listening, reflecting, thinking and planning. The trick is to get the right balance between acting too soon, failing to take necessary action, and waiting to decide how to act. In Example 1.3 a manager in a voluntary agency describes her strategy for taking time out when demands are high.

EXAMPLE 1.3 Sitting and thinking

Maria says she learned a lot from a previous manager when she was the deputy of a day centre for people with disabilities. In a crisis, when Maria would be 'running around and looking for help', she was often surprised to see her manager just sitting there.

'Aren't you going to come and help me?' she'd say.

'There's nothing that won't wait; this five minutes won't make any difference, but it gives me time to think about what I'm going to do,' the manager would reply.

Maria now uses this strategy herself, asking whether she can call back in a few minutes when she is not sure how to respond to a difficult telephone call. 'That little bit of space maybe stops me reacting in a negative sense.'

(Source: manager consultations)

Several approaches can help in acquiring a sense of balance between acting and reacting, three of which are explored here.

Clarifying the primary task

Keeping a focus on what your organisation is here to do is a useful starting point. Burton (1998) argues that the first act of managers at all levels is to clarify the primary task of the organisation. The idea of a primary task is introduced by Bion (1968, 1980) in relation to group processes and the changing task of groups as they develop. Burton uses the concept in a more static and directional way to pinpoint the reason for the organisation's existence: the proper focus of its effort (Burton, 1993). The important question then is 'What is this organisation here to do, and what is my part in it?' (Burton, 1998, p. 48).

For the purpose of highlighting priorities, it is best to keep the definition of the primary task as simple and short as possible:

> For instance, a home for older people could define its task as 'To provide the accommodation and care which will meet the needs and choices of older people who cannot continue to get those needs and choices met in their own homes'.
>
> (Burton, 1993, p. 125)

Burton goes on to suggest that once managers have identified the primary task, it can be used as a benchmark to check activity. Everything can be tested for its relevance to the performance of the task. Anything that is not connected with achieving the primary task should be rejected. A clear definition of the primary task can help managers to check that the service also works towards appropriate outcomes.

Single-handed managers in small independent organisations may feel there is not just one primary task but many diffuse ones, all of which require action by the manager. A return to clarifying the core reason for the organisation's existence may none the less prove useful.

Reducing demands and constraints and extending choices

Managers can also explore the different kinds of pressure they experience. Stewart (1991) describes a model to analyse the job and increase the feeling of control and effectiveness, which allows managers to get a 'helicopter view' of their job. Managers, she argues, restrict their options in two main ways.

1 Exaggerating the work they must do and feeling unduly busy and unable to do less pressing but important things.

2 Exaggerating the constraints that limit what they can do.

Stewart's model is described in Box 1.2 and Figure 1.1 shows the relationship between *demands*, *constraints* and *choices*.

BOX 1.2 Demands, constraints and choices

Demands

These are the tasks that cannot be ignored. They may form part of the job description: allocating work, writing reports for senior managers, meeting performance targets, supervising other staff, for instance. As well as these minimum demands that anyone in the job would meet, people create their own demands. They do work that they think they must do, even though another person in the same job would not do it.

Constraints

These are the limitations on what managers can do, including resource limitations and other people's attitudes. They form the outer boundary to the job.

Choices

This is the area of opportunity that lies between the core of demands and the outer boundary of constraints. This is where managers make a choice to pay more attention to some tasks than others, or to take on a particular piece of work.

Jobs vary in how flexible they are, and the relationship between demands and constraints can change and affect what choices are available, perhaps because of sickness, financial changes, a change of senior managers or a new policy. While demands have to be fulfilled competently, effectiveness lies in the use of opportunities for choice. Many managers do not recognise that they have choices or they have a restricted view of the choices open to them.

(Source: adapted from Stewart, 1991, pp. 14–6)

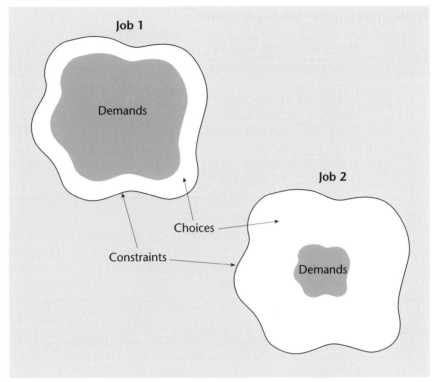

Figure 1.1 **Demands, constraints and choices** (Source: Stewart, 1991, p. 15)

Stewart argues that many managers do tasks that are not strictly important for them to do. These activities constitute 'play areas' for managers, and they do them perhaps because they feel comfortable doing activities that demonstrate their competence, even though they might appropriately be delegated to someone else in the team. This was noted in the earlier discussion of why new managers may find it hard to delegate. However, it is not only new managers who prefer to do tasks that make them feel competent.

Stewart suggests that managers also may restrict the choices available to them: strategic thinking about the job is hard to do and involves taking a broader view of its scope. The key question managers can ask themselves is 'What *should* I be doing?' (Stewart, 1991). Reference to the primary task may prove useful here. Between the boundary of constraints and the core of demands there is the area of choice. Managers can find ways to reduce the demands and constraints and extend the opportunities for choices.

Turning intentions into obligations

Mintzberg (1975) observes that effective managers gain control of their own time by turning their obligations to their advantage and turning the activities they want to do into obligations. By using demands or obligations as opportunities to achieve something that you want to do anyway – for instance using a discussion item at a meeting to lobby for a cause you want to promote – you become more effective. On the other hand, turning what you *want* to do into an obligation is a good way to make sure that you do it. Applying this approach to managing care creates possibilities, such as follows.

- If you want to spend some time with practitioners, commit yourself to meeting with them.
- If you need to spend more time in planning, arrange a time to do this with a colleague.
- If you do not get enough time for reflection, meet with peers in an action learning group.
- If you want to innovate, set up a project and get others to report back to you.

This may sound obvious, but it is surprising how easy it is for some activities to slip off the agenda because no one is pressing for them to happen.

Key points

Ways of increasing a sense of control, of acting rather than simply reacting, are to:

- clarify the primary task of the organisation

- extend choices through reducing demands and constraints

- turn obligations to your advantage and turn activities you want to do into obligations.

1.6 Managing your day

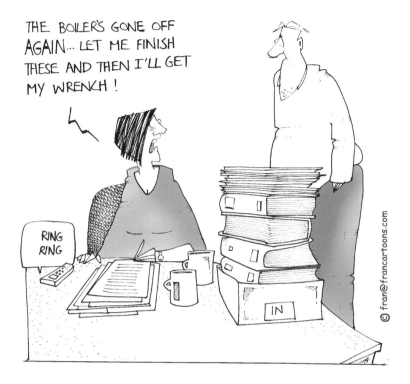

If something has not been done, the manager may have to do it

Most managers' work is characterised by 'brevity, variety, and discontinuity' (Mintzberg, 1975, p. 50). Tasks are started and rarely completed in one sitting, since interruptions are constant. Management theorists who have observed managers at work conclude that this picture, far from suggesting inefficiency, is what a real manager's job involves: talking to people, building networks, reacting to others' initiatives, jumping from issue to issue and continually responding to the needs of the moment (Mintzberg, 1975; Kotter, 1999).

There have not been any large studies of this type looking solely at managers of care services. The diaries kept for us by frontline managers confirm a picture of days full to bursting with many competing activities and unexpected events to respond to, such as staff shortages and service users' concerns. Often they reported taking administrative work home with them to finish off, as in the following diary extract by Bronwyn, a manager of a voluntary sector project offering therapeutic services to children and families where there has been abuse. A small qualitative study of operational managers in social services suggests that the managers studied were working with very short-term time horizons, almost entirely caught up with immediate pressures – effectively 'now managers' (Conway, 1993, p. 20).

BRONWYN'S DIARY

Monday

Should have been on a course but did not attend. Felt very bad about this but I had so much to do that I was starting to feel in panic mode. Spent the day catching up on paperwork at home and glad that I did. Feedback about the course was very positive and I now regret that I didn't go. Feel at the moment that I can't do right for doing wrong.

A conflicting picture emerges here. Discontinuity is apparently an inevitable feature of a manager's day. However, if managers are totally caught up in immediate pressures and unable to plan ahead, they lose the opportunity to get an overview and to act strategically. They may be managing but perhaps only just: managing in the sense of surviving (Aldgate and Dimmock, 2003). They are likely to feel at odds with their work at such times, as reported by Bronwyn. Time for planning is important, as a manager of a children's home notes:

> When you first become a manager, you need to have some space for yourself, to think and plan and reflect for yourself and not try to tackle everything. I think I was very keen to just change everything – set yourself a couple of goals. I've done that now.
>
> (Manager consultations)

How much scope is there for planning? Are managers inevitably pushed into a reactive mode? Although our managers' diaries show 'busyness' and unplanned activity, there are indications that they find time to plan and reflect. The regular onslaught of new work needs time for appraisal and planning, and opportunities to think about different ways of doing things, as Bronwyn's diary suggests.

BRONWYN'S DIARY

Wednesday

Team meeting day. The number of referrals has increased at an alarming rate. Spent most of the meeting allocating, making decisions about appropriateness of some referrals, trying to find creative ways of meeting the need for the work. Fortunately the plans drawn up the day before will help towards this.

Made date for a team day to discuss new proposals – need to book venue away from office to be able to devote the day to the task without disturbance.

Need to arrange equal opportunities and child protection yearly refresher courses for team. Team came up with a number of suggestions.

Bronwyn's diary extract mentions training 'refresher' courses, specifically for equal opportunities. If some service users are not getting a good service because of insensitive, perhaps racist, responses, the primary task is not being properly addressed. Workers themselves can also be the target of racism. The diary extract below by Surrinder, a family centre manager, highlights the importance of commitment from senior management to training in this area.

SURRINDER'S DIARY

Friday

Once the shortlisting had finished I went into another meeting with a development officer to look at our plans to follow up on the Macpherson report. [The report from the Stephen Lawrence Inquiry (Home Office, 1999) which underpins many of the requirements of the Race Relations (Amendment) Act 2000 (Home Office, 2000).] The meeting was productive. Had lengthy discussions about how we would look at issues around empowering and enabling staff to challenge and deal with racism. We talked about the sensitivity issue, and how it may bring up a lot of stuff for certain people. The development officer felt that it needed more commitment from senior managers to allocate more time specifically for looking at racism, especially when half the population in our area is black. I found meeting with the staff development officer very beneficial for me personally, because a lot of issues that I had were flagged up as issues that the department needed to address, e.g. number of black workers in senior management (service manager level). I felt like I was actually being listened to and validated in what I was saying.

When managers can find time, like Surrinder, to contribute to planning in such important areas that affect day-to-day practice, they are helping their organisation to learn from the dilemmas and challenges of practice. This is crucial work.

Stewart argues that, between the demands and constraints of the job, there is an area of choice. Enlarging this area gives the opportunity to place priority on some areas of work above others. There are many conflicts in deciding on how to prioritise. The classic difficulty is between the *urgent* and the *important*. Some things are urgent, and therefore tend to come high on the list, while others may be less urgent, at least in terms of meeting a deadline, but are of central importance in achieving what you, and others, want and expect from your job. These important matters are more likely to involve you over the longer term, have the potential to develop your work, and are the more strategic tasks. This is where the helicopter view is needed of what your organisation is here to do and what you should be doing.

A key discipline for managing your day and prioritising effectively is through good management of your time.

Time management

You can develop your approach to time management in the following ways (The Open University, 2000, p. 52).

- Decide how to spend your time in order to be more effective at work. What are the areas of choice? What should you be doing?
- Analyse how you currently spend most of your time at work.
- Reflect on how the first two differ and what you want to change.
- Decide how you will change your use of time.
- Review your progress occasionally to ensure that your approach is still appropriate. If your work has cycles of activity – around the end of the financial year for instance – it is worth reviewing at different times in the cycle to take account of highs and lows of pressure.

If you think you are not doing some of the tasks you consider important, it will be helpful to analyse in detail how you are using your time. Keeping a brief log of how time is spent on one or two typical days will give you essential information for analysis. Think about how it is different from how you would like it to be. You can then think about what opportunities there are for managing your day more effectively.

Managing your day does not mean keeping a distance from your working context or never getting involved in unplanned activities. Many of the managers we spoke to thought that it was important to be easily available to their staff, sometimes sharing office space, and if necessary getting involved in some of the difficult decisions they were making. Managers of fieldwork teams and other office-based practitioners may be in open plan accommodation and very visible and accessible. In residential and group care contexts managers are particularly exposed to the momentum of other people's days. They need to engage with the service users and what is going on in their lives in a way that might not happen in other kinds of setting. If something has not been done, the manager may have to do it, or at least make sure that it gets done, as Surrinder found in her family centre when the cook was off sick.

SURRINDER'S DIARY

Monday

Before even getting to work this morning I was assessing potentially what the situation would be like in relation to staffing levels. I had a funny feeling that the cook would be off again.

About 9 a.m. I received a phone call from the cook – she would be off today and was seeing the GP later on. There was no deputy officer in charge all week as she was in training, so I knew everything would be left for me to deal with.

The first 45 minutes were spent sorting out another unit to cook the meals, then I had to organise which staff member would go and collect the dinners.

Once I had sorted out the dinners, the food deliveries started to arrive. No cook to receive them and check if the fresh fruit and vegetables were OK. I received all the stock and then delegated to the domestic assistant to put it away.

Finished in the kitchen and went to my office in the hope of working through my 'to do' list. No sooner had I sat down, I received a phone call from a parent stating that her child would be off because he had diarrhoea again.

Urgent situations have to be responded to but it should be possible to set aside some time for longer-term strategic work, as well as more routine matters such as statistical returns. Harris and Kelly (1992) suggest some better work habits so that unplanned activities compete for a smaller proportion of the day. They are summarised in Box 1.3.

BOX 1.3 Better working habits

- Reserve a quiet hour at the beginning of the day.

- Arrive early rather than stay late.

- If you have your own room, keep the door open for periods of the day and closed when you want to signal that interruptions (including telephone calls) are not welcome.

- If you do not have your own room, find a separate room or office for tasks that require concentration or privacy.

- Screen your incoming work: for instance, a clerk or another worker could take the initial contact, so that you can then decide what needs to be done next.

- Establish a system of set times for supervision sessions and other predictable commitments and keep to them.

- List the activities you want to do during the next few months. Decide in which week action will be needed on each of them. Allocate time to the action required.

(Source: adapted from Harris and Kelly, 1992, p. 15)

Key points

- Many managers' work requires them to respond to the needs of the moment – discontinuity is a feature of the working day.

- It is important to find time to reflect and plan.

- Good time management and working habits can help to prioritise tasks.

1.7   Problem solving and decision making

The complexity of frontline managers' work is also one of its strengths. It is a creative role with opportunities to bring about change. The quality of people's lives can be improved. The work can bring genuine job satisfaction – much of it from witnessing others' achievements. In this section we look at some of that creative problem-solving activity and identify some of the regularities in what often appears complex and hard to analyse.

Managers *act* and *react* in dealing with problems and making decisions. There is a need to take account of important information in a reactive way, as well as 'taking action' when making decisions. Doing nothing is also a decision, as is referring a matter to someone more senior. Responsible decision making involves drawing on several different aspects, including knowledge and experience:

> An accountable person does not undertake an action merely because someone in authority says to do so. Instead, the accountable person examines a situation, explores the various options available, demonstrates a knowledgeable understanding of the possible consequences of options and makes a decision for action which can be justified from a knowledge base.
>
> (Marks-Maran, 1993, p. 123)

However, this description might give the impression that decision making is a rather reflective and logical process. Often, harassed managers may feel that decisions are made 'on the hoof' and that time to explore different options is a luxury. Action is sometimes needed to generate information and possible options: what Pedler *et al.* call an 'action before planning' approach (1994, p. 105). Alternatively, a decision may be perfectly logical at the time it is made but the situation then changes. Information that is needed for good decisions is not always available at the right time, and managers may need to be flexible and respond to unexpected developments. A firm focus on the values and principles of social care practice will be important.

Mintzberg (1975) describes a way of conceptualising managerial decisions, as shown in Figure 1.2 (overleaf). We shall use this as a framework for exploring roles in managing care.

Decisional roles

Drawing on studies of a wide range of managers in action, Mintzberg suggests that managers have ten related roles, which can be sorted into three main categories. The first is *interpersonal* roles; these combine with *informational* roles and the two sets combined enable the manager to play four *decisional* roles (Mintzberg, 1975).

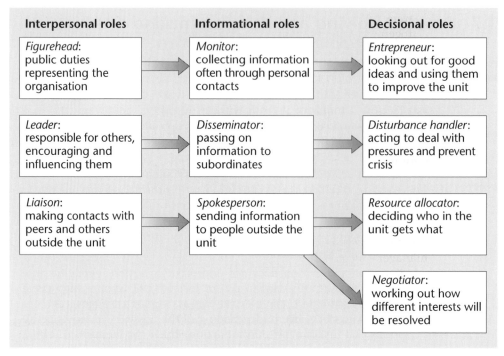

Figure 1.2 **The manager's roles** (Source: adapted from Mintzberg, 1975, pp. 54–9)

In Figure 1.2 interpersonal and informational roles involve the manager variously in roles within the unit and outside it, in relation to both people and information. Mintzberg considers that the blend of roles any manager plays will vary from one person to another, and that the wide variety of problems that managers face means it is difficult to offer a prescription for how to approach them.

We look at many of the roles identified here more closely in other chapters of this book. For now, we look in more detail at the decisional roles and how they might be interpreted in the context of managing care.

Entrepreneur

Managers seek to improve their units and adapt them to changing conditions in the environment. The entrepreneur role involves looking for good new ideas, which may emerge as a decision by the manager to back one for development through a project – this might be delegated to a team member to do. Here the manager is initiating and *acting*. An example of this is the decision taken in the early 1990s by Jane, now manager of a local Mind association, to work in partnership with other agencies, including a local community arts organisation:

> It was pragmatic because we had few resources: we wanted to make friends and influence people. I realised as a single development worker that it was absolutely impossible to fulfil my role on my own ... Those

were very early days and very raw, people were literally just working together, with a common agenda to promote some positive images around mental health and to work with a local community mental health centre ... Crucially to work with service users to actually develop activity ... and the arts has been a really positive vehicle in that regard.

(Manager consultations)

Entrepreneurial decisions may be ones that the manager, in consultation with service users and staff, can make fairly independently; they may be opportunistic; or they may involve some negotiation with other agencies, with more senior managers or with funders in order to get something new up and running.

In the voluntary sector, managers often have to run ever harder to keep core work funded. If their own jobs and any administrative costs come out of a percentage of funding for specific projects, there is always pressure to initiate project work, which then also has the effect of increasing the manager's workload. Close work with other organisations may make it possible to spread the load a little.

Disturbance handler

Managers sometimes have to respond to pressure, change or events beyond their control – this is often called 'troubleshooting'. These are the times when a manager is necessarily *reacting* to the situation. Extracts from Bronwyn's diary provide an example of her supporting the workers' decision about a child care problem and handling the resulting anger.

BRONWYN'S DIARY

Monday

... Difficult meeting with another mother. Very unhappy about a decision taken by the workers about the future direction of the work with her daughter. I explained that I endorsed the decision one hundred per cent and explained the reasons why. She left, still very angry.

Didn't spend a good night thinking about this.

Tuesday

... Phone call from mother who had left the project very angry the day before. Anger had not abated. Spent 20 minutes talking it through to find a compromise that would enable her to accept decision was in the best interests of the child – unsuccessfully. Needed a very strong cup of coffee afterwards – know this one will run and run.

Mintzberg points out that disturbances arise not only because poor managers ignore situations until they reach crisis proportions but also because good managers cannot possibly anticipate all the consequences of the actions they take.

However, there are some possibilities to anticipate. You read earlier about how Surrinder dealt with the crisis of her cook's absence. You may remember that she had half-anticipated this possibility on her way to work, and she probably had sketched out a plan in her mind about what might need to be done.

Through taking a proactive approach to planning with their teams, managers may be able to develop a framework for making decisions in complex situations. This can be a resource for team members which can enable them to proceed confidently, knowing that some of the problems they meet have already been anticipated and planned for. So there may be opportunities to prevent 'disturbance' by acting early instead of waiting for a crisis to arise and then reacting.

Resource allocator

The manager decides who gets what in the organisational unit, including the manager's own time, who takes on which work, and the form or structure of the unit. The manager also authorises important decisions about much of the core running of the unit. Some decisions, such as staff appointments, roles within the group or rotas for covering planned activities, set the overall framework, and the manager will not want to revisit them too often. Others simply crop up in the course of engaging with a particular piece of work or in dealing with daily activities.

Managers in social care may find that the resources they can allocate do not go far in attempting to meet needs. They then have to look for ways of doing as much as possible with what they have. This can be a source of frustration, as one manager of mental health services describes:

> I think, as a first line manager, the main dilemmas I faced were lack of resources, but also high expectations ... about what the service should look like, and being expected to deliver that on very limited resources.
>
> (Manager consultations)

When the major resource is the staff group, allocating work may feel positive or negative. Jacqui, a family centre manager, notes a decision to allocate work with a family.

JACQUI'S DIARY

Friday

I had to attend a case conference this morning. It was a family who have been referred to the centre so really my attendance was just for information gathering. We are required to assess the parents on their parenting skills over a period of twelve weeks. When I got back I had to spend quite a while discussing with the other managers how this will be done as we must start working with the family as soon as possible.

We identified a suitable worker to do the assessment and talked to her about it. She seemed really enthusiastic and had lots of ideas herself. It's so nice when staff members use their own initiative and it's something we encourage. We were then able to liaise with the social worker and set a date for the initial meeting with the parents.

Negotiator

Managers spend considerable time in negotiations, for instance dealing with grievances, responding to complaints, working out contracts, and simply getting the team or working unit to agree on the way forward.

Sometimes there is limited scope for negotiation, and the process is more towards communicating unpopular decisions. Jenny, another family centre manager, comments that giving an opportunity for views to be aired and listened to is very important:

> We work closely as a management team and try to take on ideas and suggestions, but if we know something has got to happen, and I know people won't be happy, I try to set up a discussion to explore why it is, and how it is going to happen. If there is a chance to air views, usually it will be tried and then reviewed ... And you can take the staff with you. Most staff here know that we are up front with them, and we tell them what is going on. It is important to have time for views to be aired and for difficulties to be foreseen and discussed.

> (Manager consultations)

She describes the need to be confident about the values you consider important, especially where the issues under debate may be ones that are outside your own expertise, for example:

managing conflict in meetings, keeping a perspective where others have expert knowledge that you don't share and being assertive about your viewpoint, not being diverted and holding on to values about user-led services.

(Manager consultations)

Again, in the decision-making role of negotiator, there is scope for acting as well as reacting.

Key points

- Much of a manager's work involves making decisions.

- The identification of decision-making *roles* can offer a tool for thinking about what kinds of responsibility managers hold, and what resources they can draw on in making confident and robust decisions.

1.8 Conclusion

In this chapter we considered some of the issues in moving from a practitioner role in social care to becoming a manager. We argued that there are links between practising and managing, and that new managers should not only be able to build on some of their practice skills but also have responsibility to maintain a commitment to practice in managing other people's practice. The transition requires new managers to attend to their own learning, and to support those they manage in learning and developing. Organisations have an important responsibility here too.

This chapter highlighted the complexity and 'busyness' of the manager's day, using the linked themes of acting and reacting. There are some ways in which managers can get an overview of their work, the choices that are open to them, and the priorities they want to make. Making decisions is a *skill*; it can also be viewed as one of the important *roles* of managers.

Chapter 2
Managing the team

Adrian Ward

2.1   Introduction

This chapter is about what is involved in managing a team for better practice and better ways of working together. This focus is often called 'team building' but, rather than seeing it as a one-off exercise (on an 'away day' for example), it is viewed here as an integral and ongoing part of the work of any manager or team leader. Through attention to building – or perhaps 'growing' – the team, a manager can enable people to work together more effectively.

The chapter draws mainly on the group care context for its practice examples since in such settings the need for teamwork is especially compelling, and the issues are therefore brought into stronger focus (Ward, 1993).

This chapter covers certain key elements that enable people to collaborate in the workplace: how teams are formed, and how people can be helped and supported in joining a new team; what managers need to think about in order to 'get the work done' in the team; how individuals can be retained and helped to develop in their roles in the workplace; and, finally, how whole teams can be supported and enabled to grow. The emphasis in this chapter is very much on a 'human relations' approach to teamwork and team building, rather than on a more administrative or technological approach. This is deliberate: my own experience, whether as a practitioner, a manager or a lecturer, has taught me that what counts most in teamwork is communication and collaboration. Unless people can talk together they cannot really work together; and unless they can work together they cannot really produce good results as a team. This is why the first section of this chapter has a strong emphasis on the 'lived experience' of teamwork.

The aims of this chapter are to:

- explain why teams matter
- argue for a 'human relations' approach to teamworking
- consider issues of staff selection and induction as aspects of team adaptation to change
- discuss the manager's role in creating a sense of working together as a team, building on the strengths and different abilities of staff.

2.2   Why teams matter

Why is it crucial for managers to focus on teams? It may be helpful to consider this question by thinking about your own work setting as you read this section. In what sense do people feel that they belong to a team, and what does that mean to them and to you?

Defining 'team'

The meaning of 'team' and 'teamwork' is contested and controversial. Different definitions stress requirements such as co-ordination, mutual accountability, diverse professional backgrounds and synergy (the idea that more can be achieved collectively than by individuals acting alone) (Shonk, 1992; Katzenbach and Smith, 1993; Pence and Wilson, 1994; Colenso, 1997).

The definition used here is *a team is a group of people who work together on a common task*. In some settings they work closely together throughout the working day, while in others they operate relatively independently of each other, but most teams have some sense of group responsibility for a shared or parallel task. This notion of a shared task is important. If there is no identifiable shared task then it may be questioned whether a team exists or whether it is simply a collection of individuals who happen to be managed by the same person.

An emphasis on the team as a group underpins this chapter. Whether or not the team regularly meets as a group, it can be argued that it still *behaves* as a group – in the sense that group processes involve a need both for a shared purpose and for attention to how people feel about being part of the team. Team members affect each other for better or worse, and influence each other's performance and morale.

Who are the team members?

This might seem obvious but think about the boundaries of a team you are familiar with, and who counts as being in the team and who does not. Do secretarial and administrative staff attend team meetings, and are they full participants or are they kept in their 'service role'? In a residential unit, what about the cook? Everybody knows that the cook has a central role in most residential homes, but often the cook is not counted as a full team member, even though she or he may have more daily contact with the residents than some of the other team members.

Other issues may arise where there is more than one team involved. In some multidisciplinary settings, for example, there may be social work, health, education and other groups of staff operating in their own groupings as sub-teams that also need to collaborate across these boundaries as a larger team. Some people may work away from the main site. Individuals from different disciplines and organisations may operate as one team but also have loyalty to a 'home base'. Such situations can easily give rise to rivalries or other tensions between the sub-teams, or to conflicts of loyalty within individuals about where their main identification should lie.

The *criteria* by which we decide who is in the team and who is not may produce different results. For instance, people's contracts and a list of their responsibilities may contrast with who attends the team meetings, who uses the same room or building, or who contributes to getting the work done.

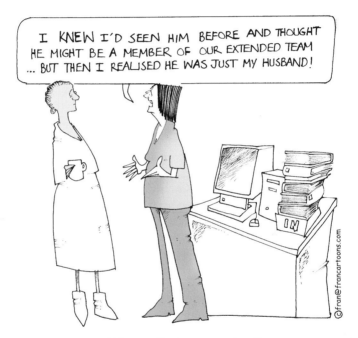

Who are the team members?

Think about where you might draw the boundaries of any work team you belong to. Is the manager a team member? What about the people who use your services? There are no ideal answers to such questions, because teams and circumstances vary so widely, but it is usually instructive to ask the questions and to consider the implications of what you find. Similarly, there is no ideal team composition or 'dream team'; there are only collections of real people with their own histories and relationships with each other, trying to get along together to get the work done.

Payne (2000) argues convincingly for what he calls 'open teamwork', by which he means an even more inclusive approach, incorporating what is usually thought of as 'networking' into the traditional concept of teamwork. According to this view, relationships in the team are the basis for team members working with outside community, service user or professional networks, going out and drawing them into the team's work. Teams are an integral part of networks, and relationships in the wider network need fostering and nurturing in the same way as they do within the core team (Payne, 2000). This approach is especially valuable in the modern context of multi-professional care, in which many professionals have to collaborate closely and communicate effectively with colleagues in a broad range of other professions as well as within their own. The importance of this inter-professional teamworking is shown by inquiries into child protection tragedies, many of which point to serious problems in inter-agency and intra-agency work (Lord Clyde, 1992; Department of Health, 1991a; Social Services Inspectorate (NI), 1991).

Why do teams matter?

Teams matter because people matter and because teams are the main way in which people are organised into getting the work done, and where they may expect some support for their work. Word soon gets around about whose team is best to work for. If the team climate is poor, people leave. Research evidence (for instance, Stewart *et al.*, 1999) generally confirms that effective teamwork contributes to best results in terms of productivity and efficiency, as well as on the more human dimensions of staff morale and reduced absenteeism, although the difficulty of obtaining accurate data in this area has also been noted (Miner, 1982).

Teamwork is not an optional extra; it is essential if people are to communicate well with each other, give of their best and work effectively together. However, it does not happen without planning and effort. It is an activity requiring awareness, support and nurturing. People need this individually so that they feel personally engaged with the task of the whole organisation and clear about their own contribution to it. People also need to learn to work as a group and to support each other, identifying where necessary with other colleagues, trusting each other, and so on. They need leadership in developing and sustaining their team-membership skills (see Collins and Bruce, 1984). For these reasons, managers and team leaders require the skills to nurture a teamwork approach.

All of this matters in industrial settings such as car factories for the sake of safe and effective operating. It matters even more in human services organisations for the sake of humane, safe and effective care. In fact, it is more complicated here because the focus of the work is not the creation of physical products but the support of vulnerable human beings. These people are not the neutral and passive recipients of services, to be manipulated into shape as sheet metal can be. They are personally and emotionally affected not only by their circumstances but also by the quality or otherwise of the services delivered to them. Staff, in turn, are personally affected for better or worse by the experience of providing such services, and by the nature of their interactions with the users (Menzies Lyth, 1988; Bosk, 1979).

Teamwork is not straightforward and it certainly cannot be assumed that teams will always be supportive or benign. For example, sometimes a team which appears on the surface to be strong and well integrated turns out to be quite ineffective at its given task, because the apparent integration has been 'bought' at the price of collusion and inefficiency. In some parts of the prison service, for instance, team 'solidarity' among the officers is extremely strong, but this can become a problem rather than an asset, because the focus of these strong teams may have become primarily targeted on the 'control' and 'punishment' aspects of their task rather than on the rehabilitative or even therapeutic aspects (for instance, see Dodd, 2001). Conversely, a team in which the working atmosphere seems tense and conflict-ridden may in fact be highly focused on 'delivering the goods'. The tensions may derive more from the nature of the work or the needs of the service users than from any genuine divisions or animosities between the people involved.

What these two examples illustrate in different ways are the intricate connections between the task of a team, the feelings team members may have about that task, and their ways of dealing with those feelings, both individually and collectively. The human relations approach, which explores these sorts of issues, is summarised in Box 2.1.

BOX 2.1 The human relations approach to organisations

The human relations approach uses a combination of systems theory and psychodynamic understanding to interpret the ways in which people behave in organisations, and the ways in which these behaviours affect each other. It focuses especially on:

- the 'primary task' of an organisation – what it 'must perform in order to survive' (Rice, 1965, p. 7)

- the function this task may perform on behalf of society as a whole – for instance, Miller and Gwynne's study (1972) looked at the function care homes may perform for society

- the anxiety this task may create in the staff.

The systems element in the human relations approach points to the ways in which groups and sub-groups in organisations (as well as the individuals involved) may affect each other. Organisations are made up of interlocking parts (teams) which are interdependent. Influencing one part is likely to influence all the other parts (see Bilson and Ross, 1999; Miller, 1993; Syer and Connolly, 1996).

> The psychodynamic element encourages a focus not only on the conscious elements of such interactions but also on the subconscious elements (see, for instance, Obholzer and Roberts, 1994a; Hinshelwood and Skogstad, 2000).

The group care context provides many helpful examples that demonstrate the human responses of people as they interact with each other and their work, and the place of teams in the wider context of the organisation, its purposes and the concerns of its service users. This context is considered next.

Teamwork in the group care context

In group care (that is, residential and day care) teamwork has two key distinguishing features: the *interdependency* of team members and the *network of interactions* between staff and service users (Ward, 1993).

In many group care settings the team needs to be more interdependent than elsewhere because members often have to rely directly on each other for immediate collaboration and mutual support during their everyday work. This might be for advice on how to handle a difficult incident, or perhaps for practical help in physical tasks such as lifting somebody. In many fieldwork settings, by contrast, people tend to carry their own caseloads independently of each other and mostly rely on each other more for occasional support and informal consultation than for sustained co-working. This greater interdependence of the group care team has widespread implications for the organisation and delivery of the service: for example, in terms of the arrangements for supervision and staff meetings (Payne and Scott, 1985).

Likewise, group care teams tend to evolve a complicated pattern or *network of interactions* between staff and service users. In fieldwork, most of the service users tend to be seen on an individual case basis, with the same (usually solo) worker. In group care, however, each person is likely to relate to more than one individual worker, and even in those settings where there is a key worker (as the main co-ordinating person) or similar system, each worker may work simultaneously with many different service users within the same group throughout the day. There are important implications here for team members in terms of the way they need to be able to communicate with and trust each other.

Key points

- A team is a group of people working together on a common task.

- If they are to be effective, they need to collaborate and communicate.

- Collaboration and communication do not happen by chance. Team members and their manager need to work at it and to develop their skills in mutual support.

- The group care context shows the importance of teamwork.

2.3   Becoming a team

This section is about how teams evolve and develop, and how managers and team leaders can promote healthy and positive functioning in teams.

It can be helpful to think about where a particular team came from and how it formed and evolved rather than to discuss an abstract notion of the team. For example, what is the history of how your team came into being? If you are the manager, were you promoted from within the team or moved from another part of the same organisation, or were you appointed from outside the organisation? This history will affect how people view you as a manager and how you view your own relationship with team members and with the organisation as a whole. Consider the three promotion histories outlined in Example 2.1 and their possible influence on relationships in the team.

EXAMPLE 2.1 Contrasting promotion histories

1   Shreeti was the newly promoted deputy manager in a family centre. She had worked in this centre for five years, having joined the team during a period of great stress and turnover of staff. At the time she had helped to 'steady' morale in the team by showing patience and resilience, and by reminding people of the importance in their work of paying close attention to the needs of the children and families attending the centre.

2   Maureen became deputy manager of a resource centre for people with learning disabilities when Colin, the manager, was instructed to appoint her by his senior management team at headquarters. She had been manager of a small 'independent living' project in a nearby town, but this had closed at short notice after a prolonged and difficult conflict with the neighbours in which Maureen felt she had not been well supported by senior management. She was transferred at only two weeks' notice, and both she and the team (and Colin) resented the imposition.

3   My own experience on being appointed manager of a children's home was that the existing team was split between loyalties to the previous (and charismatic) head, who had left some months before, and to the acting head, who (although less popular) had at least held the place together through a time of great turmoil. Although at one level people appeared keen to make a new start with me as the new leader, at another level there seemed to be a great wish to return to the 'golden age' of the original manager, rather than to consider doing things differently.

The shared and positive history of Shreeti's work in the team contributed to the welcome which all team members gave to her appointment as deputy. In contrast, Maureen's appointment was flawed from the start, which caused a great deal of pain on all sides, most of all to Maureen herself. Colin, her manager, felt imposed on and somewhat resentful. His task as manager of the unit was not helped by having effectively no choice in the appointment to such a key role as deputy manager. People are not trapped or limited by their histories, however, and Maureen ultimately proved herself in the new setting, showing that, however clumsily her appointment had been handled, she herself had much to offer in the post.

In my own, somewhat complicated situation the difficulty was to promote the idea that tasks could be done well and to high standards without necessarily doing them exactly the same as previously. Practice seemed to have become rather fossilised and routine, whereas, as team leader, I wanted people to work with current situations in new and more responsive ways. I thought some of the staff team were being quite resistant to change, whereas their view was probably that they *knew* how the job should be done and they just wanted to be allowed to get on with it.

As discussed in Chapter 1, becoming a manager involves a transition; here the focus is on the team aspects of the transition. Being promoted to be a manager in your own team can be difficult. It may take some time for former peers to accept that the new manager now has authority over them; likewise, the new manager may feel awkward about asserting authority over people who may also be friends. Once a new manager can make their own appointments, the pattern of relationships in a team can be shifted. A new worker will not know the history at first hand and may be more likely to accept the manager's authority, and to act accordingly, which in turn may influence how the whole team operates. Some managers feel that they are only really in charge once they have appointed their own staff (Coulshed, 1990).

It can also be difficult for a new manager who is appointed to manage a team they do not know. People may be very established in their ways of doing things, and they may be reluctant even to consider doing them differently, sometimes out of feelings of loyalty to the previous manager, sometimes out of a perceived need to survive by 'hanging on together'.

These changing dynamics and evolving histories of teams are not easily portrayed in models. A framework based on the review by Tuckman (1965) is widely used in discussions of teamwork. It describes a progression through a series of stages called 'forming', 'storming' and 'norming', until at last the team is 'performing'. However, this framework is based on studies of how small groups work. It captures some recognisable processes for newly formed teams. Yet it may have limited application to the situation of a working team whose tasks and purposes are often defined by the wider organisation – or organisations – within which it is situated, and whose membership changes as the team continues but the manager and members come and go (Payne, 2000). The alternative model in Figure 2.1 sees team building as a cycle of development.

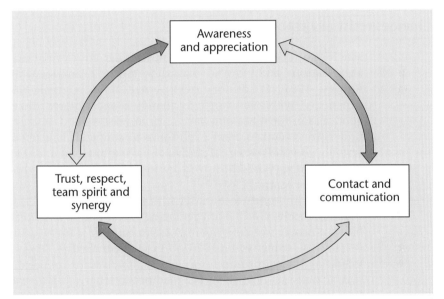

Figure 2.1 **Cycle of developing teamworking skills** (Source: based on Syer and Connolly, 1996)

Syer and Connolly (1996) argue that team members need to develop *awareness* of themselves and each other, and of their differences, through giving descriptive (as opposed to evaluative) feedback. This allows appreciation of differences, good contact and improved communication. Trust, respect, team spirit and synergy (where the team get ideas that even the most knowledgeable member could not get alone) may then emerge. This in turn leads to more highly developed awareness. The notion of a cycle more easily depicts the kind of continuous process that teams go through and need to revisit as members are introduced or move on. Both models suggest that skill and attention are required from the manager and from team members.

The notion of change and how it is handled is useful. History is by no means the only factor that affects team dynamics. The composition of a team in terms of, for example, people's age, gender and length of service, or the ethnic balance of the team, may have a major bearing on the ways in which people collaborate with each other. Equally, changes in the structure of a team, or how services are organised, may affect the amount of time different team members spend working with each other and thus the ways in which they communicate and collaborate. The common factor in most of these issues is the question of change: all teams face change and development over time, and often the way in which the team recognises and responds to these changes determines the patterns and networks of working relationships.

Change: resist or respond?

Much has been written about resistance to change in teams and organisations and how to overcome it (for example, Obholzer, 1987; Bridges, 1991; O'Connor, 1993; Vince, 1996; Carnall, 1999). In my experience, where resistance to change is encountered there is usually a good reason for it at some level – or at least a good 'felt' reason. People under stress tend to want everything to stay as it is, even if that is not actually very satisfactory. The risk of having to adapt and rethink and the possibility that something will be lost in the process sometimes causes anxiety (see Marris, 1986).

'Resistance' tends to be a term that is applied to other people rather than to ourselves. As a manager facing a 'resistant' team, you may need to find out people's underlying reasons for caution or for wanting everything to stay the same and try to address these factors. This might mean tolerating the status quo for longer than you want to, because what staff may actually be looking for is a readiness to change on *the manager's* part. Once they see that you are willing to adapt and to wait if necessary, they may feel less anxious about relinquishing some of their own rigid ideas.

Key points

- A key role of the manager of a team is to enable the members to work together on their tasks.

- This involves thinking about the history of the team as a group as well as the individual members.

- It also requires the manager to promote their ability to work together as a group.

2.4   Growing the team: finding and keeping team members

There are actions that managers and team leaders can take to promote effective and productive teamwork, especially around the transitions of joining a team. Recruitment, selection and induction all illustrate the ways in which teams need to continually incorporate and adapt to change; other changes might include staff leaving or re-forming into new work groups. The questions to ask about such change include:

- What is involved?
- What do managers need to think about and focus on?
- How can they influence developments within their team?

Some of the actions managers can take are fairly straightforward and common sense. It might be argued that if they focused primarily on getting the basics right, everything else would probably fall into place. The basics include following proper procedures for recruitment, selection, induction and appraisal. On the other hand, part of what makes teamwork 'work' concerns more intangible qualities such as a supportive atmosphere, a positive culture and mutual respect between team members. Qualities such as these can seem much more elusive and hard to achieve if they are missing than the simpler procedural matters. So, in fact, what managers have to think about is both aspects: the formal and the informal. In group process terms, this is the *instrumental* and the *expressive*: the task of *what* has to be done (the instrumental aspect) but also the process – the *way* in which tasks need to be done (the expressive aspect). This distinction between the instrumental and the expressive is an important one and will be revisited several times in this chapter. It is a balancing act and most managers will recognise the need to balance or juggle many different types of task.

Recruitment and appointment

Recruiting the best people to join the team is a key activity for managers. How that is handled will contribute to the new employee's sense of being part of a team or otherwise. The team manager (in conjunction with senior management and through consulting with the team) needs to be clear about exactly what each post in a team requires, in terms of the tasks to be done and therefore the person specification for the post. It is sometimes tempting in this process to lose touch with reality and start specifying some ideal type, rather than being realistic and grounded about what may be achievable. It matters both for the new employee and for the team that the right match is found between the jobs to be done and the people employed to do them, otherwise stress and dissatisfaction may develop. Equal opportunities also play a crucial part at this stage, in terms of whether the whole recruitment and appointment process is conducted so that all candidates (and indeed all potential candidates, whether or not they eventually apply) feel they are dealt with fairly and openly.

There are specific equal opportunities issues to be addressed concerning people who are under-represented in the workforce, such as a lack of applications from people with disabilities. Active steps may need to be taken to recruit from under-represented groups in the community, perhaps as part of a wider programme of making services more accessible and better adapted to local need. There is sometimes a 'vicious circle' to be broken: for instance, where services are perceived by local ethnic or religious groups as not meeting their needs, candidates from those groups may not apply for jobs where they feel they would be in an isolated or even a 'disloyal' position. More imaginative ways of including and incorporating local people may be needed, including working with volunteers and engaging participation from people who use the service (or might be encouraged to do so) as a means of stimulating interest and exchange, and thus breaking out of the vicious circle. Regarding applications from disabled people, it may be helpful to advertise in the disability press and to link with the local Disability Council to find out what is happening in the area. Example 2.2 illustrates an approach to involving people from a nearby community.

EXAMPLE 2.2 Reaching out and engaging

A family centre, which was located on the edge of a Hindu community in a large city, was viewed locally with suspicion and even hostility, and had never managed to recruit Hindu staff, despite having a formal equal opportunities policy. In order to address these and other concerns, a long-term programme of 'Reaching out and welcoming in' was initiated by the staff team, in which many informal contacts were gradually established with local groups and religious leaders. Three years on, the centre had taken on quite a different feel, with many local people actively engaged in the work of the centre, some as paid full-time staff, others as volunteers or on the steering group.

Such an approach makes use of all the available policies and procedures to promote best practice in recruitment, but it also moves well beyond into seeking a more active engagement between teams and their communities. In this sense, recruitment procedures and equal opportunities policies need to be closely allied with the overall ethos of policy and practice, rather than being seen as totally separate formalities.

Induction

The next important stage is the way in which a new person's arrival is planned for and managed. Induction literally means 'leading in', and this is a helpful image for the sorts of activity which induction should involve, especially in that it implies there is someone doing the leading as well as someone being led. The National Care Standards Commission now requires managers of care to demonstrate that they are meeting standards in providing induction and training for new staff (TOPSS England/ CareandHealth, 2001; see also Care Council for Wales, 2002). Effective induction cannot be achieved by simply handing the new colleagues an 'induction pack' and asking them to read through it, digest it and ask any questions at the end. Procedure on its own is never enough. What matters is that the person or group implementing the procedure understands the need for it, is in sympathy with its approach, and has the professional skills and personal aptitude to carry it through. Bear in mind that new colleagues also often have to contend with the 'unofficial' induction through rumour and gossip at the photocopier or over coffee. They need to know who they can consult to check worrying information. Some managers try to pre-empt the distracting effects of rumour, especially at times of organisational change, by making sure that they pass on all the information themselves as early as possible.

It is not only junior staff who need induction: a person who has been promoted within their own organisation may still need induction and this also applies to managers. Induction enables a person to 'become' the role: to learn what is involved in it and how the organisation looks from within that role. The workplace will look different in the position of deputy from how it looks to the same person as a care worker or nurse.

Keeping staff

Finding staff and inducting them into their new role is just the beginning. Once people begin to feel established they still need support and encouragement in taking on new challenges or in resisting inappropriate demands from those who might want to extend or change the person's responsibilities. Some people become established and settled quickly, finding their way successfully into the informal networks of the organisation as well as into the formal requirements of their role. Others take longer and need ongoing support, especially when a change of job is accompanied by moving house or another significant life transition. In Chapter 12 we look further at people's needs for induction, supervision, appraisal and professional development as a continuous process.

> **Key points**
>
> • The way in which people are recruited, inducted and supported in the team is important for effective team functioning and needs to reflect the core philosophy of the team and service.

2.5   Maintaining the team and getting the work done

In the previous section I distinguished between the instrumental and the expressive functions of teams and their managers, and much of the discussion has been about the 'expressive' function. However, there needs to be a focus on the instrumental function because, after all, teams are employed with the purpose of getting the work done. This is not always simple. For example, people may not always agree or act consistently, either in terms of what exactly has to be done or in terms of who should do each part of the task. This has some bearing on the discussion of practice-led management introduced in Chapter 1. The manager needs to think of the *practice* of the team as encompassing both instrumental and expressive aspects of its work.

Allocation

An essential part of 'getting the work done' is the allocation of responsibilities and incoming work. Every team needs a system for achieving this. Different team members are likely to have different strengths and weaknesses, which ideally should be taken into account in decisions. Moreover, team members may not always agree about their respective strengths and weaknesses. Depending on how such differences are acknowledged and dealt with in the team, difficult or confusing situations can arise. The person who has been officially allocated a particular task may be the least suitable person to hold that responsibility; or somebody may be known to be the best person at handling a particular kind of situation but is never available to take on such work because of being overloaded with other tasks.

Therefore, there are many factors to be taken into account in achieving a fair and effective system for allocating work, including not only people's strengths and weakness (and their personal preferences) but also the level of urgency or priority of the various types of work the team does. Teams and individuals vary in terms of the types and degrees of pressure they can handle. They may also vary over time: periods of high stress may need to be followed by a more 'slack' period for some team members or for the group as a whole. There is enormous potential for conflict here because in most teams people are very aware of who is 'pulling their weight', who is taking on more responsibility than they can really handle, and who might be better suited to more 'backroom' responsibilities for a while.

It is important for the team to have a system for distributing work that will be perceived as 'transparent' and fair, consistent with the type of work to be done, and responsive to the demands and priorities of referring agencies or other sources through which work reaches the team. For example, in some long-term units there is a relatively slow 'flow' of incoming work, although each new case or situation may carry long-term implications for the employee taking on this work. A unit primarily focused on 'intake' or 'assessment' may have a very rapid turnover of new work requiring relatively brief attention. The allocation systems in each of these teams might need to be quite different, especially in terms of the degree of choice or flexibility that individual workers can exercise.

Team leaders or managers hold considerable power in their allocation of work and responsibilities. The ways in which they exercise this power will have a significant effect on the overall functioning of the team. In some teams work is 'picked up' by the members during open discussion in the team. In other teams the manager makes unilateral allocation decisions outside team meetings. These different patterns will clearly each have their impact on how people feel about their work – and about their manager! A further complication is that, in addition to the explicit system, there may be informal pressure on (or between) team members to take on particular types or levels of work. Depending on the kind of work being done, a variety of strategies can be used to make the process as transparent and fair as possible. For instance, workloads can be audited; a weighting system can be devised; a chart on a whiteboard can show daily activities and who is responsible; rota systems or co-working arrangements can be devised that give individuals the opportunity to work with different colleagues and get to know their strengths and weaknesses. Discussion about who should take on new work could explicitly invite team- and self-evaluation on fair and effective distribution.

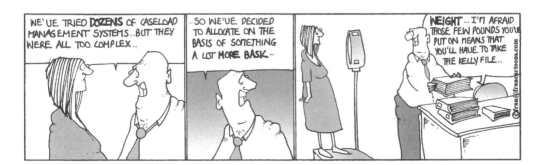

Workloads

The discussion of work allocation also raises the question of workloads. What is a fair workload, and how negotiable is this within the team? Different team members can appear able to carry different amounts of pressure. How such differences are handled represents a test of the team members' ability to work together. If one member of the team seems unable or unwilling to contribute as much (or as well) as the others, resentment may develop. As you read Example 2.3, think about what action the manager might have taken.

EXAMPLE 2.3 Silent member

In a fieldwork team, one member sat silently through allocation meetings, never offering to take work. Week by week others took on new cases, until the realisation dawned that this colleague was not taking a fair load and her tactic of silence was a success. The team manager did nothing, the rest of the group stopped volunteering for new work, the allocation pile grew, and team meetings got tense. Eventually, an experienced worker said, 'You can't expect the rest of us to take on new work while Sarah never offers to take on anything.' This forced the situation into the open and led to a discussion of workload.

The team members would have preferred their manager to have dealt with the issue of fair workloads, preferably by talking to Sarah in private. The team leader has an important responsibility in promoting openness and tolerance within the team. If this is not done, there is a risk that a pattern of scapegoating will evolve, which can lead to serious conflict within the team.

There are also risks when people are encouraged or allowed to take on too much work. As Example 2.4 indicates, they can either exhaust or overstretch themselves or unwittingly create other tensions.

EXAMPLE 2.4 Rate busting

In a children's home, a new and enthusiastic member of staff would frequently stay on at work after the end of his shift to play football with the children. This made him popular with the children at first, although he soon became less popular with the other staff, as they too came under pressure from the children to stay on after work for extra activities. Within a short space of time the new colleague became exhausted, and had to take a week's sick leave, which left everyone else to 'pick up the pieces' and do extra shifts.

The phenomenon in this example is known as 'rate busting' (that is, when somebody exceeds or 'busts' the team's work rate). Although this term originated in factory work, it is surprising how often this same pattern emerges in modern service industries. Again, managers can and should monitor and discourage this, taking care that they do not themselves provide a model of someone who works excessive hours, giving the impression to other team members that this is what is expected.

Key points

- Team managers need to pay close attention to the allocation of work as it can affect the overall working atmosphere of the team.

- There is an 'instrumental' requirement that the work gets done efficiently.

- There is an 'expressive' aspect in that people need to play to their strengths and feel that their workload is acceptable.

2.6   Nurturing the team

Managers cannot 'build' a team in a mechanical way. They can only bring people together, encourage them to work together and to learn more about the skills required for doing so, and support them through the process. At some stage they will have to take this on and do the rest for themselves, although still under the overall guidance and nurturing of their manager (see, for example, Holder and Wardle, 1981). This continuing encouragement is particularly important when people are working under extreme pressure.

Pressures on teams

The demands and pressures of health and social care are such that team members – and their managers – are often subject to enormous stresses, which carry the risk of distorting and diverting people's capacity for communication and collaboration. These are not only the ordinary strains of all working situations but also the additional factors brought in by the very nature of the work. For example, in a residential setting where the service users are struggling to cope with great personal distress or confusion, they are likely to communicate their distress to the people working with them. This happens at a less conscious level, as well as at the immediate surface level, through their unspoken expectations and the implicit messages of their behaviour. Individual staff sometimes unwittingly take on some of the hurt and pain of their service users

(Stokes, 1994). In psychodynamic terms, this kind of complex process is called *projective identification* (Moylan, 1994). Teams and larger groups of staff, especially those working in group care, can begin to re-enact some of the patterns of emotion and behaviour in the group of service users. When primitive anxieties are stirred up, there is often a tendency to try to get rid of uncomfortable thoughts and feelings and locate them in, or project them on to, others either inside or outside the team (Mawson, 1994).

If teams are to function well in such circumstances, they cannot just rely on 'common sense'. Members have a professional responsibility to be aware, both individually and as a group, of how they can work together effectively. They also need to give attention to what has to be done to keep their communication and collaboration going. This awareness and commitment need to be everyone's responsibility, and not just the manager's or team leader's. The team leader carries a specific responsibility to cultivate awareness and commitment, and to demonstrate and model it in action but, if this responsibility just stays with the team leader, it is less likely to be 'owned' by individual team members and by the team as a whole. Part of what the team leader has to do, therefore, is to promote and foster people's 'team membership skills' (Collins and Bruce, 1984; Wiener, 1997).

Systems for team maintenance

It is essential to pay attention to the detail of what keeps a team running, which may involve for example:

- actively monitoring how effectively people are communicating both facts and feelings to each other
- enabling people to check their perceptions of each other in terms of their willingness and availability to collaborate.

In a small team of, say, three or four people who are collaborating closely for most of the time, this should not be too difficult, although it takes some collective self-discipline (Ward *et al.*, 1998). It becomes much more challenging, however, to do the same in a larger team, or one with more fluid boundaries, or perhaps one where the levels of interaction fluctuate over time according to the demands of different situations or cases. Here it may be necessary to establish active systems to regularly review team functioning.

Such systems for review might include allowing some time in the pattern of regular team meetings for explicitly focusing on the team and its wellbeing and functioning. Sometimes this can be achieved by including an agenda item called 'Ourselves' or 'Team functioning' (see Example 2.5).

EXAMPLE 2.5 Team talking

In a large and busy day centre for older people, staff felt under continual pressure to meet demands, both from the individuals attending the centre and from external agencies wanting to refer more and more people. The ongoing system of staff meetings and supervision normally enabled them to cope with these pressures but, after a period of extra difficulty and a crisis which seemed to reveal serious tensions in the team, it was agreed that something more was needed. They decided to hold a session known as 'Team Talk' before their ordinary staff meetings, in which (helped by an outside adviser with experience in groupwork) they would talk about themselves as people and as colleagues, rather than about their tasks and functions or about their service users. This bi-monthly event soon became recognised as an essential part of the team's support system, and one which could then be sustained without further external support.

Developing this ongoing or organic approach to teamwork does not necessarily mean doing different things from normal but, rather, doing some of the same things differently. Thus staff supervision and staff meetings, while they are often used to focus primarily on the instrumental business of ensuring that all the responsibilities and tasks of the organisation are carried out appropriately, can also be adapted to include more of a focus on the expressive side of the work. This matters especially in group care units, where 'in one sense the whole unit is "the worker" ' (Beedell, 1970, p. 93). However, the same may be said of all health and social care teams, in which people's ability to communicate and collaborate as a group is so crucial.

Systems for team repair and rebuilding

Even in the best-run organisations, things sometimes go badly wrong, and team leaders or managers need to recognise this and do something about it. One of the skills required here is noticing what is happening to individuals as well as the team as a whole, and knowing how to interpret and make sense of this. In this respect being a team leader involves skills in working with group dynamics, like those of a group facilitator.

For example, if an individual worker becomes highly stressed, or angry about some aspect of their work, or resentful of a colleague's achievements, a manager's first instinct might be to see this as an individual problem and to tackle it only with that person. On closer examination, however, this may tell a wider story about the team as a whole, or perhaps about a sub-group within the team. Here the manager needs to focus on understanding what the team dimension of the problem is, before deciding how best to intervene. This might be explored together in the normal pattern of meetings or through a special meeting. For major communication difficulties in the team, more than one meeting may be required. The existing patterns of work and support within the team may need reviewing and redesigning. Of course, sometimes such difficulties also involve the team leader or manager as part of the problem. Here the best way forward may be to bring in an outside adviser or consultant, preferably someone without line management responsibilities to the team, to 'free up' communication and enable people to speak and difficulties to be aired in a safe environment (Furnivall, 1991).

Interpreting difficult situations in teams

Some of these situations can be very hard to understand and 'manage', especially if you are right in the middle of them, trying to do your best. It can be very difficult to know exactly why the morale of a team has sunk, why the rate of staff turnover has been so high, or why team members are squabbling. Here a different approach from the immediately obvious one may be needed. As in other 'stuck' situations it can be especially instructive to ask 'Why *now*?' (in other words, 'What else is currently going on for individuals or groups, or in the organisation as a whole, or in the local community?') and then to explore what possible connections there may be between these different phenomena. The other useful question to ask is 'What part is anxiety playing in this situation?' In other words, 'Who is worried about what, and why?'

Some of the complications arising in teams have their origins in unexpected or undetected places, such as the reactions of a key individual to some aspect of the situation that was worrying them or reminding them of another difficulty in their lives but they were not fully aware of it (Obholzer and Roberts, 1994a). Often these anxieties and patterns relate quite strongly to the underlying dilemmas and anxieties that are involved in the organisation's task. For instance, teams that are trying to prevent further abuse of vulnerable children in highly stressed families, or trying to provide some stability in the lives of adults with a lifelong history of mental health difficulties, may find themselves enacting some of the problems they encounter in this work. Example 2.6 illustrates this tendency.

> ### EXAMPLE 2.6 Power struggles in a mental health team
>
> A frequent dynamic in psychiatric institutions centres on who has the 'power' and who is 'powerless' within the team. This is a defensive shift away from the real powerlessness that the whole team shares in its relative inability to 'cure' the patient.
>
> During a staff meeting in a psychiatric unit there was a heated debate about a patient who had requested her social security cheque.
>
> *The doctor's view:* the patient was currently ill with a manic-depressive illness and would simply spend all her money on some useless article.

The social worker's view: it was a contravention of the patient's rights to withhold the cheque.

In a furious argument the majority of the nurses and other staff supported the social worker's view. The patient subsequently spent her entire cheque on alcohol and chocolates.

Neither doctor nor social worker was right or wrong – instead there was a painful choice of restricting the patient's 'freedom' or 'colluding' with madness. The whole team found it difficult to face their shared sense of helplessness about this particular patient. A focus on action and a quick decision was used as a defence against this painful feeling.

(Source: adapted from Stokes, 1994, p. 122)

'Difficult' team members

Another question that often arises is 'Why this particular person?' It is not uncommon in teams for there to be one person who appears to be the most difficult one to manage; examples of this were discussed in relation to workload in Section 2.5.

There may be many reasons why one particular person appears to be the most 'difficult'. Of course, some of them concern the individual and whatever external stresses in their life they are bringing to work with them. Other reasons may have more to do with the interactions between team members, or between one individual and the group as a whole, or even between the team as a whole and some other part of the professional context within which it has to operate. The manager's skill lies in seeing beyond the immediate 'problem person' and identifying the other possible factors. Where a major difficulty appears to be developing, therefore, the manager must try to discover what exactly is going on, and why it is happening, before deciding how to intervene to improve the situation.

Handling such difficulties may not be easy for managers, especially as it is not uncommon for people's difficulties to be expressed through direct conflict with the manager. A person who is angry about the sort or amount of work required may see this as the sole responsibility of the team manager. How can the manager then switch roles from being the 'bad' person who has imposed something on the individual that they cannot or will not handle to being a 'good' person who can help the worker to sort out the difficulty?

The manager may feel drawn into either insisting that the work must be done or 'rescuing' the person (and the situation) by backing down and allocating the work to someone else. At different times either of these responses can be appropriate but it may be that neither is of help. When one person is expressing difficulties on behalf of the team as a whole, what is needed is an honest and open debate between the manager and the team about issues such as the stresses of the work and the availability of support. However, to have such a debate the manager may need the support of an external trainer or a group facilitator, who can 'hold the ropes' between the manager and the team or individual. This need not involve the manager losing face: it can enable all sides to feel listened to and regain their morale and engagement with the team as a whole (Obholzer and Roberts, 1994b).

A positive approach

Teamwork can be challenging but managers should not assume it is riddled with difficulty and conflict. If they operated on such an assumption, they might risk creating difficulties by always expecting or even provoking them. A more positive approach is to think of teamwork as an exercise in shared creativity. What teams can offer each other (and their service users) is the mutual support and collective wisdom of a group of committed individuals. Each individual can be viewed as having not only their own potential and skills but also the key to unlocking each individual's potential, thus enhancing and extending the capabilities of the team as a whole. The extent to which these individuals can work together as a group influences their collective achievement as a team (Ward *et al.*, 1998).

According to this view, the 'whole' team can be seen as potentially much greater than the sum of its parts, because it can enable individuals to discover or develop new talents. The role of the team leader or manager can then be seen as somewhat akin to that of an orchestral conductor: bringing out the best in individuals to enhance the performance of the whole group, and thereby to stimulate individuals further to give of their best and reach new heights (see Mintzberg, 1998). How can this be done in practice? Perhaps the team leader as conductor focuses on the inter-personal dynamics of leadership and thinks about how to inspire people and help them inspire themselves and each other.

Key points

- Nurturing the team does not involve the team leader alone: it includes fostering team members' ability to care for and support each other.

- When individuals are stressed, it is worth considering whether there are team aspects to what may seem an individual problem.

- The team is greater than the sum of its parts and teamwork can be thought of as an exercise in shared creativity.

2.7 Conclusion

Teams matter because people at work need to be able to communicate and collaborate if they are to get the work done. This is especially true in the health and social care field. Several factors influence the ways in which teams operate, including the developing shared history of the team and its members.

Issues of staff recruitment, selection and induction matter in their own right but are also examples of ways in which teams need to incorporate and adapt to continual change.

I have argued in this chapter for a 'human relations' approach to managing teams. This means taking account of the expressive aspects of people's feelings about the team and their place in it, as well as the instrumental tasks of getting work allocated fairly and done to a high standard. It also means paying attention to the team as part of a more complex system.

This chapter also covered some of the ways in which managers can think about promoting and supporting better communication and collaboration in their teams. There were thoughts not only about 'team maintenance' – keeping the team on track under the pressures and demands of everyday work – but also 'team repair' – sorting out the difficulties that may arise. The overall message of this chapter might be summed up by the slogan 'people matter'. The team members are the greatest asset of any organisation and the greatest resource available to any team leader. This is easy enough to agree with but, for managers, it is a great challenge to put into operation.

Chapter 3
Leadership and vision

Anita Rogers and Jill Reynolds

3.1   Introduction

This chapter explores leadership and what it means for managers of care services. Frontline managers have a role as leaders, and they also look to their senior managers to provide leadership in their organisation. Previous chapters have already pointed to some of the leading and influencing that managers can do. This can be, for instance, through promoting to senior managers the dilemmas and concerns faced by practitioners; dealing with crises and making professional or strategic decisions; or inspiring a team to work effectively together.

There is an abundant literature on leadership: some from a management training perspective focuses on 'how to do it', while other work observes effective leaders in their jobs (for the former, see, for instance, Blanchard *et al.*, 1986; Goffee and Jones, 2000; and for the latter, Kouzes and Posner, 1987; Hartley and Allison, 2003). Government policy for modernising services places great emphasis on the need for leadership, although not always with a clear definition of what this means. The requirement to be a leader can appear daunting, bringing to mind the 'great men' of history. Early theories about what being a leader means often focused on the traits of leaders as though leadership was a characteristic that resided in them (Goffee and Jones, 2000). More recent work has focused on the potential for leadership to be developed in a range of people and distributed throughout organisations (Hunt, 1991; Tichy, 1997; Greenleaf, 1996). This implies that it is the job of leaders to encourage leadership from others – the followers. There may be some tension in leading from the front, attempting to inspire staff, while at the same time promoting their leadership skills.

The aims of this chapter are to:

- distinguish different aspects of leadership and the processes that support or constrain it
- consider how managers can adapt their preferred personal style to meet the needs of different situations
- discuss frontline managers' scope for creating and contributing to a vision of care services
- explore issues of power and participation in leadership.

3.2   Defining leadership

Hartley and Allison (2003) look at the role of leadership in the modernisation and improvement of public services. In defining leadership they distinguish between three different aspects: the person, the position and the processes (the three Ps).

Research has often focused on the characteristics, behaviours, skills and styles of leaders as *persons*, and the role of individuals in shaping events and circumstances. This tends to attribute exceptional capacity and power to individuals, and ignores organisational constraints and the contribution of 'followers' in accepting and promoting leadership.

The *position* of a leader may be important in giving authority, but does not guarantee leadership, which is more than simply holding an office such as chief executive. In contrast, a person with no formal position may none the less be a leader because others regard them as influential.

Leadership as a set of *processes* occurs among and between individuals, groups and organisations. This version of leadership is concerned with motivating and influencing people, and shaping and achieving outcomes. The role of the leader in relation to these processes is not to have exceptional capacity to provide solutions to problems. Instead it is to work with other people 'to find workable ways of dealing with issues for which there may be no known or set solutions' (Hartley and Allison, 2003, p. 298). When agencies work together in partnership to provide services that are 'joined up' and more logical for their users to access, the leadership processes need to work across organisational boundaries. No one person or their powers of position are sufficient to make things happen.

To this set of distinctions we add a fourth P – *purpose*. While person and position say 'who' is involved and processes describe 'how' things are done, purpose explains 'why'. The purpose provides the reason for doing things and is tied to underlying values. It involves setting a vision and determining strategy. The purpose connects with the primary task of individual organisations, although when collaboration between different agencies is needed then the purpose of a joint programme goes beyond the remit of any one agency.

Example 3.1 gives an opportunity to consider these different aspects. A social worker describes one of her managers as the best leader she ever worked with.

EXAMPLE 3.1 A manager who demonstrated leadership

Sheila articulated what we were there for. She put the clients first. She allocated work openly, allowing team members to work to their strengths. However, she never put pressure on anyone and she protected the team from inappropriate pressure. Sheila would stand up for you. She wasn't a pushover. She was nice, polite, but with quite a deliberate edge. She knew how to intervene and with whom.

Sheila was firm, with a transparent strategy that had a client focus. She led from the inside, not on high. She was part of the team, but there was never any doubt that she had the authority of a manager and she wasn't frightened to use her authority. She had a disciplinary expertise and won a lot of respect for her professional knowledge.

Sheila could interpret the changing political context to the team, without deskilling them. She would arrange half a day of staff training to look at a new policy direction, giving time for information and discussion and an opportunity to take ownership. Together we were able to look at ways to respond, using our skills and resources.

An example of her openness to creative ideas was a project for under-fives on one of the estates. A group of women from different agencies worked to discover what would be useful for these children. The group put together a bid for resources to fund an open, free play day. This was a real community project that the families wanted, not something imposed by social services. Sheila supported this project fully, allowing time for meetings, contributing her expertise in the bidding process.

Her manner was pleasant and she treated people with respect. Good practice has a lot to do with respect for the client group and the knock-on effect for workers. She was concerned for our welfare. Three days a week she chatted over lunch with us, never about work. She came to see me at home when I had a virus.

She was a good communicator, positively or negatively, and always dealt with people straight, not behind their backs. She gave good feedback, saying for example: 'From the client's perspective, there is a better way of doing this.'

Sheila was reliable. If you spent days doing paperwork, you got it back the next day with comments. It was a professional interchange: 'to develop yourself ...' or 'have you thought of ...?'

People helped each other on the team and there was little turnover of staff.

Thinking of person, position, process and purpose, you can see that Sheila kept her focus on the central purpose: service to clients. She reinforced and infused this sense of purpose in such a way that it was a key reference point for her and the team in their decisions and actions. Sheila had personal authority that came from her behaviour as well as her professional expertise. She also had the authority of her position. She demonstrated many characteristics that enabled her to build trust and commitment in her staff. She modelled integrity, respect and care. Sheila established and maintained processes that modelled and reflected her concern for clients, working with other agencies to provide community-based services. She extended that concern to staff through her methods of allocating work, her lunch hour chats and staff training days. Sheila was present, available, and technically and interpersonally competent. She could maintain and interpret the bigger picture while managing the detail of day-to-day work.

The description of Sheila in Example 3.1 infuses the different aspects of leadership with a sense of a particular style of doing things that is rooted in the values of care services. Some research- and practice-oriented literature builds up a picture of leadership for health and social care services that is consciously *distributed* among others: encouraging leadership and participation from staff.

Alimo-Metcalfe and Alban-Metcalfe (2000), in their study of leadership, conducted a survey of managers in the NHS and local government. They note the 'staggering complexity' of the role of leadership in these contexts. Their study suggests that an important function of leadership is what it can do for staff, but that this is more than simply meeting the staff's needs:

> The 2,000 staff who participated in this research project are also saying that leadership is fundamentally about engaging others as partners in developing and achieving the shared vision and enabling us to lead. It is also about creating a fertile, supportive environment for creative thinking, for challenging assumptions about how health care should be delivered.
>
> (Alimo-Metcalfe and Alban-Metcalfe, 2000, pp. 27–9)

Writing on residential care, Burton (1993) argues for a democratic style of management, where leadership, responsibility and decision making are shared. He points out that social services organisations must have an overall objective of helping users to achieve some measure of management of their own lives, to increase their control, power and choice. To this end, the workers in the organisation also need to develop their capacity to manage their own work. A key phrase is 'taking the lead'. Someone not in a designated management role may do this by expressing an insight or suggesting an initiative. Others respond, possibly testing or resisting the leadership, but change takes place. A different person may take up the leader role. 'If anyone becomes stuck in the leader role the progress and creativity of the group will also become stuck' (Burton, 1993, p. 77). In this view of leadership the most important task of the designated leader is to foster the leadership of others.

Through looking at the different aspects of leadership it is evident that leadership does not rely on position alone; it is not only managers who can be leaders, and indeed managers may deliberately seek to encourage leadership from others. The next section explores further the question of whether managers are inevitably leaders, and how compatible managing and leading are.

Key points

- It can be helpful to distinguish different aspects of leadership through looking at the person, position, processes and purpose.

- Leadership can involve encouraging the leadership of others – an overall term for this is *distributed leadership*.

3.3   Managing and leading

Some writers see management and leadership as two entirely separate approaches that draw on two different world views, different skills and different priorities. Zalzenik (1993) suggests that managers and leaders are fundamentally different in personality. He argues that leaders tolerate, indeed create, chaos, foster disruption, can live with a lack of structure and closure, and are actually on the look-out for change. Managers, in his view, seek order and control, which means achieving closure on problems as quickly as possible.

This is a rather restricted description of what a manager does. However, managing and leading can be in conflict with each other. When government policy or senior management calls for increased accountability and a focus on performance outcomes, this constricts the options available. More senior managers may expect their frontline managers to do as they are told, using a rather narrow definition of managing, instead of wanting them to show leadership. This kind of controlling approach to managing, which relies on the power of the position to get things done, is at odds with a human relations approach that prioritises organisational learning and professional development, such as is outlined in Chapter 1 and Chapter 2.

Distinctions between the different functions of management and leadership are identified in Table 3.1.

Table 3.1   **Comparison of management and leadership**

Management	*Leadership*
Produces order and consistency	Produces change and movement
– planning/budgeting	– vision building/strategising
– organising/staffing	– aligning people/communicating
– controlling/problem solving	– motivating/inspiring

(Source: adapted from Northouse, 1997, p. 9 and Kotter, 1990, pp. 3–8)

Bennis and Nanus also identify a contrast between managers and leaders: managers 'do things right' and leaders 'do the right thing' (1985, p. 21). It is not easy to achieve a balance between these alternatives and people may not always agree with their senior managers about where that balance lies:

> Leadership matters, it needs enthusiasm and charisma. I have learned to lead and to be happy in that role and with my power. I know when to be directive and when to be participatory. People know where the boundaries are. I do try to take an approach which looks at everybody's needs and try to model empowerment, although my supervisor says there are times when I should just tell them to 'get on with it'.
>
> (Manager of a residential care home for children, manager consultations)

Managers may also have different sets of priorities, and the priorities of senior management have an impact down the line. One senior manager in social services acknowledges this as a dilemma for frontline managers:

> I think it's a real dilemma for firstline managers that senior managers can actually delegate work to them and say 'I want this done now actually'. I will listen to what he or she thinks is the priority and hopefully we can come to some agreement ... but that is not always possible ... I do realise that it is my decision ultimately.
>
> (Manager consultations)

Leadership and management can be seen as distinct functions, or different roles, rather than as requiring different types of people. Mintzberg (1975) describes being a leader as one of ten roles that a manager performs (see Chapter 1, Figure 1.2). Three interpersonal roles – figurehead, leader and liaison person – interact with three informational roles – monitor, disseminator and spokesperson. These combine to act on four decisional roles of entrepreneur, disturbance handler, resource allocator and negotiator. Effective managers combine all of these roles. While the functions and roles of leadership draw on different strengths, training and outlooks, in the real world of care services individuals can and do embody the roles of both manager and leader.

Key points

- Being a leader can be just one of a manager's roles.
- The requirements of leading and managing can conflict.

3.4   Leadership styles and situations

As a manager, or someone entering into a management role, you are faced with a multitude of demands from different sources. Your senior managers want you to mobilise staff to meet targets efficiently and cost-effectively. Many studies, as well as a number of interviews conducted for this book, remark that staff want their managers to be present, available and supportive to their practice and to their growth and development (for instance, La Valle and Lyons, 1996; Waine and Henderson, 2003). You may recognise that you are more comfortable with some activities than others, and that your attention more naturally focuses on certain kinds of tasks and approaches. Some different styles are listed in Box 3.1. This draws on an application for organisational settings of the Myers-Briggs Type Indicator of personality preferences. The full version lists 16 types of preferences and our list is therefore not a comprehensive summary of personal style. Use it as a tool to focus your awareness of the particular strengths you bring to your leadership and management roles.

BOX 3.1 Different preferred styles

You are most comfortable **conforming** to established policies, rules and schedules and you take pride in your patient, thorough, reliable style.

You are most comfortable **responding** immediately to problems and you take pride in your open and flexible style.

You are most comfortable when **communicating** organisational norms and making decisions by participation, and you take pride in your personal, insightful style.

You are most comfortable **building** new systems and frameworks and pilots, and you take pride in your ingenuity and logical, analytical style.

(Source: adapted from Hirsch and Kummerow, 1987)

Different people have different preferences – and function best when they can adopt a style that allows them to express their own preferences. The message here is that it is best to go with your strengths.

However, a preference for a particular personal style is not the only factor in effective leadership. In day-to-day work, effectiveness often depends on how well a leader can balance the demands of both the instrumental (the tasks at hand) and the expressive (the human relations factor), that is, the needs and requirements of everyone involved in accomplishing a task. This is sometimes described as a *situational* approach to leadership: the preferred leadership style may have to be adapted to fit the demands of the particular situation being faced, which includes the needs of service users.

If you are a manager, one of your key functions is to gauge the levels of competence and commitment of your staff to accomplish the tasks in hand and achieve desired outcomes. You may find that the people you manage have variable levels of competence, depending on the situation, and variable levels of motivation too. This situational variability requires you to adapt your style, as the manager of a mental health voluntary organisation describes:

> I'm not afraid of leadership, I'm extremely aware of my own strengths and weaknesses, and the influence that I can bring to bear in the situations in which I find myself. It's an extremely important part of being a manager for me to be mindful of that and to use my skills and talents responsibly, knowing when to lead from the front, and knowing when to enable and empower and let go.
>
> (Manager consultations)

It takes time to develop a comfortable leadership style that also fits with the needs of the situation and no one can expect everything to fall into place from the start. Burton (1993, p. 81) comments on the fantasy held by and about many new managers that they will be 'Supermanager': the person who is unfailingly patient and kind, yet utterly decisive and clear thinking. It can be difficult to say 'no' when senior managers, colleagues and staff have high expectations that the new person will sort out longstanding problems. Example 3.2 describes the hopes and expectations of one new manager.

EXAMPLE 3.2 Expectations of a new manager

Anita has been appointed to manage a community mental health team where the care co-ordination process is being initiated. The aim is to have a more integrated approach, with health workers and social workers offering a more streamlined service. Anita notes that:

1 Her manager expects a sense of vision from her that will pull the team together and help them to move forward.

2 Her team members will also expect help to move forward, but they may actually want to stay where they are – in which case she will be the scapegoat when things don't go the way they want them to.

3 An initial meeting before she starts work gives her the sense that people are expecting her to wave a magic wand: 'We haven't been managed ... it's somebody else's fault that this team is in a mess.'

4 Senior managers have expectations that Anita will attend particular meetings and contribute to ongoing planning.

5 There is a strong commitment to multidisciplinary mental health teams from senior management but 'They haven't actually thought that far ahead – I suspect it's all going to be ad hoc at the moment.'

6 The team expect her to manage them. Team meetings are chaotic and one area that Anita hopes to improve through having agenda items and a fixed time slot.

7 The director of nursing wants above all else that Anita should keep the primary care trust happy – they are major stakeholders.

Anita's hope for her first three months in post is to:

- get to know her team and find out what makes them tick
- get a feel for the area that she is in, and the kind of work that comes through
- find out what the service users' main complaints are and what they are happy about in relation to the service
- talk to the primary care groups and check their expectations.

(Source: manager consultations)

Anita's main aims are to get to know who the key players in her area are and what makes her team tick. Even such an apparently modest aspiration can be quite demanding in an entirely new situation where none of the familiar resources and networks are available.

There are several *contingency* or *situational* models of leadership that attempt to understand the relationship between style and situation and we look next at one developed by Hersey and Blanchard (1988). The first step is to evaluate staff and assess their competence and commitment to perform the given task (in other words, getting to know them and finding out what makes them tick).

The leader then adjusts direction and support according to the needs of the workers. *Directive* behaviours often involve one-way communication that directs, focusing on what is to be done, how it is to be done, and who is responsible for doing it. The leader gives direction and establishes desired outcomes, methods of evaluation, role definition and tasks. *Supportive* behaviours, on the other hand, help people feel comfortable about themselves and the situation. These involve two-way communication and include listening, giving praise, perhaps asking for input and help with problem solving.

Balancing direction and support can sound a rather mechanical approach to working with people. In reality, most managers probably use a more intuitive approach to meeting the needs of different staff, but it is helpful to identify the different elements of situational leadership. These may actually be ideal types – that is, rarely encountered in exactly this way and forming instead a cluster of attributes. Figure 3.1 (overleaf) is a matrix of a leader's responses to staff situations, and an explanation of the different ideal-type responses follows (Northouse, 1997).

- A *high directive/low supportive* approach is appropriate for staff who have high commitment but low competence. This is a relationship that focuses on instruction.

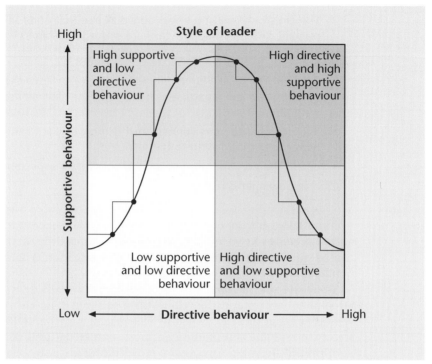

Figure 3.1 **Situational leadership** (Source: Blanchard *et al.*, 1986, p. 74)

- A *high directive/high supportive* approach may be more effective with staff who have some competence but reduced motivation to accomplish the task. Leader behaviours include coaching, giving encouragement and asking for input. However, the final decision about what the aims and outcomes should be, and how to accomplish them, remains with the leader.

- A *high supportive/low directive* approach is for staff who have competence but low commitment. This approach involves listening, praising, asking for input and giving feedback. Staff have control over day-to-day decisions, but the leader is available to help with problem solving.

- A *low supportive/low directive* approach is most effective with staff who have a high degree of commitment and competence. After agreeing what is to be done, the leader lessens involvement in planning and day-to-day details and even intervenes less with support (Northouse, 1997).

The leadership style changes over time from directing to coaching to supporting to delegating as performance improves. Managers may adapt their approach with staff for different tasks for which they have different competence or emotional reactions. Anita (in Example 3.2) may want to take a high directive/high supportive approach as she gets to know her new team, but in her approach to team meetings she may tend to be high directive/low supportive until she feels that the meetings are accomplishing what they should. Managers may also want to adapt their approach for different workers.

One of the authors (Jill Reynolds) worked as a project leader in a reception centre for refugees. The housekeeper sometimes needed urgent advice on what were quite challenging problems. Perhaps repairs were needed to the dilapidated property – originally a workhouse – or a hygiene problem was identified in relation to food storage. The approach that seemed to work best was to ask the housekeeper what her preferred way of dealing with the problem was. Often she could work out a solution, but would want to use Jill as a sounding board. The approach that Jill took with her was a low directive/high supportive one. With the interpreters, who were refugees themselves and new to the UK, Jill aimed to be quite directive and offered a lot of support.

Although the situational approach is used extensively in leadership training, it does have some limitations. There are few research studies that justify the assumptions and monitor the effect of the approach on performance. There are some practical difficulties in adopting a different approach to different members of a staff group, while also thinking about the overall level of development of the group as a whole (Northouse, 1997). It is important to be perceived as being fair and acting in the same way towards everybody. You might question whether a high directive/low supportive approach is ever the right one in care services. Even an unqualified worker in a new job is likely to appreciate some recognition of their input and ideas as well as encouragement to develop competence.

An alternative way to conceptualise leadership style that takes into account variability in situations is shown in Box 3.2.

BOX 3.2 Emphasis in leadership

Leadership style varies according to the degree of emphasis on:

- **compliance** with rules and procedures

- **delegation** of responsibility to others

- **standards** set and monitored in all aspects of the work

- **rewards** for excellence rather than for seniority or due to favouritism

- **distance** maintained through aloofness or reduced over time through building warm and trusting relationships with team members.

(Source: adapted from Coulshed and Mullender, 2001, p. 100)

According to Coulshed and Mullender (2001), managers can monitor their own approach by asking themselves the following questions.

- Are procedures sufficiently well organised that people can be left to get on with their jobs, but not so constraining that initiative is hindered?
- Are staff encouraged to take responsibility and 'own' their decisions and initiatives without too much risk of mistakes?
- Are standards set too high or too low (or not at all)?
- Is everyone regularly praised and rewarded, and criticised fairly?
- Is there a friendly and comfortable working atmosphere in which people can ask for support or advice when they need it?

There are no definitive answers to the right degree of the different emphases listed in Box 3.2. The variation in management and staff situations means that managers need to appraise their own setting and work out the relative importance of, for instance following rules or delegating responsibility and developing people. In doing so, they are adopting a practice-led approach. Ideally, this will take into account the needs of staff and the primary task of the staff group as well as managers' own preferred style.

Example 3.3 describes an approach taken in a children's home to managing the food budget. It is in contrast to arrangements – not uncommon – where responsibility for bulk ordering lies with central management. The example illustrates leadership as a set of processes. The children and staff need varying levels of support and direction to engage with the process, which is a learning situation for everyone.

EXAMPLE 3.3 Sharing responsibility for food

In a children's home with an annual budget for food, residents and staff have full control together (within their budget) over what food they buy, how they prepare and cook it and how they eat it. The job of managing the catering is taken in turns by different workers, with help from colleagues and from the children and young people. Who takes on this very difficult job is decided at either the staff meeting or the community meeting, or both, and comments, suggestions and major decisions regarding food and everything to do with it are regular items of discussion in both formal meetings and informal gatherings. The food budget is frequently examined and is available to everyone.

Most of the children are expected to take part in the shopping and cooking at some time. They are used to budgeting on a large household scale; they handle substantial sums of money and account for how they spend it. The residents learn social and practical skills – catering, budgeting, decision making – which few of their friends and contemporaries are likely to learn in their smaller family households.

> Although the food is important to everyone, not all the staff and residents are expected to take part in its selection and preparation. Some children are not ready to shop or cook. Staff move in and out of some of the domestic, household managing roles but the whole staff group are wary of reproducing stereotypical 'women's roles', particularly in connection with managing the food. The boys who live there, quite as much as the girls, have the advantage of knowing about running a (very large) household and sharing responsibility for seeing that it is a good, comforting and nourishing environment.
>
> (Source: adapted from Burton, 1993, pp. 78–9)

In this example some staff may need little direction or support in the practical matters of budgeting, shopping and cooking. On the other hand, they are also engaged in coaching the children, and this may be a more complex aspect for which they need a higher level of support. Some children will be active in learning household management (high direction and high support); others will simply take part in consuming the results. The men and the women in the group may support each other in resisting a tendency to see the management of food as 'women's work'.

The approach taken in the children's home is based on a vision of how residents and staff should be involved with such important decisions as those concerning food. The strength of the situational approach to leadership is that it recognises that leaders need to be adaptable. Situational leadership models do not explicitly focus on the role of vision and purpose, although our discussion of Example 3.3 shows that they can be applied to settings where vision plays an important part.

The advice to new managers from the manager of a mental health voluntary organisation is to trust in people, work to their strengths and share their vision:

> Keep enthusiastic, believe in people, trust in people, work to your own strengths, have a vision, share your vision, and take it forward with people, and start every new day as if it is the first.
>
> (Manager consultations)

Goffee and Jones (academics and organisational consultants who have developed and tested theory in workshops for managers) offer even more pithy advice on leadership style to the managers they coach: 'Be yourselves – more – with skill' (2000, p. 70).

> **Key points**
>
> • Managers do best when they adopt a leadership style that expresses their personality preferences and allows them to play to their strengths.
>
> • A situational approach to leadership emphasises the importance of a flexible response according to the needs of the situation, the organisation and staff development.

3.5   The place of vision

Engagement with purpose and vision is often described as *transforming* or *transformational* leadership (Burns, 1978; Bass, 1985). The implication is that people can be inspired to lift their attention above everyday affairs. Through developing shared values and a sense of doing something purposeful, transformational leaders can alter the way staff see themselves and their organisation (Martin and Henderson, 2001). Transformational leaders are not just concerned with meeting the current goals of the organisation, the service or the system, but in 'upping the stakes' and changing the goals. Values, meaning and purpose are at issue here as the leader articulates goals that others have been only dimly or not at all conscious of (Bennis and Nanus, 1985).

There are some difficulties with the literature on transformational leadership: it is speculative and argues from conviction rather than from evidence. There are criticisms of the moral aspirations of transformational models in relation to the business world; efforts to make work happier and more fulfilling may be in conflict with an overriding goal to make profits (Harvey, 2001). In relation to care services, it is perhaps more obvious that if staff feel fulfilled and valued, the relationships and care for the users of the service will flourish. The relevance of transformational models for care services is that they highlight some important core values that are central to the provision of good care: honesty, openness, respect for individuals, community of interest, mutual help, empowerment and developing other people.

Whatever the state of knowledge about transformational leadership, it is a concept that has passed into common understandings of the relationship between leadership and vision. In the context of care, the manager of a residential care home for children captures some of the essence of a transformational leadership model as follows.

It's about people having a vision; they need to learn how to create visions and look to the future. It's very important when you are coming into residential care. You are constantly evolving. When it becomes comfortable in a residential home people want to stay there, but if you stagnate it falls apart ... all sorts of different other elements come in, because you need constant recognition, constant achievement, you've got to be having a vision. You've got to be aware of what's going on in the child's world.

(Manager consultations)

Creating and implementing a vision is an important aspect of leadership. Vision is a picture of the results you want to create, an ideal sense of what is possible, a statement of destination. Some managers may feel their scope in contributing to the formulation of a larger vision is limited. They see their primary responsibilities as attending to the day-to-day operations and the practice of their staff. However, Henderson and Seden (2003) suggest that, increasingly, frontline managers are becoming involved in strategic planning, perhaps because they have important information about the needs of service users and issues for practitioners. If they are not formulating the vision, they are designing pathways for its implementation. While this can be difficult, as it pulls frontline managers away from a

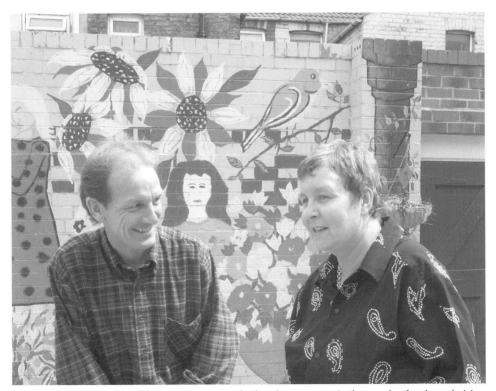

This mural by mental health service users and a local arts group is the result of a shared vision

focus on practice and operations, it is also exciting, as it allows them to help shape the service and to inform senior managers about what the important issues are. There are opportunities here for managers to be practice-led: leading from their practice base and helping the learning of the organisation. Evans (2003) describes a programme that gave managers an opportunity to reflect on practice in their teams and pass on the results of their 'team self-audits' in order to influence strategic planning by their authorities.

We argue that managers play a role in the vision sequence whether in the formulation and strategy, or whether in tying the vision into practical aims and objectives, and remaining vigilant for better ways of doing things. Even as a new manager of a mental health team (Example 3.2), Anita hopes the team can become enthused with a vision for the service:

> My new manager will be expecting from me, among other things, this sense of vision, this integrated way of working which is new to the area I'm going to and one of the things I sold myself on at my interview. Pulling the team together and helping them to move forward.
>
> (Manager consultations)

Vision can hold a team together, as described in Example 3.4. Martin, an experienced manager, recollects the importance of the shared aims or goals that put vision into practice in a newly combined team of probation officers and social workers. The vision he describes was to improve a poor system and give better service.

EXAMPLE 3.4 Sharing a vision

I think the key to it is having an aim or a goal that everyone shares. If you have that then people are less worried about the fact that the person sitting opposite them gets two more days' holiday or that they get paid extra, because they are all focused on the same goal. My main experience of this was managing a joint agency team in youth justice where probation officers and social workers came together. Now, historically at that time those two were poles apart. The fear was, 'Oh, we don't want to work with that lot', and my own perception was that probation officers often thought they were a bit better than social workers. 'Oh, we're officers of the court you know', they used to say, and social workers were a bit fearful of the probation officers, because they saw them as almost like cops, soft cops. So there were those fears.

So this group of people came together. Now if you let them, I think they would have focused on the issues around terms and conditions of service. But what we all wanted to do was improve the poor system, give a better service to the courts, give a better service to the young offenders and their families we're working with. Now it's interesting in that team that no one wanted to join it at the outset for all the reasons I've mentioned. But a year down the line, when there was a proposal put forward to disband the team and go back to the old way of working, everyone defended the team to the hilt. Now I think that's because we focused on the goal more, and it's the issue of offering support to people, and suddenly, pay, leave and pomposity wasn't an issue.

(Source: manager consultations)

Shared visions are compelling, bringing out courage people did not realise they had. They take time to develop because they require people to listen to each other and allow new insights to emerge about what is possible – part of the process sometimes described as becoming 'a learning organisation' (Senge, 1990). Martin points out that an essential feature is the team approach to problem solving, and that this may be more effective than trying to design the ideal system, for instance for developing interdisciplinary working in mental health:

You can either try to resolve every problem before you set the thing up, or you can get people together in a meaningful way at an early stage, and then ask them to solve it. In relation to community mental health teams, there are so many problems around – the documentation for example – and I've just got a feeling that if we sit these people together, they will actually resolve a lot of those issues for us, whereas managers ... can probably spend a year talking about it.

(Manager consultations)

It is especially difficult to build a shared vision in an atmosphere of tension and distrust. People can become disenchanted with the gap between the vision and the current reality. People can lose their connection with each other, forget to reinspire each other about what they really want to create, and lose the relationships that such conversations nurture. Managers, as leaders, can provide the inspiration that continually refreshes the vision.

In more prosaic terms, vision may simply be the overview that managers can provide, as Beverley, a practitioner with a voluntary child care project, describes:

Practitioners get very caught up in practice, and I think the manager's role is to have that overview, and to think, 'We haven't looked at that policy recently, that procedure recently. We haven't looked at what frames our practice, and it would be really useful for us to carve out some time, to review that.'

(Manager consultations)

> **Key points**
>
> - Creating and contributing to a sense of vision is often seen as central to leadership at all levels.
>
> - At times of tension it can be helpful for managers to involve different people in building a shared vision.
>
> - The managerial role gives managers an opportunity to maintain an overview of the work of the unit.

3.6 Managing power

Power is the currency of leadership, determining what gets done and how. Without power, leaders cannot lead (Bennis and Nanus, 1985). Important questions are:

- Who has power?
- How do they use it?
- Who has access to the positions that provide an opportunity to use power?

In this section we discuss some elements of charismatic leadership, in which power often appears to be held by an individual because they possess a strong personality and a compelling vision. In contrast, so far we have been exploring the possibilities for leadership activities to be distributed throughout organisations or partnership arrangements; some implications of this are reviewed next.

Charismatic leadership

Max Weber made a detailed study of charismatic leaders in which he defined charisma as:

> a certain quality of an individual personality by virtue of which he is set apart from ordinary men and treated as endowed with supernatural, superhuman, or at least specifically exceptional qualities.
>
> (Weber, 1947, p. 329)

More recent work has extended thinking on charisma to look at the relationship between the charismatic person and the institution or agency. For effective leadership, other people have to become engaged with the leader's project. If the agency is to continue with the leader's approach, it must embody and express the charisma in its routine life. The structure of the agency then becomes the carrier of the charisma (Starratt, 1993).

Many of the qualities and behaviours we have already ascribed to transformational leadership are also those of charismatic leadership: strong interpersonal skills, the ability to imagine a different and better future and to communicate a vision, courage, willingness to take risks, self-confidence, passion and energy. The essence of charisma is the capacity to generate excitement, enthusiasm and subsequent loyalty to the mission and the leadership. The power of the leader is, of course, grounded in the power of those people who associate with, follow and support that leader (Starratt, 1993).

Such leaders can have immense power in an immensely powerful dynamic. Charismatic leadership often emerges in times of crisis, when there is more latitude to take initiative. It can also be found in entrepreneurial settings characterised by opportunity and optimism (Conger and Kanungo, 1988). Some charismatic leaders can shift the context, creating conditions of crisis or opportunity. Many of the care services that are now taken for granted would not be in place today without the original vision and drive of pioneering men and women who saw a better way of dealing with social or health problems and found an opportunity or campaigned for change. Think, for instance, of Florence Nightingale, Barnardos, the Leonard Cheshire Homes or the Terrence Higgins Trust.

There can be a dark side to charisma (Conger and Kanungo, 1988). Because of the leader's powerful capacity to enhance people's self-esteem, self-efficacy and energies, followers can become dependent on the leader. Their self-worth becomes a function of the leader's approval. While leaders can use charisma to articulate and help to bring about a vision that serves the group or the community, they can also use charisma to serve primarily their own interests, to the detriment of the group. A stark example is Frank Beck, a manager in the 1970s and 1980s, who was convicted of 17 counts of physical and sexual assault on children and young people in four different children's homes. A student chose a placement in his home because he was 'a charismatic leader who led from the front' (Kirkwood, 1992, p. 211). At Beck's trial the judge said, in his summing up: 'You exploited authority and the undoubted power of your personality to satisfy your lust' (p. 2).

Even in less overtly dangerous situations, problems can arise because of:

- a grandiose vision and unrealistic expectations to serve the vision
- poor investigation of facts, poor assessment and use of resources
- selective communication that underestimates difficulties
- manipulation of people and relationships.

Love–hate relationships between leaders and followers can result: you are 'in' if you are performing miracles; you are 'out' if you are doing less. Charisma can be a double-edged sword. Within its very strength and power there is the potential for abuse or crisis in any organisation whose members find difficulty in making their own contribution to the common vision. A caseworker with a voluntary organisation commented:

> Our organisation is strongly associated with the name of our Director. She is regularly interviewed by the media and has raised huge amounts of donations. She has built the organisation over the last 20 years from a small group of volunteers to a staff of over 90; we own the premises we operate from. Some of us have tried really hard to get better practices and policies in relation to equal opportunities, but it's a hopeless battle. And although she's now well past retirement age, she is still not handing over responsibilities, or involving others in senior management decisions.
>
> (Manager consultations)

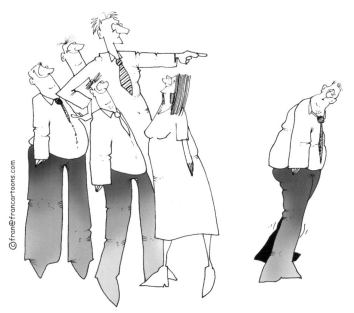

Charismatic leaders sometimes foster love–hate relationships with their staff

Nadler and Tushman (1988) refer to 'magic leadership' to describe the catalysts who start up innovative organisations or revitalise them when they flag. Weber first identified the problem of trying to find a successor to a charismatic leader (cited in Conger and Kanungo, 1988, p. 15). Nadler and Tushman comment that one person cannot sustain the magic over an extended period, and argue that it is more effective if organisations develop skilled leaders at all levels. The right mix of people in senior management positions can ensure better day-to-day leadership to keep an organisation from crisis. At worst, they can provide the next 'magic leader' to pull the organisation through.

Leadership and diversity

If charismatic leaders are best advised to share power and promote the leadership of others, who are the leaders-in-waiting who should receive this encouragement? The words commonly used to describe leaders – for instance 'great men', 'superhuman', or 'heroes' – suggest exceptional qualities. They also imply that leaders are predominantly male. A theme of US literature in the 1990s was 'leadership diversity' (see, for instance, Arredondo, 1996; Morrison, 1992). The focus tends to be on how organisations can promote more women, black and foreign-born people to positions of power. Discussion can, of course, be extended to other people who have traditionally had less opportunity to enter the workplace or take on leadership positions, such as those with disabilities or mental health problems, and gay and lesbian people (see, for example, Read, 2003). The arguments for doing this centre around better human relations practices, value-based assumptions of equity and fairness, a better reflection of the populations served by the organisation, and the potential loss to the organisation of the creativity of people from diverse social, racial and cultural backgrounds.

In a British context women are disadvantaged in gaining senior management positions in care services. The workforce study by Ginn and Fisher (1999) found that women comprise between 86% and 95% of the workforce but only between 60% and 71% of managers. A survey in 2002 of local authority social services departments by the Social Services Inspectorate (SSI) shows some increase in the numbers of women in the top three tiers of management since 1997, a move from 42% to 48% (Social Services Inspectorate/Association of Directors of Social Services, 2002). Proportionately more women continue to be positioned at the third tier level than are rising to become directors or second tier managers. Ginn and Fisher suggest that the picture is not of direct discrimination but a combination of factors. Lower qualifications play a part, but the influence of a full-time service career dominates overall; a career history with substantial full-time service is less easy for women to achieve while they have principal responsibility for child care in their personal lives.

It is possible that women offer a different kind of leadership. There are some indications that women tend to put aspects of staff care such as supervision and support above administrative concerns in terms of priorities (Eley, 1989). Grimwood and Popplestone (1993) argue that women managers in social care are more oriented to taking care of their staff and paying attention to detail.

Deborah Tannen has done research into the different conversational styles of men and women. Common conversational rituals among men often involve an oppositional stance using banter, teasing and expending effort to avoid feeling inferior in an interaction. Common conversational rituals among women are often ways of maintaining an appearance of equality, taking account of the other person's feelings, and expending effort to downplay the speaker's authority so that she can get the job done without obviously flexing her muscles (Tannen, 2003). Tannen gives examples that show how women in management positions can be quite unobtrusive in making sure that things go smoothly, which can mean that their excellence then goes unrecognised.

A review of international studies of gender differences in management behaviour and style shows inconsistent results: some studies found women to have a more supportive style, or to be more relationship- and participation-oriented; others found them less relationship-oriented or that there was no difference (Vinkenburg *et al.*, 2000, p. 128). The authors conclude that despite calls for feminine leadership qualities, few actual differences in personal factors and behaviour have been consistently and empirically confirmed by research. This leads them to argue that although there are persistent stereotypes about gender differences, there are no reasons not to promote women who are motivated and capable into top management positions.

In relation to black and ethnic minority women managers in the UK, it is difficult to obtain accurate data and perhaps many systems do not routinely collect this information. The 2001 SSI survey found only 5% of women managers were of non-white ethnic origin and the majority of these were at the third tier and in London. One review notes that there is some evidence that the position of black and ethnic minority women managers may actually be worsening (Bhavnani and Coyle, 2000). Bhavnani and Coyle's own study, evaluating training and development initiatives designed to meet the needs of black and ethnic minority women managers working in the NHS, found that training programmes were unequivocally valued. However, a large proportion of the women who took part in this study felt frustrated about their chances of career progression, and thought that white managers failed to recognise their capability. The authors argue that thinking on equality in organisations needs to encompass a view that when people from diverse backgrounds hold power, it can add value to the organisation itself. This idea requires a wider strategy of organisational development and change, and positive action to recruit from under-represented groups is insufficient.

> It is not enough to increase numbers and expect women to blend in. It is also not enough to recruit black and ethnic minority women based on an assumption that their main virtue lies in what they can offer as knowledge of their 'own people'.
>
> (Bhavnani and Coyle, 2000, pp. 230–1)

They go on to suggest that, like other diverse groups, black and ethnic minority women bring different and competitively relevant knowledge and perspectives about how to actually do work.

Coulshed and Mullender (2001) similarly comment on the subversion or hostility that members of oppressed groups may encounter when they make it into management. Black managers may find that white subordinates do not know how to relate to them as authority figures, for instance double-checking their advice with white staff. Coulshed and Mullender argue that if the only change made is to allow disabled workers, women, black people and other oppressed groups to be more fully represented in welfare organisations, this has severe limitations:

> it can mean entering an agency's workforce on the terms set by those who got there first and who have already determined the agendas of assumptions, priorities and even of language. This can lead to tokenism, harassment and continuing oppressive treatment.
>
> (Coulshed and Mullender, 2001, p. 223)

They point to the value base of social care provision, and the responsibilities of organisations providing services to consider issues of gender, ethnicity, culture and religion, age, disability and health, class and poverty, and issues affecting gay and lesbian people. These are now essential considerations in the delivery of services at the practitioner and service user level. Coulshed and Mullender argue they provide a challenge for change at the levels of management and organisational design.

The following questions can help to provide an appraisal of the state of affairs in agencies or community groups in relation to diversity and opportunity.

- Who benefits from current arrangements (in service delivery, in my organisation, in my work group)?
- Which group dominates this social arrangement (for instance a committee, a working group, a department)?
- Who defines the way things are structured around here (in my agency, my community)?
- How do practices, processes and systems promote or restrict inclusiveness (those that characterise my profession, my day-to-day work, my relationships with senior and subordinate people)?
- How does the language commonly used shape attitudes and action, and where does it come from?

Enabling participation

Issues of sharing power and leadership suggest that some specific practices need to be adopted. 'Distributed leadership' is an overall term for a variety of different practices that emphasise participation. The practice of participation in decisions can vary from consultation, where people are asked for their views and the manager makes the decision, to delegation, where authority and responsibility are given to the individual or the group. Delegation might seem a more effective means of truly distributing power, but it tends to be used selectively, often when less important decisions are involved, the manager is short of time and the person delegated to is viewed as capable of taking on the responsibility (Hollander and Offerman, 1993).

The account in Example 3.5 is from a project worker in a young people's centre, who was asked to step in when the manager took a year's leave.

EXAMPLE 3.5 Developing a participatory approach

When I started as a manager it was an ideal time really to sit down with staff and look at things they wanted to change. How happy were we with how the centre was run? And there were a lot of changes made. It helped people, because we were all making these decisions and ... all staff members were taking part in these discussions ... I do believe it helped people gain ... more of a sense of ownership of the service, and I think when you have a sense of ownership, then you work more effectively.

I do think it was part of my particular style of involving people. If we make decisions as a team, then we'll make the right decisions, because everybody's having input. Sometimes people see things differently. So if we all have input, the right decision will be made. So in some ways, it was out of fear, I think (I don't want the buck to stop with me), but in a bigger way, it was out of ... the way that I work anyway, in a facilitative, democratic way.

This is a service that challenged existing services. We were offering it in a different way which respected young people and had them involved right from the beginning. We got the project externally evaluated. We won a national award for good practice as well as three local awards for good practice. Then you start to get some sort of status within your community. You start to sit on other committees.

(Source: manager consultations)

According to Smith (2000), some of the skills and behaviours involved in enabling shared leadership and more participation in decisions are:

- show others how knowledge and experience in decision making can be acquired
- participate in deciding with team members what courses of action to take
- listen rather than talk most of the time
- encourage team initiative and accept risks and occasional failures
- invite or encourage people to take on responsibility for a development
- value contributions
- interpret organisational politics for the team.

While the idea of participation in leadership is attractive, especially in work founded on egalitarian principles, the reality many managers describe is that full and continuous participation can be cumbersome, time-consuming and inefficient. If a manager retains the responsibility for decisions and actions in the team or agency, this may discourage the distribution of power because any negative consequences will fall on the manager (Hollander and Offerman, 1993). Once again, the personal styles and competences of those involved, both managers and staff, the nature of the immediate situation, the nature of the task, the culture, structures and processes of the organisation, and the underlying purposes are all factors that shape the effectiveness of a participatory approach.

Key points

- While charisma is often associated with individuals, effective charismatic leadership has to be embedded in the life of the organisation.

- Leaders can use charisma to serve their own interests to the detriment of the group.

- If people from a more diverse range of social backgrounds are encouraged into management positions, there may need to be more recognition of the different skills, knowledge and expertise they bring.

- The value base of care provision gives some impetus to a paradigm shift towards distributed leadership and increased participation.

- Enabling participation takes time and requires skilled leadership and attention to the development of participants' skills.

3.7   Conclusion

At the beginning of this chapter a description of Sheila, a team manager, was offered as an exemplar of good leadership. This example shows many of the elements of an approach that seeks participation and develops the leadership of others. Standing back slightly and conceptualising the elements of the leadership process reveals that leadership involves a dynamic interaction of four key elements: the person, the position, the processes and the purposes. This chapter has explored the varying nature of leadership, and the evolution of the thinking and practice of leadership, from a set of characteristics, behaviours and processes emanating from special individuals to a phenomenon that resides wholly in the community.

As you progressed through the chapter, you will have seen the complexity of leadership. There is no one model of leadership, but the various approaches and emphases discussed here offer perspectives on a multidimensional phenomenon. If you are a manager, you show leadership when you effectively assess the capacity of your staff to fulfil the mandate of your organisation, and then provide the necessary direction, support, participation or autonomy to get things done. You show leadership in your enthusiasm for the work you all do, and for the structures and processes you help put in place to sustain that commitment. You show leadership in your availability, in your individual attention to your staff, in your genuine care. You show leadership when you look around and say to yourself and others, 'This can be done differently', or even better, 'Let's take a look at how we can make it happen'. You may be doing one or all of these at any given time. In demonstrating this kind of sensitive agility, you are demonstrating leadership.

Chapter 4
Managing change

Anita Rogers and Jill Reynolds

4.1   Introduction

In health and social care services managing means managing change. In many ways change is the very fabric of social care. Care provision is often required in the first place because of changes in people's lives which lead to a need for care and support services. Managers trying to improve the quality of care have to consider whether changes are needed, what they might be and how to introduce them. The level of change may be incremental and developmental, and in taking any initiatives managers are actively engaged and *acting*. Changes in social policy at a government level and their implementation locally through strategic planning also bring changes for frontline managers to implement. This sort of change often means a role for managers in which they are *reacting*, although in many organisations and charities a frontline manager may take an active lead in preparing business plans for the management committee or for the trustees.

Whether the change is large-scale and policy-driven or small-scale and local, the aim should be to improve the services being offered (even when containing costs is a strong consideration). Change is never a one-off event; it is a continuous process. If you are a frontline manager, you probably have to accomplish a number of disparate functions simultaneously, keeping old systems running, managing transitional arrangements, and bringing new structures into being.

This chapter looks at the context of change in managing care. Various examples explore the possibilities for being active and reactive when introducing changes. You will get more from this chapter if you keep in mind a change project of your own, for analysis and planning. Choose something that is always likely to be required, for instance improving how meetings are run or how work is allocated. Try to strike a balance between something that has a good chance of success and something that will make demands on you and involve you in new learning. The chapter focuses on knowledge, strategies and tools that will help you to plan and implement change, and to develop your capabilities to manage the unpredictable and unplanned aspects of change.

Change models can help you to think about different elements that need to be planned for. A wealth of different models have been devised for the purpose of managing change, and in this chapter we draw on a small selection that can usefully be applied to care settings. If you want to know more about other models, *Organisational Change* by Iles and Sutherland (2001) gives a helpful overview.

Above all, change involves people, and skill in communicating with and engaging people in planned change is fundamental to successful change. Working with a change process aimed at an enhanced quality of service and life for clients and workers requires a range of competences, attitudes and skills that allow you and your colleagues to challenge assumptions, develop common understandings and exercise new behaviours.

The aims of this chapter are to:

- recognise that the task of managing care is subject to change and adaptation
- apply some theoretical models to an example of changing care provision
- explore different reactions, barriers and blocks to the implementation of change
- note common features of successful change initiatives.

4.2 Understanding the dimensions of change

Studies of change initiatives in organisations have yielded a number of models that attempt to answer the following questions.

- How can we understand complexity, interdependence and fragmentation?
- Why do we need to change?
- Who and what can change?
- How can we make change happen?

(Adapted from Iles and Sutherland, 2001, p. 22)

These questions can help practitioners and managers organise their thinking and action. We follow them through in this chapter, focusing in this section on the complexity and interdependence of the care sector, and looking at the further questions in subsequent sections.

The skills of working with people are relatively stable and consistent in comparison with the kinds of change that commerce and industry have experienced since the 19th century. A lesson to be drawn from these sectors is that change is pervasive, many thrive on it, and most changes bring opportunities as well as difficulties (Taylor and Vigars, 1993).

While there is some continuity in the skills needed for social care, the structures within which those skills are practised and the policies for social care provision have been the subject of reform since the introduction of public and charitable services. For harassed managers, changes introduced as a result of the changing political landscape can sometimes feel like a constraint on the smooth running of the organisation. At times, the intensity of proposed change can produce negative reactions even when the general direction of policy is seen as positive, as described by a training co-ordinator in a voluntary organisation:

> The last six months has seen a tidal wave of consultation papers ... There are a number of problems here. First, the turnaround period for the return of comments on most consultation papers has been extremely short, certainly not sufficient to give all concerned time to make a considered and informed response. Second, the sheer volume of the material that has been dispatched is causing chronic consultation overload and fatigue. Third, it is evident from an examination of these consultation papers that one part of the Scottish Executive is often not checking the content of a paper with another relevant part of the Executive before dispatch. This raises questions as to the 'joined-upness' of government action! Fourth, the speed with which responses are sought encourages the view that the Scottish Executive may be engaged in a pseudo-consultation exercise.
>
> (Manager consultations)

Managers and workers are always operating on several levels at the same time. From the perspective of the frontline manager, changes can be 'top-down' and imposed, stemming from policy requirements or from within the organisation. Some top-down changes have a legislative requirement, some changes come as guidance, and some changes are advocated as good practice; they all have different implications. Changes can also be 'bottom-up', introduced as a result of evaluation by service users, or lessons absorbed from practice, or because of the manager's own agenda for change – to raise standards of work in the team for instance. Managers work with multiple priorities which all compete for time. The ideal solution is to find ways of harmonising imperatives from above with those arising from practice. Example 4.1 (overleaf) summarises an approach that did just this.

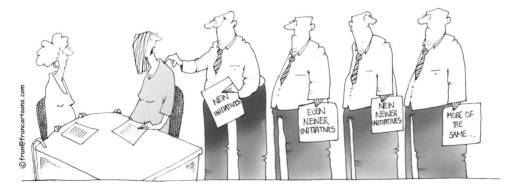

The intensity of proposed change can produce negative reactions

EXAMPLE 4.1 Reviewing the home care service

A review was held of the home care service managed by a local authority to check whether it represented 'best value' or whether changes were required. Home care workers were feeling under threat as neighbouring authorities were making staff redundant and contracting out services. The review needed to be fair, rather than merely critical, and to show the importance of the service to the council and where there was room for development.

In order to get service users' views and raise morale at the same time an innovative method of gathering information was used. A competition was held where service users or their carers could nominate their home care worker for an award. They had to describe in under 50 words what their home care worker did that was important and why they deserved to win. Four main categories of nomination emerged:

- going the extra mile – personal commitment
- personal characteristics – a cheerful or friendly manner
- performance of tasks – on time, doing what is wanted
- support for carers – valuing of the above by carers.

The comments from service users about what they valued were in sharp contrast to the language of management imperatives for greater contract specification, regularisation of hours and conditions, measurable outcomes, performance indicators, 'best value' and formal standard setting. The information from the competition challenged the direction being taken by the management. The competition gave an opportunity to publicise through the media what the service was 'really' about and emphasise that it was highly valued for its personal relationships and care.

(Source: adapted from Bilson and Ross, 1999, pp. 149–53)

Bilson and Ross (1999) describe this example as using a systems approach, by which they mean a form of practice which considers human beings in their environment. They point out that the people planning change are part of the system that is under consideration: change affects those who propose it as well as those who are the subjects of plans. Bilson and Ross argue the importance of openness to new and different understandings of the work such as those offered through the competition entries. They remark that tensions and creative opportunities are generated when systems change and adapt. In the terminology used in this book, the example is also practice-led. The reviewers sought to discover what service users and carers thought was best practice.

In the current contexts of care it is hard to imagine what an absence of change might be. How similar does a situation have to be to justify saying that it has 'stayed the same' and how different does it have to be to say it has 'changed'? Whatever your view, it is likely that a new state of affairs will be 'the same' as the old in some respects, and 'changed' in others.

Does keeping to the same course require skills that are different from those required for changing course? Almost certainly not when keeping to the same course means doing so in a changing environment with a turnover of staff and service users, while changing course means doing some of the same things as previously, although with different outcomes. Indeed, the notion that change will transform all current practice can cause alarm, as suggested in these words from a group of managers and practitioners confronted by their department's latest round of 'major changes':

> I wish they would come and look at what we are doing now and find out why we do it this way before they sweep it all away with the next round of change.
>
> (Smale, 1996, p. 5)

Smale argues that anyone who wishes to introduce change should ask 'Who sees what as a problem?' and be clear about 'What needs to change?' while also addressing 'What should stay the same?' (1996, p. 5). Continuity can be particularly important for users of care services. However, managing change and attending to continuity is not something special that managers do that is separate from the ordinary job of managing. Managing *is* managing change.

The terms 'change' and 'innovation' are sometimes used differently. Change is often seen as something unpleasant and imposed from above as a result of policy and agency requirements, while innovation is seen as good, but perhaps a luxury which can be dispensed with if necessary (Smale, 1996). In this chapter we use 'change' to cover both imposed change and initiatives arising from frontline practice, since we want to draw attention to some common features in the issues that need consideration.

This is not to imply that there is a blueprint or formula for introducing changes that only needs to be followed to ensure success. However minor changes may seem, change is never a one-off event; nor does it follow an orderly sequence of stages. It is always a continuous and uncertain process which takes place in a specific context (Pettigrew and Whipp, 1991).

Key points

- Managing change is central to managing care.

- Initiatives for change can be top-down or bottom-up.

- Managers have to reconcile pressures for change from different sources and find out where interests coincide.

- Managing for continuity needs to happen alongside planned change.

- There is not a formula for managing change, but there are some patterns in the issues that need to be considered.

4.3   Why change?

In Chapter 3 we considered the place of vision and its importance as a quality of leadership. The impetus for change often comes because the people involved can see how things could be improved. Frontline managers and their team members are likely to be involved at a variety of levels of change with different degrees of engagement. Example 4.2 describes some possibilities for change in different contexts of care provision. Some are simply ideas that people have had, some are definite intentions, and others are well under way.

> **EXAMPLE 4.2 Ideas for change**
>
> 1   Michael is a housing trust manager working with people with learning disabilities in small group homes. He would like to involve residents much more directly in the selection of staff, for instance through membership of the interviewing panel. So far he has encountered resistance to this idea from the personnel section of his organisation.
>
> 2   Susan worked as a cook in a residential home for older people for many years. She wanted a change and to be more involved in direct care work, and was successful in getting a job as care assistant. She was keen to develop activities for the residents, but nervous about asking whether she might. Her manager suggested that she might like to do this within her new role. Susan was very excited at the idea of introducing new activities that everyone could take part in.
>
> 3   Beverley works for a large voluntary agency on a project offering therapeutic work to children and families who have experienced sexual abuse. She would like the service users and project workers to be able to make an earlier contribution to the project's processes of review. At present, service users are simply asked for their views on services. Beverley would like them to have an input in planning the evaluation, so that they have more say about what is to be evaluated.
>
> 4   Mandy is the project co-ordinator of an independent young people's centre. She often wants to challenge the way other agencies work with young people. Within the project, young people's rights to information and choice are respected, and they are involved in the centre's management. Mandy believes that the positive example set by the project is having an influence elsewhere.
>
> 5   Anita has just taken on the management of an integrated mental health team. She finds that team meetings are completely unstructured, and wonders whether they waste people's time. She would prefer to have items listed in advance on an agenda. The psychiatrist appears to like the unstructured approach, which allows him to come and go during the meeting. Anita decides to seek the views of the rest of the team: if they want a different format she could tell the psychiatrist they want to try it for a while and evaluate it.
>
> (Source: manager consultations)

A common aspect of all these examples is that someone has said, 'There must be a better way of doing this.' This is a sensible starting point, although this perception alone will not be enough to bring about change. Some of the ideas may remain just as good ideas for some time to come without anyone taking further action, perhaps because the concerned individual has other priorities, or estimates the barriers to change to be too great at present. Sometimes what appear to be 'new' ideas have been tried before and replaced by current arrangements. Smale (1996) suggests that change often happens because new ideas have resonance with the ideas people already have.

Throughout this chapter we follow the story of The Beeches, a centre for people with learning disabilities, to illustrate change processes. Example 4.3 begins the story and takes the perspective of Peter, the project manager, on the background and the assessment of the issues, and the early steps in planning and implementing change in a service for people with learning disabilities.

EXAMPLE 4.3 The Beeches – why change?

The Beeches is a health trust service for people with learning disabilities. The accommodation is a large old house that was initially acquired to provide a community-based facility for people who had been in hospital over a long period. The aims of the service are to provide assessment and treatment for people with special needs who may have a mental health problem as well as a learning disability. Staff include nurses, health care assistants, occupational therapists, care workers and a speech and language therapist, and there is input from visiting psychologists and psychiatrists.

Many of the residents need long-term care and, in the absence of alternative provision, have remained at The Beeches. Over the years it has become increasingly difficult for the assessment and treatment aspects of the service to be combined with the provision of care for long-term residents. The need for continuing care for some means less space and staff time for working with new entrants who might be in acute distress. The mix of people with different needs is causing problems for residents and staff. Staff 'feel like they have three hats on': they might be trying to develop care arrangements in the community for one set of people; providing long-term care for another; and looking after people with diagnoses such as manic depression as a third group. Peter, the project manager, comments on the effects on residents:

> If you have peers around you who you don't relate to, that can also affect your mental state. You look at these people and you think 'Well, am I like these people? Is this how I'm presenting myself?' and that can cause even more problems.

There are debates between health authorities and social services, in relation to the funding of places, about whether the needs being served are health care or social care.

The building itself is unsuitable for the residents, some of whom have physical disabilities. Much of the accommodation is on the first floor and access is a problem. There are safety issues because at times staff work in relatively cramped accommodation with people who need physical assistance. Also, it is in a rural setting, surrounded by woodland, with no bus route. This hinders the potential for helping residents to develop their daily living skills and participate in community life. In addition, psychiatrists cannot get beds for their patients because the facility is full.

A new general manager has been appointed who is very keen to make improvements. A recently published White Paper, *Valuing People* (Department of Health, 2001b), sets out government plans to provide new opportunities for children and adults with learning disabilities to live full and independent lives as part of their local communities. The team has started to discuss how they can return to and develop their core function of assessment and treatment.

(Source: manager consultations)

Looking at this sketch of difficulties at The Beeches you can probably see a number of things the new manager might want to change, but you may be wondering where they should begin. Is the building the problem, or is it the particular mix of people the service is trying to assist, or is it the aims of the service? A model for thinking about change can help you to identify different elements that are problematic for people at The Beeches and work out what further information you might need. It can work like a road map to help you make sense of what is there and find ways of getting to your destination. There are a variety of frameworks that can be used and we will introduce different possibilities as we look at various aspects of The Beeches. An important skill for managers to develop is trying out different models and frameworks and assessing their usefulness and relevance.

Examining different elements

Nadler (1983) proposes a model for understanding organisations. He points out the importance of the relationship with the external environment and, within the organisation, the interplay of informal relationships, the distribution of power and the behaviour of leaders. Figure 4.1 is based on his work.

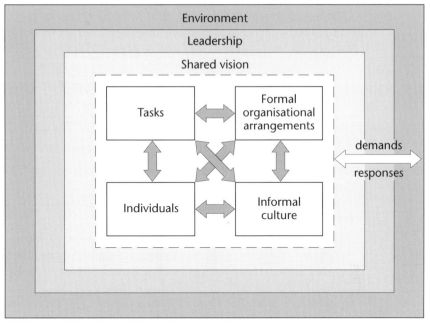

Figure 4.1 **An analysis of different factors for organisations involved in change** (Source: adapted from Nadler, 1983)

In the wider *environment* there are systems which influence the organisation and are in turn influenced by it. In Figure 4.1 the organisation is shown as sitting within the environment and there is no clearly defined boundary between them. There is a continuous process of demand and response. The environment can constrain or facilitate change.

Internally, the organisation involves four components:

- the *tasks* – the jobs, the characteristics of the work itself and the quantity and quality of service provided

- the *formal organisational arrangements* – lines of accountability, information systems, monitoring and control mechanisms, job definitions, formal pay and reward arrangements, meeting structures, operating policies, and so on

- the *informal culture* – less easy to describe or alter, but often a key to how the organisation works; it is 'the way we do things around here', the norms, rituals, values, beliefs, networks and power bases

- the *individuals* – who bring different attitudes, skills, knowledge, experience, personality and behaviour; matching individuals' needs to those of the organisation is particularly important at times of rapid change.

(Adapted from Martin and Henderson, 2001, p. 116)

The two further elements of this model are in part also internal components of the organisation, but they have a close relationship with the external environment too, and so are placed in Figure 4.1 in a way that shows this relationship. They are:

- the *shared vision* – a better future for service users, staff, the organisation
- *leadership* – purposeful, focused action that includes listening, coaching, encouraging and modelling.

(Adapted from Martin and Henderson, 2001, p. 116)

How might these different elements work together in the case of The Beeches?

Environment

The White Paper *Valuing People* draws attention to the importance for people who need intensive treatment and support to be able to access local services rather than having to live in residential care far from home. *Valuing People* refers to the English context: there are similar initiatives in Scotland and Wales (Scottish Executive, 2000; Learning Disability Advisory Group, 2001). The location of The Beeches is unsuited to these aims of community participation.

The lack of clarity about responsibilities in health care and social services is also targeted for change through Learning Disability Partnership Boards, which have representatives from a range of interested bodies, including people with learning disabilities. There may be funds available for the development of services. There will also be the views of a wider set of interested people to take into account: for instance, people with learning disabilities (and their families) who are not receiving a service, psychiatrists frustrated by the lack of available help for their patients, and perhaps others working for different services.

Tasks

The service appears to be unable to fulfil its primary task of providing assessment and treatment, although we do not have many facts about the extent of need. Are there other facilities for this purpose within reach? What other provision exists in the area for the continuing support and care for people once they have been assessed? The existing service does not seem to be designed to provide the long-term care that many of the current residents need. What other facilities are there for this kind of care?

Formal organisational arrangements

Although the needs of the clientele span health and social care, administratively The Beeches is a health service facility. Problems concern the funding of places and categorising service users' needs according to responsibility for payment. Should the social services department be more directly involved in the organisation of this facility or in planning for people with complex needs? The Learning Disability Partnership Board may offer a means of resolving this.

Informal culture

Does the service have just one culture or several? How do the qualified and support workers operate together and are there divisions between those who are based on the site and those who work there on a visiting basis? Does the new general manager work off-site? Are they part of the informal culture or excluded from it? How do the residents or patients contribute to the informal culture?

Individuals

What we know is mediated through the view of Peter, the project manager, who suggests that there are problems for residents and staff, and that the new general manager wants to make improvements. Other people will have different histories and experiences of working or living at The Beeches. For those who have lived there since it first opened, it represents home and, apart from the suggestion that the mix of people does not work well, we do not know how they might respond to any change. It may be difficult to discover more about their views if they have severe communication difficulties, but there are models for involving such people in planning (Edge, 2001). Clearly, there are problems that have frustrated Peter and other staff in their efforts to give good care. Which things work at the moment and should stay the same to provide continuity for residents and staff, and which things need to change?

Shared vision

Again, we know only that the team are talking about the kind of service they would like to be part of. If dissatisfaction is very strong there may be an impetus for them to work together on this. Alternatively, there may be pressure from the trust to change to meet aims set out in the White Paper.

Leadership

There are several potential leaders: Peter himself, the new general manager, one of the consultant psychiatrists, and perhaps others. Will they be able to co-operate in pressing for change? Are their ideas about what is needed the same? What different kinds of power do they have to make things happen?

There seem to be some positive features in the environment that may make this a good time for trying to improve the service, but there are also a number of questions and a need for more information about how different elements might work together to help or hinder changes. A shared vision will be important, but it may not matter at this stage if it is not clear in detail. What is currently needed are some ideas to provoke discussion and an opportunity for a wide range of people to engage in building a vision together.

Key points

- The impetus for change often starts from someone's vision that there is a better way to do things.

- Not all ideas for change are taken up.

- Using a model to identify different components of a situation that calls for change can reveal gaps in knowledge and areas to explore further.

4.4   Who and what can change?

Analysing the issues and assessing the readiness for change is only the first step in managing a change process. Effective change requires that someone takes a lead, and some writers refer to this as *leading change* rather than leadership, in order to highlight the need to resolve not simply single issues, but a pattern of interwoven problems (see, for instance, Pettigrew and Whipp, 1991, p. 166). Whoever is leading change, or has a strong desire to see change happen, needs to think strategically about how to engage other people. Box 4.1 (opposite) suggests some action points when planning change.

The points listed in Box 4.1 provide a useful checklist but should not be thought of as a step-by-step sequence. Ideas are more likely to be adopted if they come from more than one person – hence the importance of involving others in discussion from the earliest stage and developing ideas together. People have their own ideas and are not just neutral receivers waiting for messages about what needs to be done. So, once you have started to involve others, expect the change process to take on a life of its own. A 'simple linear' model of change – one that moves smoothly through a sequence of actions – distorts reality. It is not possible, or even desirable, to control all the actions of the people who need to change in order to implement practice and service delivery changes (Smale, 1996).

BOX 4.1 Planning a change

- Involve people – service users and colleagues – in discussion from the earliest stage, and do more listening and note taking than talking.

- Gather more information about the need for change considering the environment, the tasks, the formal and informal arrangements and the individuals.

- Clarify your aims.

- Identify the aims and concerns of the people likely to be affected by the change and think about how to protect their interests.

- Work out what the motivation is of the people you need to co-operate.

- Set targets linked to a timescale.

- Check that the time and cost involved make change feasible.

- Review the means and obstacles to change, the probable consequences (wanted and unwanted) and the risks.

- Clarify who is leading the change and 'managing' any transition period.

- Plan your moves in detail.

- 'Sell' the change to people not directly involved and check they agree.

- Plan a clear communications strategy so that internal messages override those from outside.

- Take action.

- Review the results, acknowledge success to build everyone's confidence, and plan the next stage.

(Source: adapted from Taylor and Vigars, 1993, pp. 166–7)

A key issue identified in our examination of the situation at The Beeches is the feelings of the service users about their current environment and what they might want. How do you explore possibilities of change when there are severe communication problems, and when the welfare of a whole set of people, each with their personal reactions, can have an impact on the wellbeing of others? Staff at The Beeches carried out a careful and lengthy observation of the individuals in their care, looking for what appeared to work and what caused difficulties, deciding what established routines needed to be continued, and formulating individual care plans in discussion with families.

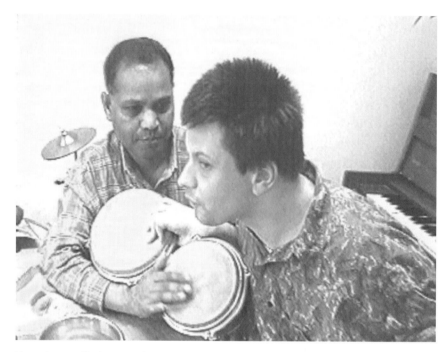

How do you find out and record people's preferences when they cannot talk and explain? (Source: Acting Up)

The photograph above shows a resident at a home where multimedia profiling is used to put day-to-day details of residents' preferences into a visual format to show support workers what is required. Residents themselves have the opportunity to play a more active role in reviewing and responding to their care plans as they are made more accessible and user-friendly. Activities and support needs are documented using a camcorder. Video clips are then edited on to computer and held in each individual's multimedia profile, giving the opportunity to point out the non-verbal communications the resident is using.

In Example 4.4 we summarise another approach used to help people with a learning disability and high support needs to be in control of important decisions in their lives.

Example 4.5 (overleaf) draws again on Peter's account of change at The Beeches to identify the nature of the changes planned there. The staff were committed to making sure that they could offer assessment and treatment to those who needed it, but it took a while to work out how this could be effected.

EXAMPLE 4.4 Recognising people's choices

Beverley lives in a residential home. She does not use verbal communication and can go for weeks without responding to people around her. She uses a number of ways to communicate:

– sounds, noises

– physical tension

– natural gestures, eye pointing

– uneasiness

– sadness, anger, aggressiveness

– restlessness

– gestures

– flickering eyes

– passiveness, lack of interest

– mimicry

– using objects

– awareness, reactions

– screaming, shouting

– joy, happiness, laughing, smiling.

Beverley screams loudly in a variety of situations, and care staff did not know what she was trying to communicate. They recorded what was happening (as below) and asked others who knew her well to record their interpretations and observations.

When this is happening: sitting at the breakfast table

Beverley does this: looks upset and screams loudly

We think it means: I want to eat alone

We should do this: have breakfast at a different time

The staff found that Beverley would use the same behaviour to send a variety of messages, such as wanting to be alone, wanting attention, or because she was unhappy about something. They acted collectively, responding in a consistent way to the screams depending on the context at the time. They checked their interpretations, looking for other signs that they had got it right. They discussed together what they found. They began to see patterns in Beverley's behaviour. This approach has given Beverley more control over everyday choices and has given the staff insights into how she communicates.

(Source: adapted from Edge, 2001, pp. 21–2)

> ### EXAMPLE 4.5 The Beeches – who and what can change?
>
> There was widespread agreement that change was needed but initially some uncertainty about what it should be. 'Not necessarily everyone knew exactly what needed to happen, and I think that's when people became quite apprehensive,' explained Peter. People knew things were not functioning well but, because they had got used to the current state, they felt comfortable with it.
>
> One of the difficulties was estimating the length of time service users might need specialist facilities, and whether some people should be receiving long-term care rather than the assessment and treatment service. 'We grasped the nettle,' said Peter, describing the decision to move some people with long-term needs as well as project staff to Middleside, another existing residential facility, as an interim measure. A small number would remain at The Beeches and they would be joined by service users and staff from Middleside, the aim being to group together people with similar problems and needs. This involved a merger of the two staff and service user groups.
>
> A linked question was whether it was feasible to provide assessment and treatment within the county or better to use facilities in neighbouring counties. Peter commented: 'We're actually saying, "No, we've got people who are highly skilled, committed to do that job, so why on earth can't we provide that service?", but that means a huge commitment to service development, and financial cost.' A newly built assessment and treatment centre is now planned, which means a second move once it is ready for use and a division of staff into the assessment and treatment team and the long-term care team, who will remain at Middleside.

The decisions for change are presented as a sequence that involves a transitional state: the merger with the project at Middleside, which would develop as a centre for people with autism, with a separate bungalow for people with sensory impairment. This would be followed later by a move to the new centre for assessment and treatment which was not yet built. However, the need for this two-stage approach was not clear at the start. Initially, the staff team hoped they would make one move to the purpose-built premises. Once a large-scale change of this sort takes shape in people's minds, the current situation becomes increasingly untenable. New buildings take a long time to complete and in the meantime the needs of the group currently being helped have to be addressed in the best way possible.

Making change happen

Example 4.6 describes Peter's perceptions of what was involved in making change happen.

EXAMPLE 4.6 The Beeches – making change happen

1 *Dealing with people's anxieties takes time:* 'The unknown, that was my biggest obstacle, explaining to staff, "Look, it's going to be better, I promise you. You might be moaning to me about how awful this place is, but actually when push comes to shove, you're more scared of moving." That became a real problem.'

2 *Delays in making a move:* 'Speed is of the essence, but you've got to get it right, and that can be quite a challenge for people to realise, "Well, we can't move yet because we haven't got it right."'

3 *Communication is important:* 'One of the biggest things I used, and one of the more simple things really, is involvement, saying to people, "Look, this is what we're looking at designing, give us some input, what do you think?" Whenever I know anything, my staff know it as well.'

News is written in a communication book – this helps information to cascade down. Meetings are held regularly for the qualified clinical team, with additional house meetings that include all staff so that there is an opportunity to consult over questions of design and new roles for staff.

4 *Communication with service users and their families has to be sensitively handled:* 'If we told one or two of the clients we were looking after weeks and weeks in advance it could cause more problems for them, so we had to be very clear on where, what and how we told them, and we did it through the clinical team.'

Families also need to understand the reasons for the move and to be introduced to new staff.

5 *Training needs analysis must take account of present and future:* the two-stage move means that there are training needs for the transitional move. The majority of those being offered care at Middleside are people with autism, and the staff group working with them need to have a team understanding of appropriate ways of working together. At the same time, many of the staff group there will be involved in the assessment and treatment work before their move to the new facility. This aspect of their work also needs attention: 'We're not bombarding people with information, but I think it's important they have a very steady flow, so that when we get to our new building people aren't sitting there scratching their heads, saying, "What on earth do we do now?"'

6 *Staffing and recruitment implications:* 'Everyone was told that they would have the right if they want to move on to the assessment and treatment service. However, I'm sure that when you're working with particular client groups, they're the sort of client groups you prefer to work with, and I am certainly very aware that some, for example, would want to stay with people with autism, or would want to work with people who perhaps have more long-term care needs.'

The team will need to recruit new members to fill gaps in either the Middleside centre or the assessment and treatment centre.

Peter's account so far identifies a number of elements that support successful change initiatives, including:

- engagement and commitment from key groups
- development and use of a variety of communication strategies and processes
- specifying the change and exploring the pros and cons
- beginning to designate new roles, responsibilities and tasks
- encouraging staff to have a positive outlook.

Looking again at Box 4.1, there are other aspects on that checklist that have not yet been discussed. They are addressed in the following sections.

Key points

- The leadership of change is likely to involve not just one issue but a pattern of interwoven problems, not all of which can be predicted at the start.

- People wanting change need to engage others in building the vision together and to continue to communicate well.

4.5   Examining reactions, barriers and blocks

People engaged in a change process are likely to have different degrees of commitment to the change. Table 4.1 (opposite) shows the range of responses and uses of Senge's (1990) distinction between *commitment*, *enrolment* and *compliance*.

Not everyone will be fully committed, supportive and active in the change process but a 'critical mass' should be enough for change to succeed. It may be more important to discover what level of support is actually needed from individuals to develop that necessary critical mass rather than trying to persuade everyone to fully commit themselves (Senge, 1990). Some people will be more significant than others in influencing attitudes. Smale (1996) argues that commitment to innovation is a contagious process which can be speeded up by making connections between key people. The categories in Table 4.1 can be used to gauge the level of commitment needed from all parties to a change proposal of your own, and to make judgements about the degree of support you need from them.

Table 4.1 **Commitment, enrolment and compliance**

Level of engagement	Response to change
Commitment or enrolment	Will *make* it happen Will create necessary structures, systems and frameworks Will act fully within the spirit of the frameworks
Genuine or formal compliance	Will *help* it happen Will be proactive within the spirit of the frameworks or at least will do what is asked
Grudging compliance or apathy	Will *let* it happen May be opposed or may not care Will do enough to preserve position
Non-compliance	Will *oppose* the change Do not accept there are benefits and will not do what is asked

(Source: adapted from Martin and Henderson, 2001, p. 131;
Iles and Sutherland, 2001, p. 47)

Example 4.7 shows some of the comments made by team members from The Beeches now working at Middleside during the transitional stage of the change process.

EXAMPLE 4.7 Middleside – reactions to change

I had some mixed feelings about moving here. The apprehension was really surrounding just what it would be like here, and we knew we were going to mesh two staff groups.

We were given the opportunity to choose where we wanted to go, but at the same time we were told that we would be put where our skills were felt to be most appropriate. So everybody had that kind of fear that they weren't going to get what they wanted.

I feel very positive about the move for the clients who came with us. We've managed to improve the quality of life already, we've increased levels of activity, we've increased the time interacting with people.

For the people already here, things may be less positive because we've suddenly moved into what is their home. Initially, we tried to get staff to work shifts at each other's units, so that you became a familiar face, but that didn't work out as well as it might because of staff shortages. When it finally happened, we all did just turn up one day with two clients. We talked about introducing staff and clients in pictorial form even.

There were some teething problems: not taking care plans seriously enough, people that shouldn't be taking the lead taking the lead. I felt quite uncomfortable having to challenge them. I went to the manager, and he is taking the lead in all that resettlement stuff. He's approachable, deals with the problem and then lets you know he's dealt with it.

(Rick, care assistant)

At the old unit we weren't informed as well as we could have been. Things got stuck: we'd all sit around and there were lots of different stories. Miscommunication leads to all sorts of fantasies about what's going to happen and how it's going to work. People were saying, 'Well, everybody's going to leave', so there was all that to deal with as well. Perhaps we could have had a series of regular meetings where we could have been informed a bit more clearly about where we were and what was happening.

What people are fixing on at the moment is that we've been given this timescale of a year, when quite a few of us know that a year in NHS terms is five years in reality.

Disagreeing with things here maybe has gone underground, and people are discussing amongst themselves, and that can sometimes get a bit negative. I think people are questioning 'What's my role at the moment? Am I as valuable a member of the team as I used to be?' There is quite an overlapping of roles and people doing different things, whereas before there was more clarity about who was doing what.

(Rowena, nurse)

The culture from the previous location has tended to dominate. The existing staff from this location who have stayed on, I think, have felt that their own culture has been diminished, and that's led to some dissatisfaction.

(Andrew, nurse)

The comments suggest some discrepancies. Few of the staff interviewed gave the impression that they disagreed with the changes being enacted. However, although Peter emphasises the importance of involving people in plans and cascading information down as soon as it becomes available, the experience of some of the staff is still one of uncertainty.

Rick seems to be seeking more management input during this change, and is perhaps uncomfortable confronting the kind of disagreement that is almost inevitable in a change process. In times of stability people act on common understandings about how things should be done, with little managerial input. However, change can increase demands for greater management among those who are managed, although they will not necessarily agree with each other or with managers about what should happen and what form management and leadership should take.

Rick's comments raise issues about the relationship of power, communication and decision making. He points out the ambiguity of communication when people were told they would be given a choice but that decisions would be made about where they were going.

He describes the move as positive for clients, but alludes to the difficulty of preparing them sufficiently, and a confusion of roles and responsibilities. Rick's attitude fits somewhere between enrolment and genuine compliance. Rowena's and Andrew's comments indicate the response of some staff is closer to grudging compliance.

Argyris and Schön (1996) take an alternative view to explain differing levels of engagement and commitment to a change effort. Superiors and subordinates hold both optimistic and pessimistic views of each other, but involve themselves in 'skilled incompetence', that is, defensive routines designed to avoid surprises, embarrassment and threat. One of these is 'management by mixed messages'. The rules of mixed messages are to:

- design a message that contains inconsistencies
- act as if it is not inconsistent
- make the ambiguity and inconsistency in the message undiscussable
- make the undiscussability also undiscussable.

(Adapted from Argyris and Schön, 1996, p. 100)

From this perspective, the comments of Rick, Rowena and Andrew on their own and their colleagues' responses may be less a matter of varying commitment and more a matter of trying to deal with a confusing situation and insufficient information. In such situations, as Rowena remarks, rumours grow and take on a life of their own and they also need to be dealt with. Taking steps to bring 'undiscussables' and assumptions to the surface, and proposing possible solutions to issues that affect staff is one first step to increasing involvement and commitment.

Example 4.8 presents the views of an occupational therapist who plays one of the key supporting roles in the change effort.

EXAMPLE 4.8 Middleside – reviewing the transition

There was a lot of pressure coming from clinical and staff teams that we had two different client mixes; they just weren't compatible living together. People were desperate for something to happen. When it looked like something was going to happen, people were quite motivated.

I talked quite a lot to staff, and we had staff meetings. I supported the manager on the management side as his two deputies were off sick, as well as looking clinically at client needs. Lots of people's views were taken on board. It was quite contentious. If you'd put something up that other people thought would not work, there'd be some resentment and anger and 'I wouldn't work there if you do that' sort of reaction.

There were lots of rumours about different things happening. If there were real fears that were becoming obvious, the manager would hold a staff meeting or write in the communications book. I'd tell him if there were some things I knew of and he would try to nip them in the bud as quickly as possible.

There was a lot of anxiety. Waiting was the hardest I think. People couldn't understand why it was taking so long and then you'd have staff sickness and you'd have lots of issues going on within staffing that would delay it even further. There were practicalities around building works and finance. They were saying, 'Why can't we just move, you know it's dangerous, why can't we just go?'

So lots of questions, anxiety and quite a lot of denial. Things like 'It'll never work.' You just had to ride it. People had to see it was happening.

I think it was easier for me because I was involved in the co-ordination meetings, so I'd go to meetings and have a plan, have objectives to meet. So it was very structured. I think a lot of the nursing assistants, who were only hearing things from other people who were going to these meetings and doing the planning, had the anxiety and the helplessness and feelings of anger at the major life changes coming.

You do see in hindsight that the move's obviously been traumatic. After the move people were saying things like 'Are you surviving, are you coping?' I don't think you acknowledge that at the time.

You become quite overwhelmed by your own role in it and don't see the people who are at the ground level, how they are struggling and how they are feeling.

People are still adjusting and still looking for other jobs now. It's a longer process than you think. A lot of people would say, 'Well, it's over now, we're in, it's done', and I don't think that's the case.

There's a lot of fear that staff will become deskilled in the area they're expected to be specialists in. I think that's the major concern, that we'll all become great specialists in autism, then be expected to go on to assessment and treatment, and be able to become specialists in dual diagnosis and mental health, having not done it for a long time.

(Michelle, occupational therapist)

Michelle's comments illustrate that change is a process, not an event. For workers and residents it involves much more than simply adapting to a different building and other new arrangements. It can be helpful to distinguish between change and transition. Change is situational: new leadership, restructuring, new buildings. Some psychologists use the term 'transition' for the psychological process people go through in coming to terms with the new situation (Adams *et al.*, 1976). Change is external and transition is internal, although there are many external indicators of the internal states. People in transition may move through recognisable stages, from denial and resistance to exploration and commitment, although not always in that order.

Bridges (1988) notes that change begins with endings and always involves letting go of things, which can be an unsettling, threatening process. Marris (1974) draws attention to the links between loss and change and suggests that change can be understood as a form of bereavement. Simic (1997) comments that to manage change effectively, one of the first tasks is to address the threat. It can be a number of different things, and Example 4.8 identified many of them: for instance, feeling overwhelmed and powerless, perhaps disoriented, losing a sense of belonging, losing your anchors. Efforts to introduce change are often ineffective because too little attention is given to this stage of the process.

In practice, dealing effectively with endings involves expressing open appreciation, celebrating past accomplishments, and bringing people together to acknowledge loss of the past and fear of the future. Loss may include loss of attachments, loss of structure, loss of the anticipated future, loss of meaning and loss of control. If loss and endings are not acknowledged, those involved may well be resistant to new arrangements. Michelle's account refers to sickness, anxiety and trauma. Workers are in the neutral zone of the transition process: an area between the old and the new, characterised by waiting and uncertainty. During this time, increased visibility of leaders and managers can be helpful, providing updated information, empathy and reassurance, and gathering views and information from multiple sources.

A simple mechanism for encouraging people to move towards exploration and commitment is to help them to evaluate and make explicit the personal and organisational gains and losses they expect as a result of change. Table 4.2 notes some of the gains and losses mentioned by staff at The Beeches.

By encouraging people to articulate their sense of loss and confusion and to acknowledge how they feel about this, it may be more possible to generate enthusiasm for the future.

Table 4.2   **A balance sheet for change**

	Loss	*Gain*
Personal	Becoming deskilled	New training in assessment and treatment
	Clear role and tasks	New challenges
Organisational	Confusion	Better client service

Key points

- People have different degrees of commitment to change: not everyone needs to be enthusiastic, but a critical mass is needed for success.

- Inconsistencies in communications cause confusion and rumours may spread.

- In order to engage enthusiasm for new challenges it is important to bring problems out into the open for discussion and resolution.

- It is helpful to acknowledge the losses involved in change as well as the gains.

4.6   Reviewing change

Change rarely proceeds in a straightforward, linear way; it is an iterative process in which, for example, planning and implementation can feed back into an assessment of the situation. In considering The Beeches, which has provided a real-life focus for this chapter, a *force-field analysis* can be used to take stock of the current situation as it has been represented in the various accounts, in order to make adjustments to the change management process. This is in effect an interim evaluation process. A force-field analysis can also be made at an early stage in planning change to preview the support and potential problems an initiative may encounter.

Force-field analysis is a diagnostic tool developed by Lewin (1951) to assess the forces driving change against the forces opposing change. The forces represent the perceptions of people involved in the change. Although intuition might suggest that increasing the driving forces for the change is desirable, it is important to note that for every action, there is an equivalent and opposite reaction. In other words, increasing the driving forces can lead to an increase in the restraining forces. It is more efficient and effective to 'decrease' the restraining forces.

In Figure 4.2 we have used Nadler's model (Figure 4.1) to organise ideas about the driving and restraining forces in relation to The Beeches. The forces are charted using arrows to indicate their direction and relative strengths.

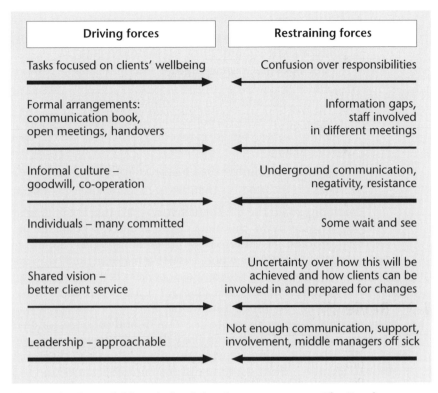

Driving forces	Restraining forces
Tasks focused on clients' wellbeing	Confusion over responsibilities
Formal arrangements: communication book, open meetings, handovers	Information gaps, staff involved in different meetings
Informal culture – goodwill, co-operation	Underground communication, negativity, resistance
Individuals – many committed	Some wait and see
Shared vision – better client service	Uncertainty over how this will be achieved and how clients can be involved in and prepared for changes
Leadership – approachable	Not enough communication, support, involvement, middle managers off sick

Figure 4.2 **Force-field analysis of the change process at The Beeches**

The staff involved in The Beeches change initiative seem to be united by a shared vision: a better and more appropriate service for clients that will ensure higher quality of care. There is a clear understanding and acceptance of why change is needed. The difficulties are in optimising the staff experience and involvement in the implementation process and, by implication, in the planning. There are many unanswered questions about the roots of the difficulties, which may originate from: the scarcity of resources; uncontrollable delays caused by building works; too much responsibility for change vested in one or two people; insufficient planning or knowledge of how change processes unfold.

The workers themselves identified the following strategies that could improve the process.

- Attend to staff needs and the philosophy of the service early in the process. Consulting with staff involved can ensure that goals are shared and targets are realistic.
- Place staff support and supervision high on the agenda. Set priorities and stick to them.

- Create ongoing mechanisms, such as formal and informal monitoring systems, to ensure continuous dialogue between those responsible for initiating change and those on the receiving end.
- Clarify roles and responsibilities and offer suitable rewards and a range of options, particularly when designating new roles, responsibilities and positions and when allocating new teams.
- Provide clear information about new career structures and workers' responsibilities, future career prospects and access to training and development.
- Take the time during the change to acknowledge personal reactions.
- Focus on the progress that has been made and celebrate achievements.

Questions about the most effective way to bring about change continue to plague analysts in this field. How is success or failure in introducing change to be measured? Why do some initiatives appear to work while others fizzle out? When policy is being implemented, why does the pace of change differ across different authorities? Is there a set of conditions that indicate receptivity for change? Can we predict likely results by identifying prevailing conditions?

Since the specific contexts, content and processes of change vary and are interdependent, it is unlikely that any simple analysis can be made to predict likely consequences. Pettigrew and his colleagues have attempted to identify a variety and mixture of causes of change and to explore these over time in different contexts of structural change in the NHS in the 1980s. Their findings suggest that there is a set of eight linked conditions that produce receptivity to change, although these may be rather specific to their context and period of study (Pettigrew *et al.*, 1992). They are not a shopping list that can be pulled together to create an instantly favourable environment. The conditions identified are in a dynamic relationship with each other, and receptivity builds up over time or, equally, may go into reverse. They are summarised in Box 4.2.

BOX 4.2 Factors in receptivity to change in the NHS

The quality and coherence of policy

This is the policy generated at local level; broad vision is more important than a blueprint at the outset. However, it does need to be broken down into actionable steps.

Availability of key people leading change

Key people in critical posts need to work as a team. Movement of key personnel can drain the initiative of energy and purpose.

Long-term environmental pressure

This is a sensitive factor and extreme pressure can affect the situation in different ways: a financial crisis can be an opportunity, but may equally be a threat.

Supportive organisational culture, especially the managerial subculture

There are key features such as flexible working across boundaries and an open, risk-taking approach. Such features develop from the values of key leaders in the area.

Positive pattern of managerial and clinical relationships

Relationships between managers and clinicians work best where negative stereotypes have broken down and there is good understanding of each other's roles.

Co-operative inter-organisational networks

The most effective networks are both informal and purposeful, but also fragile and vulnerable to staff turnover.

Simplicity and clarity of goals and priorities

If there are too many 'priorities' they become meaningless. 'Shrink' the problem at the outset or break it into manageable pieces once the change process is under way.

Fit between the overall change agenda and the particular locale

Some organisations find it easier to achieve change than others because of the kind of arrangements that already exist or because of other features, for instance the local political climate or the nature of the workforce.

(Source: adapted from Pettigrew *et al.*, 1992, pp. 277–86)

Key points

- A force-field analysis can be useful for measuring support for and resistance to change as part of the planning process or as an evaluative tool.

- There are no simple recipes for assessing the likely consequences of introducing change.

- Some common conditions feature in contexts that have been receptive to change.

4.7   Conclusion

While individuals have different attitudes to change – at one extreme constantly seeking change and at the other avoiding it at all costs – change is a disruptive and often unpredictable occurrence for everyone. It rarely takes place in a straightforward fashion but is a meandering process with stops, starts and jolts in between. You may be half-way into a change initiative, but with new information and new learning gained, you may have to revisit your initial assessment and goals. Change requires attention to structural and procedural issues, and models, frameworks and tools can give guidance here; and it also requires attention to inevitable human concerns.

Because transition is inherent in change, as a worker or a manager you will have to live and work in what is almost the past but not quite the future. This will require you, at times, to juggle what seem like two roles, two sets of responsibilities and perhaps several competing sets of tasks. As a manager involved in change, maintaining openness, flexibility and tolerance of ambiguity can strengthen the possibilities of a successful outcome. A realistic optimism, and an emphasis on maintaining core values in providing care, can help practice-led managers to reframe the aims or effects of change. For example, at a political level, many community care changes since the 1980s had reduction in costs as a target and have aimed to diminish professional power. Those managing changes now might want to emphasise the possibilities for power and resource sharing with other colleagues and community groups, and the potential for individual client empowerment. Change in social care is linked with improved quality and, for the outcome of change to be successful, the people affected – service users and workers – need to experience that the quality of service has improved.

Chapter 5
Supporting evidence-based practice and research-mindedness

David Shemmings and Yvonne Shemmings

5.1   Introduction

In this chapter we point to the role of managers in advancing their own and others' *research-mindedness* and encouraging practice that is *evidence-based*. By research-mindedness we mean a spirit of enquiry about research through the deployment of critical and analytical skills. This includes awareness of the scope and limitations of research, an ability to treat critically the claims that are made in research studies, and the policy changes based on them, and a sympathetic attitude to research in managers' own practice settings (Fuller and Petch, 1995). We believe that the development of research-mindedness is a necessary precursor to establishing evidence-based practice. People who base their practice on evidence use findings from formal research, perspectives gleaned from consultation with service users and carers, the application of theoretical frameworks, and a range of sources of practice wisdom. What we hope to convey is that, for this to happen, there needs to be a culture within which frontline managers take an active part by emphasising the need to keep up to date in their own field.

Why is it so important for managers and practitioners to be research-minded? After all, research is often criticised for using up large amounts of money to tell us what we know already. Research in social care has always been a poor relation of health services research, attracting less funding. There are concerns about both the quantity and the quality of research studies in major social work journals, and the dissemination of key findings has tended to be poor and uncoordinated (Trinder, 2000a). The nature of the evidence in social research is complicated and not always easy to interpret since so many different factors play a part.

The simple argument for research-mindedness is that practitioners and managers are expected to know what they are doing. They are paid to intervene in people's lives on the basis that what they do will be well judged and based on an informed appraisal of alternatives. They are working in conditions of complexity and uncertainty but they should at least know the basis on which they *think* they know what they are doing (Brechin and Sidell, 2000). They need to articulate the kinds of knowledge they draw on, including knowledge gained from research. Research matters because it can offer important guidance for improving services and interventions. In a more defensive spirit, it can provide material to satisfy needs for accountability. Funders of services want to know that they are getting the best value for their money. An argument for continuing provision or for change needs to be supported by evidence of the impact of services on people's welfare.

There are welcome developments in the nature and quality of research available. For instance, there is an increasing number of sound research findings on the provision and delivery of social care. Statistical surveys at national and local levels can give important information about trends. Findings from inspection and audits provide information about service performance (see, for example, Davis, 1999). The evaluation and testimony from service users, carers, children and their families about their experiences offer important learning and guidance (see, for instance, Read and Reynolds, 1996; Hatton *et al.*, 1998; Shaw, 1998; Qureshi and Henwood, 2000; Thornton, 2000). Moreover, there is an accumulation of practice knowledge built from considerable experience over time (Scott, 1990).

There are also various initiatives, each aimed at raising the profile of evidence-based practice, both at the level of practice and with policy makers and managers. First, the Social Care Institute for Excellence was established, which is aimed at co-ordinating information and initiatives concerning evidence-based practice. The appointment of a first chairperson who has campaigned successfully for disabled people's civil rights indicates a likely emphasis on what works best for users (Beresford, 2001). Second, organisations such as Making Research Count and Research in Practice were established to provide practitioners and managers with help to access, appraise and use research findings. Finally, over the past few years, the Department of Health has produced a series of reviews of its own commissioned research studies, subtitled 'Messages from Research' (there is a complete list on the Department of Health website). (The web addresses of these organisations are in the References.)

What follows in this chapter is applicable to managers working within the wide range of care settings. You do not need a detailed knowledge of research methodology (that is, the theoretical perspective underpinning the choice of research method) to work on this chapter. However, if your knowledge feels a little rusty you could refer to Gomm *et al.* (2000), who present examples of different styles of research studies together with helpful explanations of what you need to understand about the method used. The Electronic Library for Social Care has a glossary for research terms (see the References).

The aims of this chapter are to:

- discuss what evidence-based practice is, and why it is developing so quickly
- review contested areas about the concept of evidence-based practice

- explore the extent to which practitioners and managers currently use research to inform their practice
- suggest ways of implementing change and consider how managers can contribute to it.

5.2   What is evidence-based practice and why is it developing so quickly?

Evidence-based practice is one of the fastest-growing developments in social care at present. This is not surprising because, at first sight, 'the argument that practice should be based on the most up-to-date, valid and reliable research findings has an instant intuitive appeal, and is so obviously sensible and rational that it is difficult to resist' (Trinder, 2000b, p. 3). Evidence-based practice also complements parallel concerns for the increasing accountability of social care agencies by fixing their attention on 'what works best'.

Problems emerge, however, when defining what 'reliable research findings' actually are. Similarly, to ask the tantalisingly straightforward but inevitably naïve question 'What works best?' means tackling what is meant by 'works' and who exactly it works for – the service user, a child, the family, the neighbourhood, or society in general? Also, what is meant by 'best': does it mean 'most effective', 'most efficient', 'most likely to deter others', 'most liked by service users, other members of the family, the neighbourhood, and so on'; or, does it really mean 'the cheapest'?

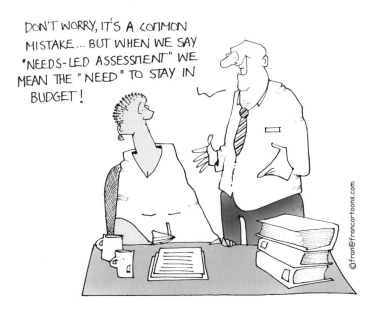

There are important debates about both who should do research and who should be the focus of it. Holman, for example, raises both points when he states:

> users should be financed to undertake their own studies ... so that the deprived study the privileged ... a research group of social service users could study directors of social services departments and large voluntary societies.
>
> (Holman, 2001, p. 14)

There is an increasing number of research studies designed and done by people who have experience of using services (see, for example, Faulkner and Layzell, 2000; Mental Health Foundation, 1999). Whoever does the research, the quality of their findings will depend heavily on the skill of the people doing it and their ability to subject their own assumptions to rigorous scrutiny. We shall explore some of the complexity surrounding what constitutes 'evidence', taking the view that definitions need to be expanded along the lines of the comment in the opening paragraph of this chapter, before evidence-based practice leads to lasting changes in professional practice.

Although originally referring to medicine, the following definition by Sackett *et al.* (1996) tends to be the one adopted by contemporary writers on evidence-based practice. Here it has been modified for the field of social care:

> Evidence-based social care is the conscientious, explicit and judicious use of current best evidence in making decisions regarding the welfare of those in need.
>
> (Sheldon and Chilvers, 2000, p. 5)

Evidence-based practice developed earlier in the health service, in particular in medicine, where it has taken off since the early 1990s. A key figure behind its inception was Archie Cochrane, a general practitioner who had been concerned for some time that medical intervention was not always based on the most up-to-date evidence. He argued passionately that, apart from the most obvious medical conditions for which there could be only one treatment, many others were subject to the prevailing predilections of the doctor (Cochrane, 1973). So, if a person goes to a surgery complaining of headaches, for example, different doctors may well approach both the diagnosis and the treatment in radically different ways. This will depend not on their knowledge of current research data but on their existing preferences, their susceptibility to fads and fashions and even their prejudices (not to mention the persuasiveness of the drug companies). Referring to the work of Antman *et al.* (1992), Reynolds makes the worrying point that the majority of contemporary medical textbooks recommend treatments for a heart attack that were proved to be worthless: 'more recently developed treatments, of proven efficacy, were not recommended' (Reynolds, 2000, p. 19).

Cochrane believed the reason why doctors were behaving in this way was not because they were complacent or that they did not see the need for up-to-date knowledge to be informed by good research but, rather, because there was *too much* research for them to digest. Using the field of mental health as an example, Geddes powerfully illustrates this problem of 'research overload':

> For *Evidence-Based Mental Health* ... over 5500 potentially relevant journal articles are read every year. To accomplish this him or herself, a clinician would have to read 15 articles each and every day every year ... If the clinician only managed to read two articles every day, after two years, the clinician would have a 10-year backlog. After 20 years, the backlog would take over 100 years to read!
>
> (Geddes, 2000, p. 67)

The aim of evidence-based practice is to overcome the gap between research and practice through a range of practical methods. The identification of research of direct clinical significance, the use of rules for evaluating research evidence, frameworks for clinical decisions, and the benefits of information technology have all made this more possible in medicine (Reynolds, 2000). Transposing these ideas to social care, the concept of evidence-based practice could have a unique part to play, as Box 5.1 shows.

BOX 5.1 The claimed benefits of evidence-based practice when applied to social care

Evidence-based practice:

- identifies research that is of direct relevance to workers and service users

- provides a set of simple rules for evaluating research evidence

- emphasises the responsibility of managers and supervisors to use their professional judgement, personal experience and also external evidence in making decisions

- refers explicitly to the welfare of service users

- expects decision making to be made explicit and thus open to question and examination

- accepts that there are different types of evidence and that some are better than others

and assumes that (as with health professionals):

- most workers need to be taught how to interpret and use research findings

- most workers (including managers) need help to use research to inform practice throughout their careers
- research findings must be disseminated to workers more efficiently.

(Source: adapted from Reynolds, 2000, pp. 19–22)

These are strong claims and they account for the interest in evidence-based practice. However, there are some questions about the direct transferability of this model to social care. The interventions in care services are of a different nature from those of medicine, and it may be less easy to identify the critical factors for success. Social care encounters are not straightforward and linear but messy and complex, located in a social and political context (Trinder, 2000a).

Example 5.1 provides an interesting perspective on an evidence-based approach in the field of mental health.

EXAMPLE 5.1 Applying evidence to social care

At a recent multi-disciplinary mental health conference the following quotation was read out, amended however, so that wherever the phrase 'case management' occurred, the name of a mythical second-generation neuroleptic drug, Lususoproxine, was substituted (lusus is Latin for joke):

> Case management increased the numbers remaining in contact with services. Case management approximately doubled the numbers admitted to psychiatric hospital. Except for a positive finding on compliance from one study, case management showed no significant advantages over standard care on any psychiatric or social variable. Cost data did not favour case management but insufficient information was available to permit definitive conclusions.
>
> (Marshall *et al.*, 2000)

The audience was then asked what should happen in the light of this evidence, and overwhelmingly suggested that the medication should no longer be used. However, when they were let in on the little thought experiment, a substantial number, though sympathetic to the principle, thought that little could be done about social care interventions since they were embedded in national and local policies, and that different rules applied. Interestingly, the way forward in the field of relapse prevention and maintenance in the community for people with schizophrenia seems to be not abandonment of case-management, but the adoption of a more intensive, proactive, multi-disciplinary version of it called 'assertive out-reach' (Marshall and Lockwood, 2000) which is achieving superior results, though with some cost implications.

(Source: Sheldon and Chilvers, 2000, p. 3)

Depending on your point of view, Example 5.1 illustrates different possibilities. It could be cited as the failure of mental health practitioners to apply an evidence-based scrutiny to the use of case or care management. Alternatively, you may think that evidence on social care interventions is more complex to interpret than evidence on drug treatments.

A significant problem with importing a model of evidence-based practice derived heavily from the field of medicine is that it relies too much on ways of looking at research that are more suited to testing new drugs. Experimental designs are not easily applied to the evaluation of what works best in social care settings. We now look at some of these dangers in more detail.

Key points

- Evidence-based practice is a developing area for social care.

- There are some difficulties in defining what constitutes evidence.

- Practitioners do not have the time to read all relevant research findings for themselves.

- In medicine some practical methods have been instituted for evaluating research evidence and disseminating findings, which may not be directly transferable to social care contexts.

5.3   Contested areas about the concept of evidence-based practice

We indicated earlier our concerns about emerging definitions of what should constitute reliable research evidence. In particular, we would question the idea that the use of *randomised controlled trials* (see Box 5.2 overleaf) should be the 'gold standard' of social care research or, as Sheldon and Chilvers (2000) put it, 'the strictest tests of professional good intentions' (p. 1). (In Box 5.2 you could substitute the words 'service users' and 'workers' for 'patients' and 'doctors'.)

BOX 5.2 What are randomised controlled trials?

The core feature of [a randomised controlled trial] is the random allocation of all potential participants to the control or to the experimental treatment. Random allocation to conditions, regardless of the personal preference of the patients, the expectations of their doctors, and of any other personal characteristics and qualities, ensures that all sources of bias are distributed at random between the control and experimental groups.

(Source: Reynolds, 2000, p. 26)

In practice this kind of approach is rarely used in social work and social care, for good reasons. We are not decrying randomised controlled trials in all contexts. When such a design is appropriate, and competently and properly carried out, the evidence it produces may be more reliable. However, the choice of research method should always reflect the research question or hypothesis under consideration. Some perfectly valid research questions cannot be explored by an experimental design using random allocation (see Box 5.3 for some examples of research questions that need different research methodologies).

BOX 5.3 Five different research questions needing five different methodologies

Research question 1

Does cognitive behavioural therapy work better than counselling with convicted sex offenders?

Appropriate method

Experimental design using randomised controlled trials – that is, the intervention is tried out with a random sample of people who are then randomly allocated to each treatment. They are then tested before and after the intervention and the results compared with a matched or very similar group of people who did not take part in the intervention. A quasi-experimental design could be used if it is thought unethical to allocate people randomly to different groups. This could be done by matching convicted sex offenders who are receiving therapy or counselling with similar people who are receiving no service.

Research question 2

What do children say about their involvement in decision making?

Appropriate method

In-depth qualitative interviews using an appropriate form of qualitative analysis: that is, a process whereby the researcher is interested in developing not so much an interview as a more equal 'guided

---

conversation', the purpose of which is trying to understand the *meanings* of the interviewee (rather than count pre-set categories).

Research question 3

To what extent do social workers read about research?

Appropriate method

Large-scale survey followed by statistical analysis.

Research question 4

In optimising quality of life, is home care or residential care more cost-effective for older people?

Appropriate method

Cost-effectiveness study – this involves a randomised controlled trial comparing different kinds of outcome for groups receiving the different forms of service. The costs and benefits are not restricted to financial matters.

Research question 5

How could people chairing decision-making meetings improve their skills?

Appropriate method

Detailed observations of their practice verified against a set of baseline skills; or a qualitative analysis of their views using a semi-structured or themed 'guided conversation'.

So, there are good – and not so good – designs available to tackle particular research questions. In practice a combination of methods is often required. Randomised controlled trials might be the most appropriate approach in *evaluative* research or in *outcome* studies, where the outcome or output of an intervention can be clearly specified in advance: for instance, the 'number of children looked after' or 'days of home care provided'. Other forms of enquiry, such as 'exploratory research' or surveys, are not best served by randomised controlled trials. Indeed, Sheldon and Chilvers (2000) themselves produced a survey of professionals' reactions to aspects of evidence-based social care, yet they did not use randomised controlled trials. Does this, by their own definition of 'gold standards', reduce the validity of their survey's findings? Clearly not and we refer to them later in this chapter. The point is that randomised controlled trials were not appropriate in their survey because primarily they were trying to establish more precisely what professionals' views were about evidence-based practice, not conduct an experiment.

There are other arguments against a restricted model of evidence-based practice (that is, one that privileges a scientific and quantifiable approach). They are summarised in Box 5.4 (overleaf).

BOX 5.4 Difficulties surrounding a restricted concept of evidence-based practice

Conceptual problems

- Evidence-based practice can be seen as an incomplete or a reductionist approach to practice, based on 'scientism' rather than science, producing partial or misleading understandings of real-world situations.

- Can the evidence be trusted?

- Are objective data possible and are practitioners (and especially researchers) always unbiased? The selection of 'outcome measures' involves highly politicised processes which may be overlooked in evidence-based practice. Reviewing findings and studies always involves *interpretation*.

- Can evidence always be applied?

- Can evidence gathered from large populations always be applied to individuals?

Pragmatic problems

- Is the evidence always available?

- Sometimes there is too much evidence, sometimes it is of poor quality and sometimes it is of limited relevance.

- Can the implications from results of evidence-based practice studies and reviews always be translated into practice?

- It is not enough to assume that applying the 'right' and discarding the 'wrong' information will lead to lasting changes in practice.

- Good ideas and sound interventions may be rejected, not because they are ineffective but because they cannot produce sufficient evidence.

- Can evidence-based practice take account of other forms of knowledge and 'ways of knowing' such as practice wisdom, the use of theory and service users' views?

(Source: adapted from Trinder, 2000c, pp. 218–35)

In addition it is claimed that some areas of social work are difficult or impossible to quantify in such a way that they can be evaluated. For instance, defining measurable or verifiable aims for reminiscence therapy with an older person will in practice present considerable challenges. So will work with a person who has Alzheimer's disease using an approach based on validation theory (encouraging individual self-expression regardless of the content of what is said). On the other hand, designing verifiable aims for 'dressing a wound' or 'evaluating a cognitive behavioural treatment programme with a mentally disordered offender' may be more straightforward. As June Thoburn, Professor of Social Work at the University of East Anglia, is quoted as saying:

> The nature of our evidence currently – perhaps inevitably – is that when you are dealing with individuals working with other individuals it is going to be very difficult to say what should happen. The thing that has the biggest impact on outcome is the quality of the relationship between the client and the worker, and how do you reduce that down to simple formulae?
>
> (Rickford, 2001, p. 19)

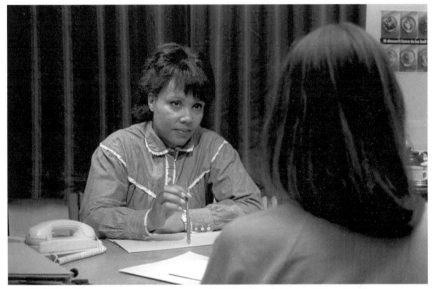

The quality of the relationship has the biggest impact on outcome
(Source: Dave Richards)

It is important to use evidence in planning interventions in social care, and to be able to articulate the sources of that evidence. However, the definition of what constitutes evidence needs to be broad so that people can see it as relevant to their work. Evidence involves the findings of one or more researchers and the interpretation of those findings. For evidence to become useful and useable knowledge it requires the addition of other perspectives: those borne of practice wisdom and service user experience (Lewis, 2003). Practice wisdom is an accumulation of knowledge about what constitutes 'best practice' through: observation and reflection on your own and other people's practice; talking to colleagues; reading articles in practice-based journals; and hearing presentations from other practitioners in case discussions and workshops. Such wisdom may seem to be based on intuition but there are arguments for seeing it as a kind of practice theory based on experience and expertise (Curnock and Hardiker, 1979; Scott, 1990; Schön, 1991).

As Thoburn indicates above, a simple formula for transferring evidence from one context to another will not work. Managers need to develop skills themselves and to encourage their development in other people: skills in critical appraisal and in critical practice in making use of available evidence (Brechin *et al.*, 2000). Indeed, the knowledge and evidence available may not be of a kind that enables practice in social care provision to be *evidence-based*. It may be more accurate and productive to think of *evidence-informed* practice. This term takes into account the point that evidence cannot be applied in practice in a way that bypasses the knowledge and experience of practitioners and service users.

Key points

- The development of research-mindedness and evidence-based practice needs to recognise that different research questions require different research methods to address them.

- A broad definition of 'evidence' is required so that practitioners can see it as relevant to their work.

- This definition needs to take account of practice wisdom, theoretical perspectives and service users' perspectives.

- It may be helpful to think of practice as being informed by, rather than based on, evidence.

5.4 To what extent do practitioners and managers use research to inform their practice?

> There was no evidence base for what we did. Nothing had been tested in terms of alternative strategies, and we made all kinds of interventions in families without really having enough knowledge about their likely impact.
>
> (Rickford, 2001, p. 18)

In this quotation Mike Leadbetter, a Director of Social Services, reflects with some discomfort on his early career as an unqualified social worker in the 1970s. How far do social workers and care workers today read and use research in their daily practice? The indications are that they tend not to use either research or theory, preferring, as Trinder (2000b) points out, to rely on other indicators, such as:

- knowledge gained during initial qualification training
- opinion (but may include prejudice)
- outcomes of previous cases
- current trends
- advice of senior colleagues and peers.

Professional values and practice wisdom are important factors that help practitioners to make judgements. However, the key point is, as with any claim to provide 'evidence' of effective intervention, they need to be subjected to a rigorous critical appraisal.

The study of research methods, research awareness and research utilisation has been a requirement of both pre-registration and post-registration nursing education since 1972. In contrast, social care workers do not have a long history of being required to use research to inform practice decisions. Only recently have they been expected to demonstrate the ability to use research at both qualifying and post-qualifying levels. However, to date, there is no requirement for them to demonstrate the use of critical appraisal skills, except at the post-qualifying Advanced Award level.

Sheldon and Chilvers (2000) conducted a survey which gives some evidence that helps gauge the level of research-mindedness and attitudes to evidence-based practice among social care professionals. From their base at the Centre for Evidence-Based Practice in Social Services, Sheldon and Chilvers sent their questionnaire to social care professionals in 16 social services departments in the south-west of England. Respondents comprised social workers, senior social workers, team leaders, occupational therapists and heads/deputies of homes. They also included other workers, such as 'foster care liaison officers' and 'community project staff'. A stratified random sample of 2285 workers was drawn up and sent questionnaires, of which 1341 (58.7%) were returned. A further 115 had to be discarded because they did not fall into the categories set in the study. The qualifications profile of the 1226 who were included (53.7% of the targeted number of individuals) is shown in Table 5.1.

Table 5.1 **Qualifications profile of respondents**

Category	*Percentage*
Qualified social workers	61.8
Qualified occupational therapists	8.7
Other	16.2
Missing responses	13.3

(Source: adapted from Sheldon and Chilvers, 2000, p. 18)

In addition to gathering demographic information on age, gender, ethnicity and job-specific details, the topics covered in the survey were as follows (there is a summary of the findings in Box 5.5):

- departmental influences on the availability and use of research findings
- existing reading habits and preferences
- familiarity with research publications
- existing levels of knowledge of research terms
- attitudes to evidence-based practice
- suggestions for the priorities of the Centre for Evidence-Based Practice in Social Services.

BOX 5.5 Summary of a survey of research-mindedness

Only 5 to 10% of respondents thought that research findings were discussed 'often' in supervision or at departmental/team meetings.

Keeping up to date was seen as a joint responsibility between the individual and the organisation, although, unlike occupational therapists, social workers saw it primarily as the organisation's role.

Nearly half the sample claimed to have read something pertinent to their work within the last two weeks but 34% had not done so during the previous two and four weeks. Nearly 20% had not read anything relevant to their work during the last six months. No particular demographic factors distinguished these groups.

Most of the material read was magazines (such as *Community Care*) and specialist books, but not evidence-based research journals.

Regarding their own field of work, 57% had never read any evaluative research (or were not sure); 65% had not read a relevant client opinion survey (or were not sure); and 95% had never read the results of a relevant randomised controlled trial (or were not sure).

Although nearly 50% said they felt either 'very' or 'quite' confident that they could critically appraise research findings, only 13% could identify a reason why a client opinion survey might have produced positive outcomes other than because of the professional intervention itself. Of the 432 (out of 1226) who said they knew of a client opinion study, only 12.7% could identify one. Although 38% said they could define the meaning of the term 'statistical significance', only 6% (of the 38%) could explain it correctly (in other words only about 2% of the sample knew what it meant).

On a more optimistic note, 90% said they viewed the concept of evidence-based practice as either 'very' or 'quite' relevant to their work (but only 7% reported frequent usage of an evidence-based approach in their work).

(Source: adapted from Sheldon and Chilvers, 2000)

A critical appraisal of this study might include the following questions and comments.

- To what extent were the findings representative of (a) social care workers and managers in the south-west of England and (b) their use of research nationally (that is, can the results be transferred more widely)? The rate of inclusion in the survey was only 53.7%, which may not provide strong grounds for confidence that the findings apply nationally.
- Not knowing what terms mean – for example 'statistical significance' – does not necessarily indicate the absence of critical or analytical skills.
- Social care workers may not have time to read journals. They may also believe they lack relevance to their practice or are unnecessarily complicated. In other words, the implication could be to encourage writers to be clearer and to think about the relevance of their research to practice, rather than to 'blame' social workers.

In spite of these caveats, the survey's findings do give some indication of the nature of the innovation represented by the attempts to increase research-mindedness and evidence-based practice. What precisely is involved here? We believe there are three main features.

1 Introducing research-mindedness and evidence-informed practice involves attitudinal change. For the introduction to be considered successful, people would be transforming their practice.

2 Sheldon and Chilvers' survey concludes that, although social care professionals see benefits in becoming more interested in using research in their work, many will experience difficulties interpreting research findings because they lack critical appraisal skills and knowledge about research methods. They are willing but may lack capability. Managers and supervisors will need, therefore, to handle the question of practitioners' capability carefully and sensitively because, tackled inappropriately, some people could end up feeling more deskilled and stressed than they do already. The claim of nearly half the sample that they had read something relevant recently is a positive finding. This enthusiasm needs to be encouraged and the skills built on.

3 Attention is needed to the context in which the innovation is introduced: that is, for some practitioners to accept their own role in becoming more aware of research. Supervisors and managers have to address whether the organisation itself is both capable of and willing to provide access to research data. More importantly, they will have to allocate some time and space to the twin enterprises of research-mindedness and evidence-informed practice.

Next we consider some practical ways of achieving this by referring to our own experience of working alongside practitioners and managers in several social care organisations.

Key points

- A survey of social care professionals in south-west England indicates that their ability to critically appraise research findings is limited.

- Managers need to handle the development of research-minded-ness and evidence-informed practice in their units sensitively, to avoid increased stress.

- Managers and their organisations have a role in making research data accessible and actively used.

5.5 Ways of supporting research-mindedness

Implementing evidence-informed practice in social care will probably be a lengthy and complex undertaking (Trinder, 2000c). We turn now to the role of managers in stimulating and supporting change on such a scale. The discussion here builds on some of the ideas introduced in Chapter 4.

One of the unique contributions of the late Gerald Smale, founding director of the Practice and Development Exchange at the National Institute for Social Work, was his review and analysis of the literature on how some ideas get translated into action in organisations while others do not. He drew several conclusions, each of which challenges received ideas of how innovation spreads through organisations, particularly when the aim is to change attitudes and behaviour.

He noted in the literature a profusion of models, schemas and diagrams, most of which were not derived empirically but, nevertheless, claimed that change takes place through hierarchical, downwardly transmitted, organisational processes (Smale, 1996). Consequently, the discourse of change management is replete with phrases such as 'trickle-down', 'cascade approach', and so on. However, while some short-term gains can be made in this way, the research, drawn mainly from the field of social psychology on how lasting change actually happens, forces the opposite conclusion: that change on a more permanent footing occurs more often when it is 'caught' – like a virus – between people *operating at the same level*.

At around the same time as Smale was working on this topic, a similar set of conclusions was being articulated by Malcolm Gladwell in the USA. As neither author refers to the other, presumably they formed their insights in parallel but in ignorance of their respective discoveries. The subtitle of Gladwell's book *The Tipping Point* (1999) – the moment when new ideas seem to spread like wildfire – is 'how little things can make a big difference'. Concentrating on the 'little things' is a key part of what managers and supervisors can do to increase research-mindedness and evidence-informed practice. By 'tipping', Gladwell (1999) is referring to the idea of a *critical mass*, a kind of boiling point. This is not gradualism or successive incrementalism; it is more akin to geometric progression. The expansion of mobile phone use in the UK is a good example. In the early or even mid-1990s they were seen as the province of pretentious and 'upwardly mobile' people. Today many people own one. The reasons for this change in buyer behaviour go far beyond the fact that the phones have become much smaller.

What managers and supervisors can take from this research and apply to the introduction of research-mindedness and evidence-informed practice is that people pay attention to those around them and their immediate environment so, providing they are the right ones, little changes can have big effects.

Both Smale (1996) and Gladwell (1999) question the use of biological metaphors when thinking about 'epidemics' and 'contagious processes': too often 'colds' or 'flu' or 'HIV' spring to mind. However, the same processes of contagion can explain why some ideas get taken up and others do not and, of particular relevance to managers and supervisors, the authors both conclude that we can deliberately start and control positive epidemics.

Having the right people around is not enough; achieving 'stickiness' is thought to be the key to successful change (Gladwell, 1999). Just spreading the ideas is a necessary but not sufficient condition because, if they are not taken up and translated into action, there will be little point to the exercise. Supervisors and managers need to work with the specific aim of getting the message to make an impact and stay – or 'stick' – in the mind. This does not just happen. Creative ways need to be found to package the information and make it interesting and inspiring. The messages of the original innovators have to be translated into a form that is suitable to their team or unit. This inevitably means 'reading' the audience accurately.

Finally, aspects of the environment in which the new ideas are likely to develop are important. The aim is to help people change their behaviour alongside their 'neighbour' at work, while recognising that people behave differently in different contexts. In addition to considering practical issues, such as whether there are enough computer links to facilitate access to the web, managers and supervisors need to think carefully about the optimal time to encourage the spread of something as radical as research-mindedness and evidence-informed practice. If a department is about to undergo a major restructuring exercise, it is unlikely to be an optimal time to introduce new ideas that it is hoped will nurture different attitudes and actions. However, it may be possible to link research to other planned changes, as in Example 5.2 (overleaf).

EXAMPLE 5.2 Researching training needs

Rowena is a mental health nurse recently appointed to work in a learning disabilities service. The service is developing its assessment and treatment work with people who have mental health problems and learning disabilities, and Rowena's role reflects these changes. As well as a day-to-day clinical role in the current residential centre, Rowena is involved in discussions about how the team will work with the more challenging client group that they are expecting. She is doing research on the training needs of learning disability nurses when working with people with dual diagnosis. This will involve her in assessing current relevant skills and knowledge in the nursing team, and setting up a training and development programme to help the team acquire new skills.

(Source: manager consultations)

Smale (1996) concludes that individual professionals will consider new ways of working after seeing colleagues they value and respect grapple with the same ideas, and then begin to experiment with new practices themselves. Watching colleagues, talking to them and using them as models is seen as an important conduit for change. His analysis translates especially well to situations when professionals support an innovation in principle. From our own experience, underscored by Sheldon and Chilvers' survey, this appears to be the overall reaction of professionals to developing research-mindedness and evidence-informed practice. They welcome the idea in principle. On paper at least, this augurs well for the adoption of new practices.

Naturally, senior managers have to be seen to 'own' an innovation. However, in both Smale's and Gladwell's analyses, rather than managers spending their time organising a succession of 'away days' and promotional events, they are better advised to work out ways of lubricating the system on the ground to support the change. They both draw on Everett Rogers' work on the diffusion of change in support of their arguments (Rogers, 1995).

In Chapter 4 Senge's distinction between commitment, enrolment and compliance in the range of responses people have towards change was noted (Senge, 1990). Rogers (1995) also found there are several distinct ways in which groups of staff accept and then take on new ideas. In his terminology, these range from the original *innovators* and venturesome *early adopters* (usually around 20% of the workforce), through the *early and late majority* (about 60%), to the *laggards* (also around 20%). Interestingly, traditional approaches to innovation and change concentrate on either the *early adopters*, who tend to change quickly anyway, or the *laggards*, who are unlikely to change under any circumstances and for whom a 'damage limitation' strategy may well be the best approach. Consequently, the challenge for managers and supervisors is learning how to get to grips with encouraging and enabling the 60% of the 'early and late majority' to adopt new practices.

This large group in the middle tends to be more sceptical and may need more convincing; but this need not be viewed as 'resistance', as unfortunately it so often is, because, as Smale (1996) points out, sometimes 'the people on the edge see the furthest' (p. 33). This may be because they are exercising their own professional autonomy and judgement. Instead of thinking of sceptics as being 'resistant', confident managers and supervisors might consider encouraging critics to voice their viewpoint – maybe anonymously, if the organisation is thought not to support open criticism – because their insights can help fine-tune aspects of the implementation.

We have been working separately in different social services departments, discussing ways of increasing research-mindedness and evidence-informed practice. Box 5.6 is a brief summary of how one of us was asked to facilitate a process to help managers and practitioners in a social services department introduce research-mindedness.

BOX 5.6 The introduction of research-mindedness in a social services department

In 1998 the Director of Greenwich Social Services asked David Shemmings to devise a plan to introduce research-mindedness within child care teams. The idea was to go beyond merely sharing research findings and, instead, aim to help teams to develop:

1 an awareness of the need for research and evaluation

2 an understanding of why and when different research methods are used

3 critical appraisal skills.

An invitation was sent to teams asking them to send a representative to attend an initial meeting to gauge interest. About 25 people came and detailed discussions were held with them. It was felt that the best approach was to take the list of topics devised by team members and summarise (a) why the research had been undertaken, (b) the main results, and then (c) outline why the particular methods used were selected. Key studies were appraised using questions from the NHS's Critical Appraisal Skills Programme (see the References).

Finally, those who attended were expected to take the material back to their teams and try to stimulate discussion.

A series of 20 three-hour sessions were planned over 18 months to cover the following topics:

● attachment theory

● the involvement of young people in decision making

- the Department of Health's Assessment Framework
- the effectiveness of cognitive/behavioural approaches with offenders
- family and domestic violence
- neglect and emotional abuse
- child observation.

During the sessions the following issues were discussed:

- different research methods
- making sense of statistics in journal articles
- using the internet to develop research-mindedness.

Attendance at these sessions was consistently high, as was the interest level in the content of each topic covered. All sessions included copies of relevant journal articles and several participants asked for these articles to be provided *before* the next session. At a midway review, those who attended provided very positive feedback about their own responses to the sessions, which included:

The sessions will help me in my role by
... helping me when making decisions
... increasing my confidence
... informing my practice as well as that of team members
... helping me to work and speak with more knowledge
... encouraging me to see what is happening in the world of research and this has already been of great help in supervision
... giving me greater confidence when challenging others.

They felt initially, however, that they had achieved only limited success when disseminating the material among team colleagues. The problem was not so much not having enough time; it was more centrally about feeling a lack of confidence to present the sessions again to colleagues. The following actions were identified to rectify this:

- increased access to and use of websites in teams
- additional resources to purchase journals
- setting up discussion groups, where research findings could be related to practitioners' actual work with families.

Feedback at the end of the programme indicated that this strategy was beginning to have good results.

There are several practical steps managers and supervisors can take to support research-mindedness and evidence-informed practice.

Practical ways to support research-mindedness and evidence-informed practice

The following ideas are from managers in four different social services departments.

Explore and question plans and decisions

When workers write reports or attend meetings, stress the need for them to provide evidence of their assessments or requests for resources. An example from the field of social care is the regularity with which 'respite care' is recommended in reports without an analysis of the growing evidence about when such provision is effective and when it is not (McNally *et al.*, 1999; Ashworth and Baker, 2000; Pickard, 2001). Another example from family support and child protection is a recommendation for 'parenting classes' but without a justification of why they are thought likely to help a particular family (yet there is a body of research available that has evaluated the specific merits of parenting classes, for example Smith, 1996). Looking at files and records gives a good indication of the level of research-mindedness of the practitioner: see Walker *et al.* (2001).

Support 'research champions'

There will be people in the organisation who have done research – sometimes of a pioneering nature – and others who are very knowledgeable. If they are viewed by their peers with respect and they have good communication skills, these practitioners are a tremendous asset when introducing research-mindedness and evidence-informed practice.

Encourage discussion

There are encouraging reports about workers spontaneously setting up journal clubs, email bulletin boards and email discussion groups. Anything managers and supervisors can do to support such activities will be appreciated. Encouraging open discussion is arguably the most effective way of bringing research to life.

Link to staff development and appraisal systems

It is obviously sensible to discuss how to increase the use of research and the creative application of practice wisdom and learning gained from consultation with service users and carers during staff development and appraisal meetings.

Modelling

What we *do* often carries more weight with other people than what we *say*. Hence, managers and supervisors (and local authority members) should model the principles of research-mindedness and evidence-informed practice. This means not proposing changes when there is conflicting evidence, and especially not when there is no evidence at all.

Allocate resources for journals and books

Taking out corporate membership of key journals is a cost-effective way of encouraging professionals to keep up to date. Membership often includes access to otherwise restricted websites, together with the added facility of being able to download the full text of articles.

Encourage the use of web-based information searches

Try to help workers feel comfortable if they look up research findings on a website during work time that it is seen as a valid and legitimate use of time. Encourage them to email website addresses to each other. Yvonne Shemmings has been working with a variety of authorities to provide practitioners with personalised, evidence-informed information in response to their practice-related questions concerning children and families. This information is available on a web-based subscription service called 'Thinking It Out'.

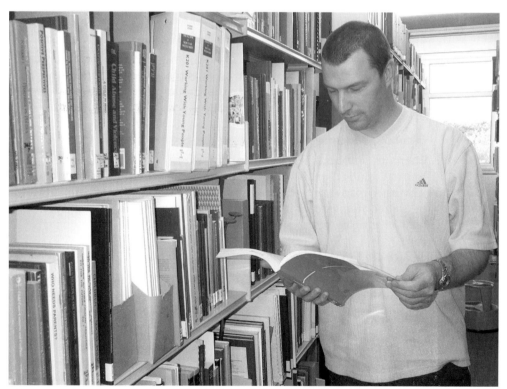

Allocating resources for journals and books helps to encourage professionals to keep up to date

Help promote critical appraisal skills

In terms of their knowledge of how to critically appraise the research they are reading, individual practitioners will be at different stages. It is important to encourage them to become more competent and confident in doing so. The various appendices at the end of Gomm *et al.* (2000) contain excellent guides on how to appraise each of the main types of study. There are also some good websites (just type in 'critical appraisal skills' in any of the internet's main search engines).

Making change happen

The list above is very practical. What it does not do is offer a conceptual framework within which to analyse strategic options. Getting practitioners to increase their research-mindedness and to recognise the importance of acting from an evidence base means bringing about change in attitudes and practice. As you read in Chapter 4, several factors create high energy conditions for change (Pettigrew *et al.*, 1992). Smale (1996) refers to the 'innovation trinity', the three main components he identifies as being central for consideration in introducing changes:

- the people
- analysing the innovation
- understanding the context.

Box 5.7 is a modified set of questions which Smale suggests people who are trying to spread new ideas should ask. Many of these questions explore the factors that are important in receptivity to change.

BOX 5.7 Questions for managers emerging from Smale's 'innovation trinity'

The people

- Who needs to make the change happen and take action for it?

- Bring 'research champions' and 'early adopters' together and then support them.

- Help it happen by releasing resources.

- Who has to let it happen?

- Who has to give their consent?

- Who could sabotage the innovation?

- Who must not block resources?

- What meaning does the status quo and the innovation have for the key people involved?

– For whom does the innovation change the purpose of their work?

– Who will experience a change in status or image of themselves?

- What is the impact of the change on individuals, working groups and the wider social system?

- Who experiences what as 'winning'?

- Who experiences what as 'loss'?

- How can you make sure people have space to mourn their losses?

- What can you do to build commitment to new practices?

Analysing the innovation

- How 'adaptable' is the innovation?

– Who perceives it as (a) better, (b) no different and (c) worse than the status quo?

– Can it be tried out before adoption?

– Can it be observed in operation elsewhere?

– Does it require extra resources – if so, what are they?

- At what stage is the innovation?

– Initiation?

– Development?

– Implementation?

Understanding the context

- What other changes can this be linked to, to gain support?

- Are the required resources available?

– Time?

– People?

- Who needs to take part in consciousness-raising events?

- Who needs what form of staff development?

- Who needs what knowledge?

- Who needs to develop which skills?

- Who needs coaching?

(Source: adapted from Smale, 1996, pp. 55–90)

Finally, there are important actions that organisations and senior managers can take to help spread research-mindedness and evidence-informed practice, as Box 5.8 indicates. Although the list may appear somewhat idealised, the intention when compiling it was deliberately to reflect 'best' practice. The six points are adapted from Sheldon and Chilvers' work and include action that would have to be taken both inside and outside social care organisations, and usually at a senior level.

BOX 5.8 Organisational implications of evidence-based practice

There is a need for:

1   A well-qualified workforce and an emphasis on qualifying and post-qualifying courses for students and candidates to review research and critically appraise service effectiveness.

2   Regular updating of knowledge and experience, by training courses which make regular reference to research, in terms of both the nature of social problems as well as the effectiveness of different approaches designed to address them.

3   A supervision system which draws regularly on research and encourages practitioners to ask 'So why are we proceeding this way?' and 'On what evidence?'

4   Senior departmental managers to act in the same way as they expect practitioners to act when making key decisions and allocating resources.

5   Professional groups and individual practitioners to take more personal responsibility for being aware of research into service effectiveness.

6   Better collaboration between social services departments and local and regional universities as well as research institutes.

(Source: adapted from Sheldon and Chilvers, 2000, pp. 8–9)

Key points

- Research-mindedness may occur more often when it is taken up by peers who can influence each other.

- Managers can be most effective in supporting this kind of development if they build on existing interest and enlist those already involved in research to help those occupying the middle ground to take up new practices.

- There are several practical steps managers can take to support research-mindedness and evidence-informed practice.

- A focus on the people, the innovatory approach to increasing research-mindedness and the context in which it is happening provides a helpful checklist of questions for planning this and other changes.

- There are implications for organisations, senior managers and wider professional bodies and academia in bringing about the widespread cultural change required for evidence-informed practice to become accepted practice.

5.6 Conclusion

Practitioners and managers tend to agree that their actions should be based on the best evidence available to them. However, because current definitions of evidence-based practice have been predicated almost exclusively on positivist research methodology and the ways of conducting medical science, it has already started to attract fierce critical comment when applied to social work and social care (see, for example, Webb, 2001; Hollway, 2001).

In this chapter we have argued for a wider definition of evidence-based practice, partly to accelerate the spread of ideas about the use of research in social care. Consequently, we have challenged the belief that randomised controlled trials should be reified as the 'gold standard' for research in all situations. Instead, we propose a more inclusive working definition of 'what counts as evidence', based entirely on the nature of the research or evaluative questions under consideration rather than on any predetermined method of enquiry. In addition, we suggest that it may be more appropriate, given the difficulties of directly applying lessons from evidence gained in widely differing circumstances, to think of practice as being informed by, rather than based on, evidence.

Ultimately, the *evidence* itself is not the most important feature of evidence-informed practice: far more critical is the ability to use professional judgement – what Webb (2001) calls 'deliberation' – about the relative weight given to *the complete array of evidence* collected. Thus, rather than trying to become experts in research methods and findings, the key role of supervisors and practice-led managers is to develop critical thinking skills within teams and then to facilitate the processes of professional enquiry and self-critical reflection on practice.

Part 2   Managing Services for People

Introduction

People are at the heart of care, yet sometimes service users experience care as too administrative and functional. Managing care involves managing a creative network of relationships between people in agencies who all have a part to play in meeting needs. Service users and carers often have difficulties in getting help with care needs that cross the boundaries of provision from different organisations, whether involving health care, social services, housing, education or other services. Since the 1970s central government has attempted to encourage joint working and a multi-agency approach to meeting complex care needs. Collaborative working is now a requirement of government policy. Frontline managers are the people with the responsibility to make such arrangements work at a local level. Their role is building the relationships that make such partnerships real and effective, so that service users are not neglected or harmed, and so that the services they can access are suitable for their needs.

In Chapter 6 'Managing across professional and agency boundaries', Charlesworth outlines the history of joint working and the different ways of defining the processes involved. She begins by considering the rhetoric about collaboration, and why it has never been easy. There are many instances of failed partnerships, and of situations where agencies have failed to act together, with the result that people's needs were not met or they were harmed. It is important for managers to understand the pitfalls and find ways to avoid them. It is also important to be positive and work creatively for partnerships that are effective on the ground. Working in collaboration pervades every aspect of managers' work. Managers use the skills involved all the time: decision making, communicating, negotiating, leading, measuring outcomes, and managing information and finances. Understanding both the different organisational imperatives that are driving other participants in partnerships and the different cultural expectations and aims is central to successful working. Working in partnership requires the ability to understand other people's motivation, to build relationships and work for shared vision and equal commitment.

These issues about the expectations and responsibilities of different agencies permeate every area of care activity, especially the question of who will pay. Managers who commission services and managers who provide them are equally concerned about providing a Best Value service. People worry about whether they can afford the services they need, so making stretched resources provide as much as possible for as many as possible concerns managers too. This means understanding and working with the financial relationships between the agencies that provide services. Taking good care of people is also about money and resources. If you have not managed a large budget before, moving into management can be a big step. In Chapter 7 'Managing budgets and giving Best Value', Gallop aims to demystify the different aspects of setting budgets and managing budget processes. He explains that the numbers give a picture of the agency and its services, so the budget is not just about figures but about how the agency works with its partners and service users. He illustrates this with examples from practising managers and from current local authority practice. In particular, he explores the notion of Best Value and what that means legally as well as at policy and local levels. Gallop argues that real partnership, between agencies and in particular with service users, increases the likelihood of achieving good value.

Another policy development affecting managers in all sectors is 'e-government', as policy makers seek to increase the use of information technology in the workplace and to facilitate access to new technologies by service users. New technology is a powerful way to make services accessible to the public, but is it a double-edged sword? Will it increase the possibilities of surveillance and government control of citizens and workers? Does it make working in partnership easier because databases can be shared, or do multiple and conflicting approaches to data mean that managers, workers and service users alike have yet more issues to consider? Will people be empowered by having better access to information that is held about them or will agencies that share databases pass information from one to another inappropriately?

Whatever your response to such questions, if you are a manager, handling information is part of your work. In Chapter 8 'Managing information and using new technology in care agencies', Ousley, Rowlands and Seden identify some of these debates. They argue that a practice-led approach to the development of information means practitioners and their managers can work to ensure the information produced assists the tasks they have to do. In partnership terms, the complex issues about confidentiality and information sharing have to be resolved.

'Co-operation', 'collaboration' and 'working together' are often emphasised in government publications about the expectations of social care agencies to protect individuals from harm. The numerous failures of multi-agency work in this arena are well documented. At the same time, much has been written about the management of risk in social care, but often still in a way which only considers risk assessment from a narrow agency perspective. Brown (with Seden), in Chapter 9 'Managing to protect', explores ideas about vulnerability and abuse in both adults' and children's services and locates the responsibilities for protection in a broad societal context, which involves managers in all kinds of care setting working together to play their part. Concepts such as vulnerability and the need for safeguards have also been challenged and debated. Some adults dislike the term 'vulnerable' because it does not reflect the strengths of their identities. Young carers might also dislike this expression when they make a major contribution to their families on their own terms. None the less, there are times when very young children, young people and adults are in a vulnerable situation and managers must act to protect. Brown argues that a practice-led approach to protection is a balanced intervention where decisions are made from knowledge about needs, vulnerabilities and risks for the people involved. She explores managers' responsibility to consider situations carefully, using the best knowledge available, so they can be as sure of the ground as possible before taking protective action. When agencies work together, each one has a different role and remit, so when they are brought together to address abuse issues they have very different responsibilities and orientations. Here again, managers in all settings need to work collaboratively to co-ordinate systems: both to respond to harm that has occurred and to bring about quality services that promote safer service environments.

Chapter 6
Managing across professional and agency boundaries

Julie Charlesworth

6.1 Introduction

The concept of different agencies and professionals working together to plan and deliver care services is nothing new: there has always been a degree of mixed provision, involving public, voluntary and private sector organisations. Many managers and professionals have become accustomed to working outside their usual teams at several different levels: for example, in consultation procedures, planning and policy making and liaison with individual clients or patients. Since the 1970s, a plethora of directives and initiatives have been designed by both central government and local agencies in order to stimulate joint working and to emphasise its role in effective service delivery. There is a growing realisation that meeting complex care needs requires a multi-agency approach where managers and professionals work together to plan and deliver services. Child protection inquiries, in particular, have highlighted this.

Service users and carers consulted during the preparation of this book (see Appendix 1) gave many examples of the problems encountered when service providers do not work well together. One man, who cares for his 93-year-old mother, described the response when she developed ulcers on her legs:

> I was told very, very clearly I was in a grey area. Now the social services used that. When the social services came to see me, she said, 'We didn't realise your mother's legs were that bad.' I said, 'Well, I told you they were when she was in hospital.' When the district nurse comes, they say they don't do legs any longer, they're too busy, they haven't got time to wash people's legs, that's the social services job. So they're arguing in my mother's house about who's going to do what.
>
> (Service user consultations)

What do we mean by partnership, collaboration, and inter-agency and inter-professional working? When is it appropriate and what skills are required to be a partner? The burning question is how difficult is inter-professional or inter-agency working? The title of this chapter encapsulates a fundamental aspect of collaboration – boundaries. A boundary implies a wall that may need to be removed or crossed over (for example, around organisations, professions, different funding regimes, changing

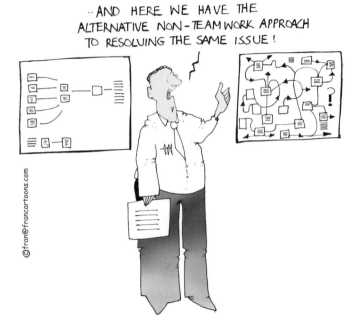

Meeting complex care needs requires a multi-agency approach

organisational responsibilities, restructuring of services and organisations) and a lack of geographical coterminosity between organisations. Managers work at the interface of these boundaries and, if their perception is that the boundaries need to be broken down, they may experience problems in collaboration.

Collaboration is not easily viewed as a discrete topic for frontline managers. It both pervades all aspects of managers' work (for example, monitoring and audit, service user consultation, managing change) and draws on a range of management skills and knowledge, such as decision making, communication, negotiation, leadership, measuring outcomes, managing information and finances. Furthermore, some of the discussion in this chapter concerns wider locality-based and strategic partnerships, which usually involve more senior managers. However, it is also important to understand the broader context of inter-agency working, as so much decision and policy making is now conducted in this way, and frontline managers have a key role to play in these arrangements.

There is a growing literature on joint working and this chapter aims to draw out from it some of the key issues and debates in managing inter-agency and inter-professional working, particularly in facilitating more inclusive, accountable and effective structures.

The aims of this chapter are to explore:

- the desirability of working together
- the blocks and barriers to effective co-working
- the skills needed for operational aspects of inter-agency work.

6.2   Putting inter-professional and inter-agency working in context

This section focuses on why organisations, professionals and managers choose to work collaboratively. It is useful to understand the broader policy context and the attempts made by central government to stimulate partnership, so the section begins with an overview of key developments since the 1970s. Collaboration has not always been a direct result of government policy: local agencies have also developed their own initiatives and best practice and there is considerable variation between localities in terms of how organisations and individuals have pioneered different ways of working together.

Background to joint working

Joint working has a relatively long history. In 1973 the NHS Act required health and local authorities to establish joint consultative committees (JCCs) for considering policy and operational issues. Unfortunately, they were deemed unsuccessful as much key decision making happened elsewhere. In the late 1970s joint care planning teams (JCPTs) were set up to advise the JCCs on strategic and service developments and to better integrate social services with health, housing, transport and education. Initially, the JCCs mostly involved statutory agencies but the voluntary sector was gradually included and, although the joint planning structures were heavily criticised at the time, they did start to provide a wider forum for discussion and consultation (Lupton *et al.*, 1998). The identification of care group structures (mental health, physical disability, learning disability, elderly people, and children and families) also helped give the voluntary sector a higher profile and facilitated the formation of user groups to feed into joint planning (Lupton *et al.*, 1998). However, the introduction of joint finance tended to dominate the JCC agenda and, ultimately, structures for monitoring and shared accountability for the outcome of inter-agency planning failed to emerge (Wistow, 1990).

During the 1980s, under the Conservative government, joint working, particularly with the private sector, was primarily about offering more choice, creating competition and reducing costs. The NHS and Community Care Act 1990 provided new impetus to developing partnerships by requiring social services departments to involve other agencies in the assessment of individuals' community care needs. At a strategic level, the concept of *joint commissioning* was introduced, again with a greater emphasis on collaborative working between health and social services. However, problems of a cumbersome legal framework, different funding regimes and costs hindered much joint commissioning activity.

When the Labour government came to power in 1997, the restructuring of public services was based on a discourse of partnership and 'joined-up' policy. This picked up, and extended, the notion of inter-agency working from the Conservative government, although clearly the ethos had changed from one of competition to collaboration. Cost cutting, however, also appears to be behind much of the government's thinking. The need to work in partnership is now encapsulated within all policy areas (health, social care, housing, social inclusion, crime and disorder, employment) and pervades all aspects of care services. Box 6.1 is a summary for England and Wales; similar expectations apply in Scotland, and in Northern Ireland where health and social care services are provided in a single integrated system. The government has recognised that these are cross-cutting issues, not fitting neatly under the remit of one organisation and that, in fact, they fall into the 'inter-organisational domain'. This is a policy space where the only means of dealing with such issues successfully is through collaboration between organisations, perhaps with one organisation acting as a 'strategic bridge' to bring them together (Huxham, 1996a). Thus, the government has now acknowledged in policy what many care workers have always known: health inequalities are linked to social and economic inequalities.

BOX 6.1 Three levels of joint working

1 Strategic planning: agencies need to plan jointly for the medium term, and share information about how they intend to use their resources towards the achievement of common goals.

2 Service commissioning: when securing services for their local populations, agencies need to have a common understanding of the needs they are jointly meeting, and the kind of provision likely to be most effective.

3 Service provision: regardless of how services are purchased or funded, the key objective is that the user receives a coherent package of care and that they, and their families, do not face the anxiety of having to navigate a labyrinthine bureaucracy.

(Source: Department of Health, 1998a, p. 6)

Defining the process

Different terms are used to describe working across boundaries, including: joint working, collaboration, partnership, inter-organisational relations, networking, alliance, co-ordination, co-operation, teamwork. These may reflect the degree of formality of the collaboration: for example, whether it involves dedicated resources or has its own budget and partnership board. There is little agreement about how the terms are used, thus thinking about the *meanings* associated with collaboration might be a more fruitful course to pursue, particularly thinking about the reasons why organisations might want to work with others (Huxham, 1996b).

It is useful to start by considering the differences between the terms *inter-professional* and *inter-agency*. In many ways they entail similar ways of working and obviously a partnership can be both inter-agency and inter-professional.

Inter-professional working can happen within the same department or organisation, for example between social workers and housing officers or general practitioners and district nurses. An advertising campaign in 2001 for NHS recruitment drew on this by showing how many professionals were involved in the care of one patient. Each professional group has its own identity, culture, training and accreditation and allegiances beyond the workplace to national professional bodies (Biggs, 1997). There are different ways in which professionals might work together (the following examples could also be inter-agency):

> The subject of interprofessional working is also broader than describing how practitioners work together to help patients or clients. It describes how professionals work together to undertake management and planning tasks, which benefit a group of patients or contribute to the running and planning of service organisations. Examples of formal groups are management teams, project teams, planning teams, training teams, multidisciplinary audit groups and quality groups. Examples of tasks include formulating a procedure for referrals and assessments to be followed by many professions, deciding a plan to reduce higher than average length of stay, deciding a joint health and social services training programme, creating a purchasing plan for a community care plan, agreeing a care management model, and working in a quality group to reduce the rate of readmissions.
>
> (Øvretveit, 1997, pp. 2–3)

However, inter-professional working does not involve everybody all of the time. In her analysis of studies of inter-professional working in child protection, Stephenson (1994) suggests that team members divide into 'inner' and 'outer' circles, depending on the amount and frequency of contact team members have with each other and the work. This raises issues concerning teamwork and whether it is as 'tight-knit' as the literature suggests in inter-professional working. Stephenson suggests that a 'network' is a more apt description for many of the team members (in the outer circle) who have limited involvement in child protection and may be brought in just for conferences. Payne (2000) suggests that such wider relationships also need nurturing (in the same way as for core team members).

Inter-agency working usually occurs because there is a need to go beyond involving known individuals or professionals and to invite wider representation and expertise, perhaps because of government guidelines, or because there may be a realisation within an organisation that previous policies have been unsuccessful owing to limited resources or expertise. Often, collaboration is initiated because one organisation needs the input – and invariably resources – from another sector, such as voluntary and community groups. One useful classification of partnership is provided by Hudson, who identified six types of inter-organisational partnerships in primary health and social care, which are summarised in Box 6.2.

BOX 6.2 Inter-organisational partnerships

1 *Administrative/governance partnerships:* the extent to which agencies share administrative boundaries, organisational arrangements and decision-making processes.

2 *Legislative partnerships:* a statutory permission to engage in joint working, and a statutory obligation to do so.

3 *Programme partnerships:* social services and health working jointly to deliver a programme of care, often based on specific tranches of money.

4 *Community partnerships:* tend to relate to areas of deprivation and seek involvement of individuals and groups in their own health care through a community development approach.

5 *Commissioning partnerships:* transfer of money between organisational budgets or some form of alignment or pooling of budgets.

6 *Performance partnerships:* where joint responsibility is taken for monitoring and reviewing either specific programmes or 'whole system' programmes.

(Source: adapted from Hudson, 1998, pp. 1–4)

In reality, one type of partnership cannot always be distinguished from another in such a clear-cut way, but it is a useful starting point from which to consider the reasons why organisations collaborate, often involving directives from government. Now that the government is emphasising the 'duty of partnership', clearly many partnerships would fit the categories of programme and performance partnerships. Many of these partnerships entail inter-professional working as well. Hudson highlights the implications for different professional groups of joint working and questions whether different occupational groupings could work from the same locations.

Ling (2000) draws attention to whether partnership working has the ability to transform organisations, particularly as they become more integrated. He questions whether partner organisations become increasingly similar (*convergence*) or manage to maintain their own distinctiveness (*co-evolution*) in working together closely.

There is also a sense in which collaborations might progress through different stages as partner organisations become more used to working together and see the benefits of developing more formal relations. Hudson *et al.* (1998) describe these in the following terms.

1 *Isolation* (no joint working)
2 *Encounter* (informal, ad hoc contact)
3 *Communication* (involving formal joint working, frequent interaction, sharing of information)
4 *Collaboration* (high level of trust, common interests, joint planning and service delivery)
5 *Integration* (organisations integrate teams or even merge, with a loss of individual organisational identity)

It is extremely unlikely that the first stage still exists, given the government's emphasis on partnership. There are some examples of the final stage of integration: for example, community trusts merging with primary care trusts, and merged health and social services functions. Whether these could still be classified as partnerships is open to question. Most organisations are probably somewhere in the middle of this range. However, partnerships do not have to progress through different levels or up the 'ladder of partnership' (Gaster and Deakin, 1998), as some organisations may feel confident enough (and sufficiently resourced) to go straight in at an advanced level.

Why collaborate?

The government agenda set the pace for collaboration during the 1990s but it was based on a history of inter-professional and inter-agency working across different services, and the drive to improve services, reduce costs and duplication, add value, increase accountability and respond to the complexity of service users' needs:

> At one level [partnership] is a rational response to divisions within and between government departments and local authorities, within and between professions, and between those who deliver services and those who use them. It is also a necessary response to the fragmentation of services that the introduction of markets into welfare brought with them. It has the potential to make the delivery of services more coherent and hence more effective. If each partner stands to gain from the

additional resources that other partners bring, from pooling ideas, knowledge and financial resources, then partnership 'adds value' for each participant.

(Balloch and Taylor, 2001, p. 1)

According to Huxham (1996b) the concept of collaborative advantage 'is concerned with the creation of synergy between collaborating organizations' (p. 14) and 'focuses on outputs of collaboration that could not have been achieved except through collaborating' (p. 15). However, partnerships often fail and this is termed *collaborative inertia* to describe 'when the apparent rate of work output of a core group is slowed down considerably compared to what a casual observer might expect the group to be able to achieve' (Huxham, 1996a, p. 241). These are perhaps obvious points but they illustrate the importance of maintaining a clear focus on the potential results attainable through collaboration and not regarding joint working as something that will automatically generate results just because it is 'a good thing' to do.

The arguments for closer working together are clear and generally accepted. People have needs that do not fit neatly under the responsibilities of particular agencies or professionals; and service users' needs are neglected when there is a lack of co-ordination. For reasons of both effectiveness and efficiency, increasing attention has been given to breaking down old ways of working and replacing them with processes and practices that have service users' needs at the core. However, problems continue to be encountered in collaboration (see Example 6.1).

EXAMPLE 6.1 The Victoria Climbié inquiry

Inquiries into the deaths of children since the 1970s have highlighted the need to improve inter-agency and inter-professional working in children's services in the UK. The Victoria Climbié inquiry, which heard evidence in 2002, revealed that a large number of agencies and professionals had contact with Victoria (doctors, social workers, police officers, a pastor, charity workers, childminders) (Larning, 2003). A breakdown in communication, lack of training, the pressure of high workloads, staffing shortages and no questioning of decisions led to a failure to acknowledge the abuse and arrange appropriate care.

So far this chapter has outlined the context for inter-professional and inter-agency working in terms of different influences, policy agendas and why organisations and managers collaborate. The rest of this chapter concerns the practical implications of collaborative working for managers and how they might anticipate and address the problems and challenges on a day-to-day basis and avoid people 'falling through the net'.

Key points

- Inter-agency and inter-professional working have a long history and have increasingly been adopted across all health and social care services.

- Partnership can be a 'catch-all' term.

- Different levels of collaboration may coexist.

- Inter-agency and inter-professional working improve the co-ordination of services and help to meet service users' needs.

6.3   The challenges of managing inter-professional and inter-agency working

There is much rhetoric about collaboration – from central government and from local agencies – but in reality it can be difficult and many people have experienced failed partnerships. More importantly, service users are often failed by a lack of communication. Experiences of the same initiative can be mixed: for example, statutory agencies may proclaim a particular inter-agency or inter-professional initiative a success but representatives from voluntary organisations, service users and carers may feel they have not played an equal role in it. This type of experience could make people wary of future proposals and unhappy about contributing time and effort if their views are deemed subordinate to those of other partners.

Although there are many examples of best practice and services where the philosophy of joint working is embedded, the government agenda has effectively made collaboration 'core business' across health and social care and something organisations and managers cannot ignore. The following quotation from a local authority policy officer captures this concern:

> I'm trying to persuade people that this partnership working isn't something that you do in addition to your day job. Partnership working becomes the way you do your day job.
>
> (Quoted in Charlesworth, 2002)

So how can managers ensure that collaboration produces successful outcomes and is inclusive and accountable? What factors contribute to the success or failure of cross-boundary working? In this section some of the main barriers to successful partnership working are outlined and some preliminary suggestions for overcoming them are explored. A focus on 'barriers' creates a rather negative tone to this section but it is important to understand more about the pitfalls so that they can be anticipated and, if possible, avoided. The following quotation sums up well the range of issues that affect joint working:

> new approaches need to be based on clarity about the roles, powers, and accountability requirements of stakeholders at all levels. They also require an understanding of the different expectations different players bring to the partnership and the factors that support or create barriers to partnership working at different stages in the process. This needs to include attention to the expectations and support needs of communities, front-line staff and service users, as well as managers and politicians. All this needs to be set in the context of the wider political agenda (for example, regionalisation, modernising local government, best value) and the demands of central government.
>
> (Balloch and Taylor, 2001, p. 7)

There is literature on why collaboration fails in research on public, voluntary and private sector organisations and, although there may be some sector- or service-specific factors, many of the issues raised are applicable to all types of collaboration. For example, similar issues occur whether the initiative is between a local authority and a voluntary organisation or between different multinational companies! This section focuses on the following barriers: developing partnership within a wider context of conflicting pressures and constraints; organisational and professional differences; power relationships; and lack of clarity about purpose and outcomes. Example 6.2 illustrates an initiative bringing together several different service providers in one location, where barriers to developing a truly integrated vision were still experienced.

EXAMPLE 6.2 Inter-agency working in children's services

Coram Community Campus at King's Cross in London brings together public and voluntary service providers co-ordinated by Coram Family, in order to integrate education, training and child care services. The initiative was intended to facilitate greater inter-professional and inter-agency working through the benefits of co-location, shared activities and resources, and developing a shared vision.

Collaboration has not proved as extensive as first envisaged for the following reasons:

- lack of opportunities for informal contact as no shared area for meetings
- lack of 'non-contact' time to reflect and plan
- staff and volunteers are too busy
- lack of communication about different organisations' plans and activities.

(Source: adapted from Wigfall and Moss, 2001)

Conflicting pressures and constraints

Successful joint working does not happen overnight, partly because collaboration is a lengthy and painstaking process even under ideal conditions, but largely because managers are operating within an environment of new structures and tight resource constraints. Consequently, acquiring change management skills takes priority in training new managers in care services! Managers say that the sheer pace of change and new legislation in the late 1990s has made their work particularly difficult and creates conflicting views on what, and how, to prioritise, as illustrated by a local authority policy officer:

> I suspect it would be fair to say that one of the major changes in what's happening is the amount of legislation around at the moment. While it's always emphasising partnership, in many ways it's been destructive because people are so focused on delivering the agendas which they have been told they must do by their own agencies, that it's kind of limiting some of the opportunities and choices and chances for partnership.
>
> (Quoted in Charlesworth, 2002)

The government is emphasising partnership but other elements of its modernisation agenda are putting pressure on successful collaboration and limiting the vision. An assistant chief executive for a local authority discusses these issues:

> So we've got this large government agenda and all these drivers on performance targets and they want to see outcomes, they want to see things that make a difference, but that is a really difficult, rigorous systematic process to go through when you're trying to engage partners. Traditionally, when we've done partnership working, we've looked for people to come together to begin to work through things and ideas begin to grow. Now the whole driver is a much more kind of disciplined approach from government. It's very difficult to put that across to people who might not have been involved at all in the subject.
>
> (Quoted in Charlesworth, 2002)

The limiting effects of these pressures can prove frustrating for service users, who hear the government rhetoric on partnership and want to see improvements to services, as a manager of a mental health service comments:

> I think what service users and carers are seeing is a willingness to change ... So I think the culture's right for change, but I also think users and carers get very frustrated with the pace of change. You know that at government level there's been a lot of talk about it happening, and it's just not quite translating down yet on the ground: we're still at the talking stage.
>
> (Manager consultations)

Even where organisations manage to embark on partnership, coping with new and changing organisational and team structures can be both exciting and frightening at the same time. Nurses and social workers discussing their experiences of an integrated trust illustrate this challenge:

> It's been sort of moving forward in the dark together, trying to work out which bits we can look to [my manager] for, and which bits we can't, and how we're going to invent structures which haven't really been invented yet to support nurses into the future.

> As opposed to being directed by either central government, Department of Health, county council policy or NHS policy, I guess we are on the cutting edge of change. But sometimes it feels like you're a crew member on a fairly large ship, which takes a little while to change direction and you just get that sneaking suspicion through the gloom that you can see the coastline. And you think, 'Well, I hope somebody's on the bridge, and I do hope somebody's got hold of the wheel, and they're about to turn this thing around.'
>
> (Manager consultations)

Despite a degree of uncertainty, they also appreciate the advantages of their new organisation and feel optimistic about staff working together to overcome difficulties:

> The joint working we get now is just superb ... It used to be so difficult to get messages to people, and there's so many things you just wouldn't bother to say to people. Whereas now, you catch their eye while you're writing up your notes, and you just start having these sort of conversations.

> I think my manager's really crucial to making the team work effectively ... We have regular community team meetings and through those we've developed that sense of team identity and support.
>
> (Manager consultations)

Freeth (2001) highlights the 'mundane' barriers such as location and timing of meetings, multiple reporting structures and requirements, and even finding suitable accommodation for teams. Lack of communication is frequently a complaint: when managers are busy and teams short-staffed, they may forget to communicate information more widely and network with new contacts. Staff may also resist performing duties they perceive as additional work when they are already feeling stretched. When several different professionals and agencies are involved in a person's care, neglecting to check that others are aware of problems or developments can, of course, have serious consequences, as shown by the Victoria Climbié inquiry (Larning, 2003). Thus, it appears that a combination of external and internal factors is potentially creating barriers to forming new collaborations or sustaining existing ones.

Organisational and professional difference

People bring different backgrounds, experiences and traditions of working to inter-agency and inter-professional working. There is often talk of the strong cultural differences between organisations, such as between health authorities and local government, many of which arise from their different management structures and the presence of electoral politics in local government. This may be less of a problem at frontline manager level but there are usually variations in the degree of autonomy that local authority managers have compared with health authority managers. Some managers may not be empowered to make decisions or commit resources at the time of a meeting, which can delay moving forward and spoil the momentum of enthusiastic joint working. It may also be disconcerting when decisions agreed in inter-agency groups have to be ratified in, or may be thrown out of, local authority committee meetings.

In an integrated organisation, differences between organisations and professionals may be amplified. For example, in England, primary care groups and trusts have had to deal with bringing together a range of professional groupings, all with different pay and conditions, employment status, experience of line management structures, and ways of working. This may lead to tensions between staff, which managers need to resolve, but the differences could also foster feelings of loss of identity. In an integrated organisation where traditional roles and responsibilities become blurred or posts are funded by different organisations, workers may question their new role. 'Which organisation do I belong to?' 'Will staff with different professional backgrounds accept my role?' 'Do I still feel affiliated to my national professional body?' These are illustrated by extracts from an interview with Anita, the new manager of a mental health team you met in Chapters 3 and 4 (see Example 6.3). Anita is frustrated that her team do not see the advantages of her health and social care background, and it actually seems to hinder the team's development.

EXAMPLE 6.3 Anita: nurse or social worker?

I think one of the main dilemmas in the job is, I don't actually feel I belong to anybody. At this moment in time I'm not sure who's actually employing me. I think it's a health post, paid for through social services.

I'm an SRN and, having a social work qualification, I thought I'd be more acceptable to the team because I've had experience of working within both systems. I think what I found more than anything is distrust by both. Social workers see me sort of align myself more towards health, which I think probably is true unfortunately. And I don't know quite how to get round that. [Nursing staff say] social workers don't understand this, this is nothing like social services. And I think trying to explain to them that, you know, I've never worked in a traditional social work setting, I've always worked in a

> multidisciplinary team ... I almost feel that in order to help them integrate
> I've really got to prove myself on both fronts.
>
> (Source: manager consultations)

Staff are often concerned about threats to their professional identity and
whether their jobs and roles will be merged. In the next quotation a nurse
from an integrated trust talks about her initial reservations about whether
nurses and social workers working more closely together would mean
people losing their jobs or identities. In fact, closer working appears to
have strengthened their understanding of each other and led to a
heightened defence of their different professional identities:

> there was an understanding of social workers and community nurses
> doing very similar jobs and they could be knocked together ... I think
> that what's happened is that we've become much more understanding of
> each other's role. We have been able to stand together with the social
> workers and defend our role, so the difference between social work and
> nursing has become amplified and more clear.
>
> (Manager consultations)

This is corroborated by another manager, who perceives that closer joint
working will lead to a better understanding of roles and benefits to
service users:

> I think what we're talking about is maintaining professional
> identity. I think people who are from the social care background need
> to advocate for what they believe in, that they believe social care can
> effect change in people, and I believe people from a health care
> background need to do the same. Now the issue is, why are we putting
> these people together? We're not doing it for the workers, we're doing it
> for the service users. They don't want to have two assessments, they
> don't want to have two organisations at each other's throats ... it's [also]
> about respecting the difference, but in a way where we work together,
> instead of competing against each other.
>
> (Manager consultations)

Where staff are resistant to inter-professional working, there may be
difficulties in getting them to take on work formerly allocated to different
professionals. This can hinder the development of a team identity, as
Example 6.4 shows.

EXAMPLE 6.4 Anita: more divided than unified?

[There's no] sense of team responsibility. Nobody will sort of take on board
tasks for the sake of the team ... Everybody is too busy fighting over whether
[a referral] should be a nurse or a social worker or it's not for us. Nobody will
actually look into it. Nobody'll actually take it that one step further. Nobody
will take responsibility for almost developing a unified response.

(Source: manager consultations)

Although Anita was the team manager, she would have liked all the team members to participate in workload decisions. A general resistance to change seems to be part of the problem here too. Perceived threats to professional identity can also lead to concerns about the status and power of certain professional groups. Anita describes her problems with a colleague who was obstructive in meetings and refused to accept her authority as a manager:

> [The consultant] said 'Well, we were fine before you came ... we worked together perfectly well as a team. Why are you interfering? I used to be able to do what I wanted before you came.'
>
> (Manager consultations)

Differences between organisations and professionals potentially create communication problems, particularly through the use of different jargon, which can be confusing enough for professionals and managers in statutory service but may be completely bewildering for service users and voluntary organisation representatives. It makes them feel excluded from discussions. As a manager of a council of voluntary service explained:

> Small voluntary organisations ... suddenly find themselves in a discussion group with people in statutory authorities who are well-versed in talking about need and care and health issues but they have their own language which is not quite the same as the everyday language that the rest of us use.
>
> (Quoted in Charlesworth, 2002)

Therefore, managers seeking wider representation in inter-agency groups need to make language more accessible in order to reduce concerns about power imbalance. The interviewee above suggested that training days to help service users and volunteers express themselves and gain confidence in inter-agency meetings would be helpful (as would sessions to train statutory authority staff to listen).

Power relationships

Power relationships cut across all aspects of inter-agency and inter-professional working. There is a paradox, however: they are the reason why partnership working takes place – to make the planning of services more inclusive and accountable by reducing power imbalances between agencies and with service users – but if the imbalances persist, partnership can fail.

What are the sources of power imbalance? The following extract, concerning regeneration partnerships, considers this issue in organisational terms:

> power imbalances apply to the relations between partners – from the public, private, voluntary and community sectors. However, they can also apply to relations within the sectors engaged in partnerships –

between one grouping within a community and another, between
representatives and those they are supposed to be representing, between
majority groups and minority interests, between those with the most
extensive networks and those with the least extensive.

(Mayo and Taylor, 2001, p. 40)

The discussion above on professional difference also started to explore
issues of power, illustrating different status, pay and conditions among
professionals, and how threats to them may engender conflict. This can
create difficulties when trying to encourage new occupational groups
(such as practice nurses) to take an enhanced role in management
structures or to take on new responsibilities. Furthermore, gender, class,
ethnicity and disability cut across power relationships and affect different
people's capacity to participate fully in policy making.

Lukes (1974) provides one of the most frequently cited discussions of
power. His concept of 'non-decision making', whereby issues are kept off
the agenda, is applied by Mayo and Taylor (2001) to partnership. They
suggest that powerful partners (government departments, private sector
organisations) influence outcomes through setting agendas and deciding
what is, and what is not, going to be discussed.

For partnership to work, all parties need to feel they have an equal voice
and be able and willing to share power. Representatives from voluntary
organisations and service user groups often express concern that they do
not have the same position in the collaboration because they do not have
financial power and they feel their position is 'tokenistic' (Gaster et al.,
1999). In fact, voluntary organisations do have a source of power because
they are needed by statutory agencies for their views and contact with
service users. If the purpose of partnership is to empower groups outside
the statutory agencies to provide better services, managers need to be
aware of power structures and imbalances and find appropriate ways of
overcoming them.

Agendas, objectives and outcomes

As Huxham (1996a) reports, the very nature of collaboration means
organisations have different aims, objectives and reasons for being
involved in working with others. This is also the source of strength of
the interaction. Huxham further suggests that there are two types of goal:
first, *meta-goals*, which are goals for the collaboration and the reason why
it exists. However, there is an inherent contradiction with setting these
goals: they need to be explicit but the more rigid they are, the less likely
organisations are to sign up to them. Second, there are *organisation-specific
goals*, which each of the organisations wants to achieve through the
collaboration but are separate from the collaboration, such as raising their
own organisation's profile (Huxham, 1996a). Both types of goal may need
to be addressed in order to achieve a successful partnership. However, the

presence of different aims and objectives can also create difficulties in building trust. Relating back to the issue of power, are people being open about their agendas?

When people embark on cross-boundary working without a clear idea of what they want to achieve, the literature suggests it is doomed to fail (Huxham, 1996a). People are often too busy to attend meetings and commit resources to a new initiative that lacks a clear focus.

Degrees of commitment to partnership also vary. The lower the commitment, the less likely the organisation is to endorse aims that involve contributing substantial resources (Huxham, 2000). In the following extract, a local authority officer discusses this dilemma:

> Police, the council, probation and health had to co-operate because under the Crime and Disorder Act we had to set up this Youth Offending Team and I can remember being involved in the early discussions and we were all saying, 'Don't we get on well together? We're talking about this, it's great, we want to do a pilot.' And then it came to the point where we had to discuss resources, you know, how many staff probation, police and the council actually part with, how much money they part with ... This is the point where the threat came in. It's all very well when it was on the cerebral level but when it went down into the pockets, it became a little more painful!
>
> (Quoted in Charlesworth, 2002)

There are no easy answers to reconciling conflicting views. Learning from experience and examples of good practice from others can help.

Key points

- External and internal pressures squeeze the time and resources for developing new cross-boundary relationships.

- Joint working involves substantial change, which may be perceived as either welcome or a threat.

- Organisational and professional differences take time to work through.

- Joint working can raise concerns about professional identities.

- Being clear about agendas and what different people hope to achieve from collaboration should help success rates.

6.4   Developing skills for partnership

The previous sections outlined the dilemmas and barriers faced by managers when working across boundaries. You may be wondering at this point whether they are insurmountable. They are certainly very challenging and some of the examples in this chapter illustrate that even the most accomplished and experienced managers are still frustrated in their attempts to improve joint working. Banks discusses the variety of tasks and responsibilities required of managers to undertake cross-boundary working:

> [middle managers] are often expected to undertake both the 'day' job and the role of change management, as well as cope with shared loyalties to two different organisations. Most middle managers are given little backing, training or time to work with new partnerships, and tackle conceptual and practical problems. These will include major headaches around negotiating pay and work conditions, resolving professional issues and arranging accountable joint budgets and joint information systems. Much of their work goes unrecognised as performance measures are largely aligned to traditional roles, not just those within partnerships, and there are few explicit rewards for partnership working.
>
> (Banks, 2002, p. 10)

This focuses on middle managers and is a rather pessimistic view but it does illustrate some of the difficulties. Managers need to be constantly aware of what might be causing a barrier or resistance. What are the cultural differences between different organisations and care workers? Why do they persist? Why are there power imbalances and how can managers ensure accountability, representativeness and cultural change?

Many of the skills required to tackle the barriers are generic management skills and qualities developed by professionals within a care context. In this section we look at the skills and knowledge needed for inter-agency and inter-professional working. First, a broader view of partnership is taken with some suggestions for embarking on partnership. Then there are some solutions to help with a manager's day-to-day work.

Readiness for partnership

How does a manager know when developing a new partnership is appropriate and viable? The discussion in Section 6.3 highlighted the problems of internal and external factors affecting the ability to collaborate. Consequently, many organisations attempt to streamline their involvement in partnerships to make better use of resources.

Researchers at the Institute for Applied Health and Social Policy at King's College London developed a 'partnership readiness framework'. This includes nine key characteristics for effective partnership against which organisations can assess themselves in deciding whether to pursue commissioning partnerships (see Box 6.3). The researchers used it in their study of an integrated health and social care trust in Somerset and found that the organisations had a 'complete alignment of apparently positive factors' (Peck *et al.*, 2002, p. 32).

BOX 6.3 The partnership readiness framework

1 Building and agreeing shared values and principles with a vision of how life should be for people who use services, likely to involve seamless care with a single point of access and the integration of key services.

2 Agreeing specific policy shifts that the partnership arrangements are designed to achieve, supported by the development of single operational policies.

3 Being prepared to explore new service options and not be overly tied to existing services or providers.

4 Being clear about what aspects of service and activity are inside and outside the boundaries of the partnership arrangements, so that there is a focus on the real added value of joint working.

5 Being clear about organisational roles in terms of responsibilities for and relationships between commissioning, purchasing and providing in order to derive a coherency that draws upon all appropriate expertise and ensures that any tension in the system is creative, including clear financial arrangements.

6 Identifying agreed resource pools, including pooled budgets, and agreeing to put to one side unresolvable historical disagreements about financial responsibility.

7 Ensuring effective leadership, including political and other senior level commitment to the partnership agenda.

8 Providing sufficient dedicated partnership development capacity rather than it being a small and marginalised part of everyone's role.

9 Developing and sustaining good personal relationships, creating opportunities and incentives for key players to nurture those relationships in order to promote mutual trust.

(Source: Peck *et al.*, 2002, p. 33)

In a similar vein, Example 6.5 and Box 6.4 (overleaf) illustrate how Milton Keynes Council gathered detailed information about its participation in strategic-level partnerships. Local politicians had expressed concerns about how many they were involved in and their 'value' to the council. Local authorities are required to carry out several Best Value reviews every year, and one of them needs to be 'cross-cutting', so the Council decided to integrate the need for up-to-date information with their Best Value review. Examples of strategic-level partnerships include steering groups concerned with health, the environment, crime and community safety, the local economy, education and drugs action teams. 'Local strategic partnerships' co-ordinate different public, voluntary, private and community groups at neighbourhood level and, ultimately, streamline the number of separate partnerships in a locality.

EXAMPLE 6.5 Milton Keynes Council's research on partnership

Main concerns

1 To identify what strategic partnerships the Council was involved with; their terms of reference; their measurable outcomes; their reporting arrangements; and the level of resources the Council devoted to each partnership.

2 To develop an evaluative mechanism for partnership working at a strategic level.

3 To use the evaluative mechanism to enable the Council to monitor its involvement in strategic partnerships.

Methods

The research involved questionnaires, interviews and meetings with representatives from the partnerships, local authority, voluntary organisations, community groups, other public sector organisations, the private sector and local authorities outside the area. Information was sought on four key partnerships in health, lifelong learning, the environment, and crime and community safety, as well as best practice in other localities and nationally.

Main findings

1 A long list of all their partnerships. Eventually a clearer idea emerged of the extent of the involvement and a firmer understanding of what strategic partnerships are.

2 There was no policy on the formation of partnerships and no monitoring procedures existed to review progress and effectiveness.

3 There were no formal mechanisms for feeding information from individual partnerships back to Council committees.

Main recommendations

1 To set up a database for information on all strategic-level partnerships (aims and objectives, representatives, etc.) and to review annually.

2 To develop adequate methods of monitoring partnerships and assess their value to the Council.

3 To apply the *Guide to Effective Partnerships* (Milton Keynes Council, 2000).

(Source: adapted from Milton Keynes Council, 2001)

The draft guide to effective partnerships includes lists of questions which organisations could use at different stages of the partnership, such as before starting a partnership, once it gets going, reviewing success, and ending a partnership. Box 6.4 illustrates the first stage. The guide covers a range of topics, such as aims and objectives, purpose, models of partnership, leadership, decision making, building trust and measuring progress. Other organisations appear to have found the guide useful. A local umbrella group for voluntary organisations used it to prioritise their involvement in partnership and make the best use of limited resources.

BOX 6.4 Questions to ask before going into partnership

Legal requirement

- Is there a statutory requirement to establish the partnership?

Clarity of purpose

- Is there a clear and shared vision of what the partnership wants to achieve?

- Is it clear what each partner organisation is trying to achieve?

- Do the prospective partners recognise and respect the objectives of individual partners?

Commitment

- Do all (prospective) partners have the backing of their parent organisation?

- Are the partners willing to commit the necessary time and resources to make the partnership work?

Accountability

- Will the partnership have clear decision-making processes?

- Can differences of opinion be resolved?

- Will the partnership have clear reporting procedures to each parent organisation?

Realism

- Is working in partnership really the most effective way of achieving your key objectives?

- Are the partnership's objectives consistent with those of the parent organisations?

- Will the partnership achieve the most cost-effective outcome?

(Source: Milton Keynes Council, 2000, p. 7)

Although this example focuses on strategic-level partnerships, which usually involve senior managers, the issues raised can affect frontline managers in several ways. First, an awareness of how the organisation fits into a wider picture of partnership illustrates organisational commitment to working across boundaries and gives an indication of vision and strategy for developing and improving services. New working relationships established at senior level may permeate down to other levels and provide new opportunities for inter-agency and inter-professional working and an enhanced role for service users. Second, it is useful to ask questions of any new or existing collaboration along the lines suggested by Milton Keynes Council's guide or the partnership readiness framework. It may be excessive to go through all these questions when collaborating with one other person in a small area of work but being clear about purpose, accountability and monitoring should help the chances of success.

Skills, expertise and knowledge

Statham (2000) reports that training programmes for health and social care workers have not traditionally focused on the development of skills for partnership. She suggests that the protection of professional identity has been considered paramount in career progression and that working at the boundaries of health and social care was considered 'risky' or even 'deviant'.

However, skills and experience in inter-agency working are gradually assuming greater importance. Example 6.6 describes an inter-professional initiative which aimed to improve inter-professional training and encourage greater networking and prospects for future collaboration.

EXAMPLE 6.6 Inter-professional skills training

The Clinical Skills Centre at St Bartholomew's Hospital in London established a joint training programme in clinical skills for nursing and medical staff. Despite changes in nursing and medical education, mergers of the Schools involved and loss of original team members, the Centre has reported success in producing relevant courses for nurses and doctors, based on 'improving participants' ability to integrate theoretical knowledge, practical experience and expertise from different professions, to plan and deliver high quality, efficient patient-centred care'.

Participants' evaluation of the course highlighted: increased understanding of the roles, responsibilities and needs of different members of the multidisciplinary team; and increased motivation to collaborate in their future professional practice. The Centre's staff reported greater collaboration in each other's working groups and committees.

(Source: adapted from Freeth, 2001, pp. 41–3)

What kinds of skills, expertise and knowledge are required? In the following extract, a senior local authority manager discusses his requirements when recruiting new partnership managers:

> [We] want people with good analytical skills ... You need skills in dealing with the community, speaking the same language, because they have a different set of languages to the professionals, and then you need skills of diplomacy, negotiation, empathy with partners, being able to look at the broad horizon and short-term project management ... But the interpersonal skills are probably the most important because you get people who in an organisation progress from being a professional to being a manager ... If you're constructive and positive and you recognise that you have a personal relationship, they're much more likely to help you and be someone you can call on if things go wrong, or if you upset them, they'll probably be prepared to live with it ... Command and control might deliver a project by pushing people to get things done by a certain date but it's probably [more] the ability to be able to use a menu of different skills on appropriate occasions.
>
> (Quoted in Charlesworth, 2002)

This seems quite an ambitious list but many managers already have such skills and attributes. Obviously, not all people involved in partnerships are managers: service users, volunteers and elected members often take leading roles in collaboration. Arranging a joint training programme, however brief, for partnership representatives is often useful in terms of learning new skills and networking with other participants during the training. Valuable skills and attributes include: being able to communicate and use appropriate language; negotiation; listening; empathy with partners; understanding and respecting difference. Ways of 'learning' these skills vary and often team members find it useful to learn together and, in the process, build a team identity, as illustrated by the following extracts. A manager involved in a Surestart initiative, working with children, commented:

> Everybody's ideas of team meetings were different. Some had never had team meetings and that was really quite difficult at first because some people didn't think you had to come ... and I think it was very difficult because you just made assumptions from what you'd done yourself and so we actually very early on sat down and wrote our own ground rules. And they've been really useful 'cos we're now sort of like two years on and we still refer back to them sometimes.
>
> (Manager consultations)

People needing to work together at a practice level used the same model of working out the rules to prepare themselves:

> When we had two people working together, they actually set themselves a co-working contract ... how they were going to deal with things, what skills they were both bringing, what their styles were, and what

would annoy them, and then at the end of each group session they would actually talk about that ... they talked very honestly about it and they got so much out of it and, at the end of it, they visibly had increased their confidence.

(Manager consultations)

Other suggestions from managers include asking team members to give brief talks about their organisations and their responsibilities. This could form part of each major meeting, as a policy team manager describes:

[The director talked] about what it meant to work in local government ... he gave them some very basic information ... They hadn't the first idea that that was how we operated and ... I was part of a selection team at the health authority ... and somehow that same conversation came up and they said: 'We would really like you to come over and do that for us as well.'

(Quoted in Charlesworth, 2002)

Extending this to 'away days' can also be useful in terms of encouraging people to learn more about each other and their expectations for the collaboration. Inviting people to meetings and training programmes is useful but time needs to be recompensed in some way and/or expenses reimbursed. Voluntary and community groups and users and carers often have limited resources. As one voluntary organisation director explains:

It's as if [the statutory authorities have] said to themselves, 'Hello voluntary sector, you're here, how nice to meet you!' With that acknowledgement has come all this extra work – we're delighted to be recognised – but it's come with no funding to achieve it and voluntary organisations based on volunteers are cheap and very economical and value-based organisations but they're not free because, somewhere along the line, somebody has to organise the volunteers, someone has to pay for the postage, and somebody has to pay for the phone calls, premises and the mileage of the volunteers and out-of-pocket expenses.

(Quoted in Charlesworth, 2002)

In addition to thinking about ways of improving communication and team building, attention is also needed to issues of leadership and trust, particularly for teams with strong differences in organisational and professional cultures and potential sources of conflict. Therefore, the situational leadership model (see Chapter 3), where the direction and support of a team might be adjusted once the manager has got to know the team, could be appropriate in a partnership setting. Leadership and vision are required in order to keep a strong focus on the aims and objectives of the partnership. One aspect of skill in leadership is to encourage the leadership of others. This is important in a multi-agency environment, where people outside statutory agencies should be encouraged to chair meetings.

The ability to build trust is crucial in achieving successful collaboration but it is extremely difficult, particularly where there is no history of partnership working or there is a legacy of poor relations (Huxham and Vangen, 2000). Stereotypes of other professionals may get in the way, as will unrealistic expectations of what each partner can contribute. Building trust is a reinforcing process in that it is needed at the beginning of collaborations to establish good working relationships, but successful outcomes are also required so that the trust is developed further and collaboration advanced (Hudson *et al.*, 2003). Of course, it is also a two-way process: you need to trust others and they need to trust you (Loxley, 1997). In addition, there needs to be inter-organisational trust (and internal organisational cultures receptive to partnership), so that when key individuals leave, the collaboration does not fall apart (Ferlie and Pettigrew, 1996).

As you have seen in the examples of managers' experiences in this chapter, some people find inter-agency and inter-professional working potentially threatening, particularly those who fear change. Skills in managing change are useful attributes in this context. Rogers and Reynolds (in Chapter 4) outline points to consider when planning a change: for example, involving people, gathering information, clarifying aims, setting targets and selling the change. Managing change is likely to be an ongoing process and it is important to remember to communicate information to team members and enable others to discuss their concerns.

Key points

- Inter-agency and inter-professional working draw on a variety of skills and knowledge.

- It is important to be clear about the purpose of partnership and why you and your organisation are involved.

- Joint training programmes, 'away days' and informal meetings can aid team building and increase the confidence of people without formal management training.

- Skills in leadership, building trust and managing change are required at different stages of the partnership process.

6.5 Conclusion

All frontline managers can probably expect to be involved in cross-boundary working and this chapter illustrated some of the problems that might be encountered during the process. It also highlighted the reasons why this way of working is considered so important. First, a lack of communication and co-ordination between agencies has serious implications for quality care. Second, different agencies can play a role in planning and delivering services and, finally, improved care services result from true partnership between providers and service users.

The examples from managers' experiences show how initial concerns about threats to jobs and professional identities have often proved ill-founded. Managers can help ease the process but, as the examples in this chapter suggest, sometimes even the most experienced managers can face resistance from their team members. This is perhaps a reminder that inter-agency and inter-professional working can be slow and can draw on a variety of management skills (and considerable patience).

It is not helpful to be prescriptive about having partnership at all levels and in all care contexts. Learning from your own and others' experiences – both negative and positive – is more effective. Looking at these examples should raise some questions, such as how would you do things differently? How would you translate an example of a successful collaboration to your own team or organisation? What kind of improvements can service users and carers expect? How can your manager aid communication and co-ordination? Reflection on experience in practice can help in developing a practice-led approach to working across agency and professional boundaries. Inter-agency working happens at different levels and there is much scope for 'bottom-up' initiatives on partnership. This is where frontline managers have a key role to play, particularly in involving service users.

Chapter 7
Managing budgets and giving best value

Les Gallop

7.1   Introduction

> I wouldn't mind so much, but I came into social work partly because it
> didn't need a lot of maths. Maths was never my strong subject. Now
> what they really want is an accountant.

These are the words of a team manager in a statutory social care setting in
the early 1990s, required by new legislation to manage a budget with
several noughts at the end. Until then, she had only really had to worry
about the team coffee fund and checking expense claims.

These words somehow capture much of the role change that first-time
managers experience. The move into frontline management, often made
over a weekend ('On Friday I was a worker, now on Monday I'm called a
manager') can feel like a move from the comfort zone of recognised
competence to an unknown world of new problems and new skills.
Responsibility for budgets is prominent in the anxieties associated with
moving into management. Money is, after all, such a symbol in our
society. In the words of a popular song, it is 'the root of all evil'; according
to Bob Dylan (1961) in another song, 'Money doesn't talk, it swears'.
In this chapter I try to analyse these anxieties about financial management.
I look at the bigger picture first in order to set the context, and then seek
to establish some key principles and consider some practical approaches.

Four main sources inform this chapter. First, my own experiences as a
manager trying to manage budgets inevitably influence my thinking,
particularly where the activities involved in attempting to understand
variations are discussed. Memories of poring over budget statements with
colleagues are vivid, wondering how our own records could be at such
variance from the 'official' version before us. Second, some texts on
budgeting and financial management are used. These are useful in
providing a guide through some of the technical parts and making links
with other management processes. Third, I draw on conversations with
former colleagues about their struggles with budgets. Fourth, I decided to
talk with current managers about budget management to gain different
perspectives on the process: a senior manager (Sandy); a manager of a
residential unit for older people (Sally); a voluntary sector manager
(Angela); a financial specialist (Brian); and a manager whose team
commissions individual care packages (Pradeep). This helped me to gain
an understanding of the 'realities' of budgets and different ways of looking
at them.

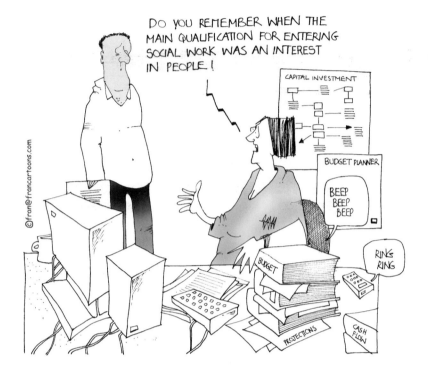

The changing context

The personal change of moving into a management position involves
questions about self-concept, as the new manager begins to develop new
relationships at work (see Chapter 1). Besides this re-evaluation of who
they are and the need to redefine working relationships, there is a related
question: 'What, in this new role, am I paid to worry about?' In other
words: 'What will sit on my desk as something new that I am responsible
for?' The manager quoted at the beginning of this chapter identified a
common new worry: money. Life has not always been like this for
frontline managers. Before the 1980s most care organisations gave
financial and resource responsibility to central sections and more senior
managers; frontline managers had very limited financial responsibilities.
Several factors combined to create the current climate of more active and
obvious frontline management:

- across employment sectors, the belief that organisations perform better
  when decision making is devolved as far down the hierarchy as possible
- increasing criticisms of the public sector as too bureaucratic, with
  decision making too slow and removed from delivery
- a general move away from highly centralised structures
- a government-led initiative to create greater diligence over public
  spending

- a continuing need for those in the private sector to reduce costs in the face of increasing competition
- the introduction of the duty on local authorities to secure Best Value (Local Government Act 1999).

The atmosphere of management at all levels has changed in response to these pressures. Now, frontline managers need to be skilful in demonstrating to levels above them that they are 'managers', and to their teams that they are in touch with the world of practice. Such emotional and intellectual balance in a turbulent world can be as demanding as physical balance is on a tightrope. In the next section I consider the origins and nature of Best Value before looking at its implications for budget and resource management.

The aims of this chapter are to:

- consider Best Value and understand its impact on the practice of management
- identify the main funding mechanisms and resources available to an agency and how to mobilise them
- discuss how to manage an agency budget
- outline some key issues for the development of services.

7.2 Best Value

Old wine in new bottles?

Although the term 'best value' exists in general English usage, here the legal sense, as in the Local Government Act 1999, is used. This different usage is probably somewhat confusing for many service users and other citizens. There are, however, some overlaps between the general and the legal sense of the term. The government's stated intention – to create a clearer public sector commitment to good-quality services – is a sentiment with which few users of services will disagree. In the words of a government circular on Best Value:

> the central purpose of best value – to make a real and positive difference to the services which local people receive from their authority.
>
> (DETR, 1999, p. 4)

Best Value was first discussed in the years leading up to the General Election in 1997 as part of the Labour Party's manifesto. It was to be a way of ending the Compulsory Competitive Tendering regime established by the Conservative government (and in part supported by the then Labour opposition) through the Local Government Planning and Land Act 1980. Compulsory Competitive Tendering was part of a larger government agenda, concerned with introducing competition into the public sector, and based on the beliefs that (a) the existing public sector was inefficient and (b) the market was the most effective regulator of service cost and quality. Best Value differs from Compulsory Competitive Tendering in the following important ways.

- The government specified which services should be subject to Compulsory Competitive Tendering: for example, cleaning and catering. Best Value is about all services provided or commissioned by local authorities. Under Best Value requirements, local authorities set targets for their local education authorities for aspects of school performance. York City Council's improvement targets for 2001–2 are set out in Table 7.1. This is just one example of the way councils are using indicators to measure what they have achieved and what they plan to achieve in the future.
- Compulsory Competitive Tendering required the specified services to be put out to competitive tender. There is no compulsion in Best Value, although it can be required in circumstances where local authorities are judged to be failing to ensure Best Value in any service.

In Table 7.1 the first two columns are what the council has achieved so far. The percentage improvements in the third column are targets for the next year 2001–2. Note that the council improved on most but not all indicators in 2000–1. The figures give a useful picture of where the improvements have been made, and what remains to be achieved.

Table 7.1   **York City Council Education Best Value Plan, 2001–2 (extract)**

Our performance	*1999/ 2000 (%)*	*2000/ 2001 (%)*	*Improvement target (%)*
The percentage of primary school classes with more than 30 pupils in reception to year two inclusive	2.6	**0**	0
The percentage of primary school classes with more than 30 pupils in years three to six inclusive	31.2	**37.5**	30
Percentage of three-year-olds with access to a good-quality, free early-years education programme	50	**71.3**	80
Proportion of pupils getting five or more GCSEs at grades A* to C	51.5	**52.6**	60
Proportion of 11-year-olds achieving level 4 or above at Key Stage 2 (English)	75.5	**73.9**	76
Proportion of 11-year-olds achieving level 4 or above at Key Stage 2 (Mathematics)	73.9	**78**	79

(Source: York City Council, 2001)

Devolved government means that the implementation of Best Value will vary between the UK countries but the key principles are the same. Best Value was at first restricted to local authorities. The NHS Plan (Department of Health, 2000a, para. 6.19), however, extends this to health bodies, and signals a commitment to joint health and social services Best Value reviews. Therefore, managers in all employment sectors in the four countries are affected by Best Value because both local authorities and health authorities must apply the principles when commissioning and when providing services. The reasoning behind this seems to move beyond the 'Which sector is best?' debate of the 1980s and 1990s to decisions in particular situations about the best value for money. It is in this sense part of the Labour government's 'third way' and a confirmation of the notion of the mixed economy of social care provision.

All managers, whether in the private, voluntary or statutory sector, need to know the rationale behind Best Value and its demands on them and their colleagues. Managers who can be active at a local level have an advantage over those who cannot. A day centre manager, for example, can consistently seek service user feedback and respond to this, rather than waiting for a Best Value review officer to come along. If managers are responsible for commissioning care packages, they clearly have a duty to both service users and the wider community to seek Best Value. Best Value is not a wholly new idea. As with all public policy initiatives, it exists within a particular set of ideologies and understandings, and builds on them, albeit with some new interpretations. Probably most significant in the recent history of the public sector are the 'three Es', established by the Audit Commission in the mid-1980s as a framework for monitoring and evaluating public sector performance (Audit Commission, 1984).

The three Es concern the cost and quality of services, although it could be argued that the way they were applied was mostly to do with cost. It is common knowledge that it is easier to work out the cost of most things than to work out their quality. Oscar Wilde (1892) wrote disparagingly of this tendency: cynics, to him, were people who 'know the price of everything and the value of nothing.'

The three Es are:

- *Economy* – delivery at an agreed level of quality at the lowest possible cost. This requires organisations and their managers to watch costs. They must ask themselves, 'Are we spending more than we need to?'
- *Efficiency* – a measure of the level of outputs from any given level of inputs. It is therefore about spending well. Managers need to ask, 'Are we getting as much as we can reasonably expect from our resources?'
- *Effectiveness* – evaluating how actual and intended results relate to each other. Questions to ask are, 'Are our services achieving our policy objectives? What impact are we having? Are we spending wisely?'

The Best Value process

With the introduction of the duty of Best Value, these considerations remain at the heart of government thinking about all public services. The modernisation agenda, signalled in the White Paper *Modern Local Government – In Touch with the Peopl*e (DETR, 1998), integrates them into the broader Best Value Performance Assessment Framework. The five broad areas for making judgements about local authority performance are:

1 national priorities and strategic objectives (the extent to which it is delivering the government's priorities for social care)
2 cost and efficiency
3 effectiveness of service delivery and outcomes
4 quality of services for users and carers
5 fair access.

Points 2 and 3 are the three Es, and point 4 reflects the government's drive for quality to be defined in relation to users' experiences. Point 5 is new and interesting in that it responds to criticisms that the Audit Commission criteria should have included a fourth E – *equity*.

Alongside this increased emphasis on internally driven review against a national framework, inspection is a further vehicle for central government to maintain understanding of, and control over, public sector services. It comes in various forms from government bodies such as the Social Services Inspectorate and the Audit Commission. Inspections are usually made against a set of standards. With the mixed economy of care now so firmly established, such inspections include the performance of statutory organisations in working with the private and voluntary sectors. Best Value is, in essence, a cyclical process covering a series of steps that looks very similar to many descriptions of the strategic management process (see Figure 7.1 opposite). Best Value requires this cyclical process of thinking.

Rogers (1999, p. 54) suggests it is 'the most holistic way yet developed for local authorities to develop their approaches to performance and quality management in a way which may involve creating a more participative form of local democracy'. At the broad, strategic level (planning), local authorities must have Best Value performance plans. These make explicit their aims and objectives, state how they will evaluate performance (mainly through the development and use of performance indicators), and identify plans for reviews of all services over a five-year period. Each review needs to consider the 'four Cs' (see Box 7.1).

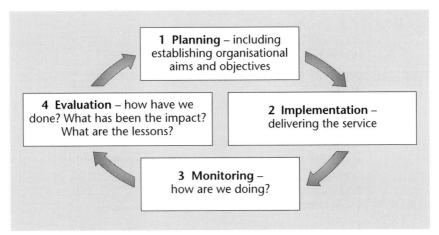

Figure 7.1   **Cyclical process for Best Value**

BOX 7.1 The four Cs

Challenge why and how the service is being provided.

Key questions:

- Is this service needed?

- If so, in this form?

Compare with the performance of others across a range of relevant indicators, taking into account the views of both service users and potential suppliers. At this stage benchmarking is an expectation; this involves comparison with organisations perceived to be in the top 25% of performers.

Key question:

- How well is the service doing relatively?

Consult with local taxpayers, service users, partners and the wider business community in setting new performance targets.

Key questions:

- What do important people think and feel about this service?

- What can we learn from them?

Competition is to be embraced as a means of securing efficient and effective services.

Key questions:

- Is it appropriate to seek other providers?

- Would a change of provider give better value for money?

(Source: adapted from DETR, 1998)

A fifth C is then anticipated: *continuous improvement*. What have we learned in the review that will enable us to improve this service?

The complexity of Best Value

On paper Best Value looks logical enough. Few people would argue with the idea of ensuring that services are needed, that they are delivered to a good standard and that managers should be cost-conscious. The idea of continuous improvement is woven into most contemporary approaches to organisational life. To rest on your laurels risks becoming yesterday's success story. However, agreeing on Best Value in practice is likely to be more complex than any model can represent.

Think about the activity of planning a holiday. You probably do not question the reason for taking a holiday: it would not prove difficult for busy managers to justify it! You might check the prices and offers of rival travel companies and consider your attitude towards them. Were they helpful in the past? Have friends used them and, if so, what did they make of them? Reputation is an elusive but important part of people's attitudes towards travel companies. At this stage your judgements are already becoming multidimensional. Cost is a factor, but the thought of a holiday that is cheap but unsatisfactory is unappealing. Such judgements increase in complexity when you consider holidays for a group. The classic example for people with children is the experience of negotiating the venue and type of holiday with them as they grow up. Quality for some parents (peace and quiet, simple surroundings) has little attraction for some adolescents. The time may arrive when definitions of best value and quality are so much in opposition that a family holiday is no longer feasible.

Making sense of Best Value in the workplace

The holiday example illustrates that judgements of value will legitimately vary. For managers, this may become evident in consultation processes. Service users are individuals and have their own views, and the same is true of staff and other people who need to be heard. Organisations and their managers need to be sophisticated when they make judgements about quality and Best Value. The 'old' attitude of 'We know best' had, if nothing else, the advantage of making judgement more straightforward. Its considerable disadvantage was that it created services based on paternalism, where the provider, not the user, defined quality. Similarly, judgements made solely on cost will not meet the Best Value test either. Pradeep, a commissioning manager, said 'Best Value is in general terms a good thing as it means I don't have to go for the cheapest, but the best at a reasonable price.'

The commitment to embrace more than one perspective opens up possibilities for more creative service development. Real partnership with service users in particular increases the likelihood of a Best Value (and best value) outcome. Cambridgeshire County Council provides an illuminating example of this (see Example 7.1).

EXAMPLE 7.1 Listening to service users

As part of its Best Value review programme, Cambridgeshire Council looked at day services for people with mental health problems. A council officer and a service user representative carried out the review jointly. The process led to understandings that cut across many of the professional orthodoxies about the role of day services. In particular, service users did not see the clear distinctions that others did between social services day services and health services, which had a more overtly therapeutic role. What they identified as most valuable was the chance to meet people with similar problems in a supportive environment. This was expressed by one person as 'It helps you cope with everyday life' and by another as 'Coming here makes life possible.'

The learning from this included the need to think of provision beyond the current hours, and to do this in a way that is user-led. It also meant that basic assumptions about the role of day services had to be revisited. Therapeutic programmes were valued, but were referred to much less by users than access to mutual support.

(Source: adapted from Allen, 2000, p. 22)

Best Value, whatever else, insists on service user involvement. This is not a new way of thinking to many for whom empowerment and partnership have been part of their language and aspirations since at least the 1980s. What Best Value does, more than earlier Compulsory Competitive Tendering, is to subject such aspirations to analysis. In this, it moves from a focus on intentions (articulated, for example, through a person's value base) to an interest in outcomes (behaviour and results). What drives this is the review process. In the next section I turn to a consideration of what local managers can do to incorporate Best Value in their day-to-day practice so that review becomes more of an opportunity than a threat.

Active management

All managers involved in services to people will over time become aware of Best Value reviews. Active management in relation to Best Value involves considering the benefits of reflecting on local performance. Where there are local business plans developed beyond the 'once a year and forgotten about' stage, it is easier to integrate Best Value into your and your team's thinking.

The set of questions in Table 7.2 is by no means exhaustive but is intended to start discussion about 'growing' Best Value locally.

Table 7.2   **Key questions about Best Value**

Activity	*Questions for unit or team*
Challenge	What would be the impact of our not being here?
	Have we gone beyond our sell-by date?
	Do we need to reconsider our core aims and objectives?
Compare	How well are we doing?
	How do we know?
	Would we buy this service from us?
	What do we know about how others provide this service?
	What might we learn from them?
	Would collaboration with others have mutual benefits, particularly for our service users?
Consult	Who are the people who should have a voice in our service?
	In what ways do we listen to them?
	Is consultation mainly an 'official' process, perhaps annual and by questionnaire?
	Does consultation also happen as we go along, as part of our routine?
	Do we have a checklist of ways to consult?
	What happens to the ideas and information that we get from consultation?
Continuous improvement	Do we have time set aside to learn from the process of evaluation?
	Who is involved in this?
	What do we do with our learning?

Best Value can provide frontline managers with a way of asking simple but important questions about their local service. Part of this reflective process concerns costs. There will always be a relationship between costs and quality, although the most expensive is not always the best. In the next section I consider the cost part of Best Value considerations, through looking at budgets.

> **Key points**
>
> - Best Value is not wholly new as a concept but now has a particular legal and policy meaning for service users, commissioners and providers.
>
> - Best Value captures much of the essence of the changing context for managing care and affects managers in all settings.
>
> - Best Value is a process and requires the ability to hold on to notions of quality and cost.
>
> - Managers need the ability to recognise, respond to and embrace a range of perspectives about what constitutes value.
>
> - Best Value is best achieved via partnership with service users.

7.3   Managing a budget

As noted earlier, managing budgets at work creates anxieties for many new managers. I try in what follows to demystify budget management. If you want to remind yourself or think in more detail about budget sheets and budget headings, look now at Appendix 2 'Understanding budget reports and accounts'. This part of a manager's responsibilities, however, cannot be separated from other aspects. Budgets are an integral part of the planning and delivery of a service. So where exactly do they fit? This section considers:

– what a budget is
– sources of funding
– the advantages and problems of budgets
– the stages in budget setting
– the responsibilities of frontline managers
– key principles.

What is a budget?

At its simplest, a budget is a financial action plan. Geneen and Moscow (1985, p. 139) say 'In business, numbers are the symbols by which you measure the various activities of an individual enterprise or combination of enterprises which make up the parent corporation'. They warn, however, that 'the numbers are not the business; they are only pictures of the business' (p. 140). Brian, a financial specialist, described budgets in a similar way:

> Accountants like to make budgets sound really complicated. In fact they are quite straightforward. All organisations are in business to achieve some sorts of goals, and budgets are just the statements of what resources they are going to use to try to achieve them.
>
> (Manager consultations)

Angela, a voluntary sector manager, drew on past statutory experience to identify the distinctive nature of budgets in the voluntary sector: 'Here, we have to be much more concerned with income at the annual planning stage; it got much less attention when I worked in the statutory sector.'

The word 'budget' has its origins in the French word *bougette*, meaning a small leather case, as used by the Chancellor of the Exchequer to carry the government's financial plans (the Budget). This has a particular application to the public sector, as the Chancellor's budget statement in part concerns setting limits to public spending.

The money – where does it come from?

Budgets and their management inevitably vary between different sectors. This is at least partly because of the different sources of funding described in Box 7.2 (opposite).

Both voluntary and private sector organisations need to raise or earn the money they spend. Statutory sector organisations have less of a sense of this relationship. None the less, there are some overlaps as social care attracts significant government funding that is spent in all sectors. The Best Value regime underlines the government's commitment to a mixed economy of care. Attracting funding through this arrangement necessitates demonstrating that services, from whatever sector they are delivered, meet Best Value criteria. How frontline managers attract funding for their units varies depending on the sector they work in. For example, some are able to consider National Lottery applications, whereas others need to turn to other parts of their organisation to do this. All managers need awareness of their own agency's processes for allocating money, particularly the budget-setting process.

I turn now to the overall budget process and frontline managers' roles within it, starting with the obvious question: why have budgets?

BOX 7.2 Funding sources

Local government

(a) The revenue support grant (the principal payment to local authorities, based on the government's assessment of spending needs)

(b) The business rate

(c) The council tax

(d) Specific grants

(e) Income from charges

(f) Miscellaneous revenue

(Source: Glasby and Glasby, 1999, p. 11)

The voluntary sector

(a) Social services, health authorities and primary care trusts

(b) Other council departments

(c) Trusts and charities

(d) Special grants and government funding programmes

(e) National Lottery or other national organisations, e.g. Princes Trust

(f) Companies

(g) Earned income and 'do it yourself' fundraising

(Source: Department of Health, 2000b; South Yorkshire Funding Advice Bureau, 2000)

The private sector

The main source of money for those in the private sector is income from business.

The importance of budgets

At first, it seems superfluous even to think about the importance of budgets. Few managers could conceive of a world without a budget. None the less, there is a danger with any taken-for-granted processes that their rationale is forgotten and they are not managed well. Budgets are a key part of the overall business-planning process. Atrill and McLaney (1997) strip this planning down to three broad and linked activities (see Figure 7.2 overleaf). You may recognise in this model much the same levels of consideration outlined in the cyclical planning process described earlier and applied to Best Value.

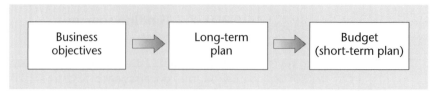

Figure 7.2 **The business-planning process**

Using this model, the budget for which you are responsible should be an end product of earlier planning. Budgets themselves also involve three broad activities:

• budget setting
• budget management and monitoring
• budget review and renewed planning.

Budget setting

Managers working in centrally controlled organisations would describe this activity as largely mysterious and occurring somewhere else. Sally, manager of a residential unit for older people, said with feeling that she has little or no impact on the process: 'Take office supplies, the amount is nominal and every year I write and say it needs increasing, but it never changes.' Others will have a part to play in the process of budget setting. Angela, the voluntary sector manager, thought that things had moved in a positive direction in recent years, since the introduction of individual department plans in addition to the overall agency plan. Department plans were the subject of discussion at all levels of management, creating a greater sense of ownership. Where the frontline manager's voice is heard, the views of staff and service users are more likely to be included. Smaller organisations may have less difficulty in ensuring that all voices are heard.

With the increasing emphasis on responsiveness and user-focused services, it is more important than ever, for both organisational effectiveness and individual service quality, that frontline managers and their staff are involved in discussions about future plans and budget allocation. The routine supervision process is helpful here. Through this, frontline staff can have a voice, with frontline managers, in future developments and frontline managers can, in turn, discuss with their supervisor ideas about improved efficiency and possible future developments. This gives the basis for a practice-led management approach to budgets and best value. The Cambridgeshire example (7.1) underlines the importance of service user involvement in review and development.

Budget management, monitoring and review

All frontline managers have budget management and monitoring responsibility. Some have budgets that support unpredictable needs; others have relatively limited responsibilities, to do with monitoring. Where the level of demand is unpredictable, estimates of likely demand are needed and the frontline manager's local knowledge, supported by information about population trends, is important. I shall return later to this part of the budget process. Budget review should involve frontline managers in the same way, and for the same reasons, as budget planning, since review and planning go together. Managers must review and evaluate in order to aid planning.

The budget reality?

Some commentators criticise the planning model in Figure 7.2 as being too rational and lacking the edge of the 'real' world in the following respects.

- For private sector organisations some, such as Grint (1995), argue that the main emphasis is on short-term returns to hungry shareholders, and that the budget does not sufficiently reflect the longer-term dimension. In such situations the pressure on managers to keep shareholders happy lessens their ability to think strategically. Grint contrasts this 'firefighting' approach to management with German and Japanese approaches, which allow for more emphasis on the longer term. The annual setting of budgets by local authorities feeds this preoccupation with the short term, both in their own units and in private sector agencies that have substantial contracts with them.

- For the public sector, the criticism has been that the annual budget process is typically incremental; this year's budget, for example, will probably look very much like last year's, albeit with a little more or a little less. Such incrementalism does not necessarily fit with the political agenda for continuing change and development. For the voluntary and private sectors, their concern with implementing the rational planning model has been that they are vulnerable to the whims of those with whom they have contracts. The overview report of inspections of relationships between the statutory and voluntary sectors (Department of Health, 2000b) found improvement in this area in many places, although with room for more improvements. Voluntary sector respondents, for example, welcomed contracts agreed for three years rather than one. Some inspections found that black and ethnic minority voluntary sector organisations were under-represented at partnership meetings, so that their needs would be difficult to include in the planning process.

Reality revisited – conversations with managers

The conversations I had while planning this chapter threw some light on the link between theory and practice. Managers from different levels in organisations were chosen to enable a range of perspectives to be heard and there was a considerable degree of consensus among them.

All took budget management very seriously. Sandy, the senior manager, expected managers to be aware of their budgets through checking reports and to discuss issues arising from them in supervision. Brian, the senior financial specialist, agreed. All the frontline managers interviewed thought this integral to their jobs. The manager of a residential unit for older people, Sally, reflected on change: 'It seems very different from when I started in home management in the 1980s. I don't remember getting involved with budgets then, it wasn't so high profile.' Now, she personally checks budget reports and regularly discusses the budget with senior staff in her unit: 'You need to take time to understand the figures on the reports, so that you know what you're reading.'

Angela, the voluntary sector manager, said her organisation had established a second finance post to run an improved management information system. Pradeep, manager of a team that commissions individual care packages, received two sorts of budget report. He would study the 'actuals' fortnightly to check on spending, but found the second sort of report on 'commitments' more useful, and often more worrying. Commitment reports tell him what he has committed from his budget, not just what has been paid for.

Few managers were satisfied with current arrangements. They would have liked more involvement and responsibility for themselves. Sally, the manager of a residential unit, argued for a simpler budget framework, not the immovable divisions into different areas (for example, provisions and equipment). This would allow her more discretion. She would also welcome a greater role in the budget review and setting process, to help take ideas on service development forward. Brian, the financial specialist, favoured more complete devolving of budgets and more frontline manager involvement in budget setting: 'The ideal would be to put budget decisions where people know best what is happening and that means local managers.' He recognised the need for prior action to make these ideas effective, including more training and support, and realistic budgets.

Angela, the voluntary sector manager, felt that the organisation had changed as it grew: 'You can run like a family firm for so long, but then you realise that you have got to a point where you cannot know everything from the centre. We devolve more to frontline managers now, with positive results which, to be honest, we still find surprising. It takes time to realise that you are not the only ones with ideas.'

The business-planning and budget-setting processes came together in a problematic way. Sandy, the senior manager, felt that the tail wagged the dog: 'The budget works incrementally and is therefore difficult to align with business planning. You end up tailoring objectives to the realities of the budget.' The finance specialist was concerned that his organisation did not have an informed grasp of what services cost and so could not engage in detailed business planning. The manager responsible for commissioning care packages was only slightly more optimistic about the relationship between budgets and business plans: 'I think that the budget planning is to a certain extent aligned to the business plan. The problem is that the business plan tends to say that we can do everything, but the budget plan doesn't.' Managers have to juggle priorities.

There was some difference between Sally, the unit manager, and Brian, the financial specialist, about handling underspends and overspends. Brian considered it legitimate to take money from a unit which was underspending and using it to cover an overspend elsewhere. Sally said this made her feel penalised for being careful with her budget. Both perspectives have validity. Clearly, large organisations need to think through the balance required between corporate and local responsibility.

There will always be gaps between models of management and practice; this was evident from the conversations I had. Interestingly, although you might expect to find a disregard for 'theory' among busy, streetwise managers, they had a positive regard for some of the theoretical ideas about budget management. Business planning is still a relatively new idea for many care organisations and there will probably be some teething problems, not least in making strong relationships between services and money in a world that is not always predictable.

Frontline managers, sitting at the boundary between the agency and service users, have a key role in helping their organisations to narrow the gap between budget principles and budget practice. The conversations with them confirmed that it is worth working at establishing an effective budget and planning framework. Money is better used if it is allocated in line with properly thought-out plans and objectives. To be effective, managers need an awareness of the reality of their organisation's circumstances and of other ways of doing things, including theoretical models.

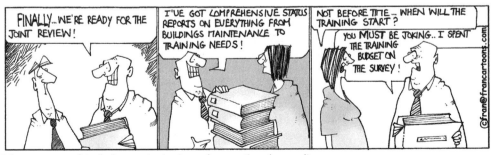

Managers need to balance strategic and operational spending

Benefits and problems of budgets

Budgeting remains a necessary evil for many managers. In Scott Adams' words, 'the budget process was invented by an alien race of sadistic beings' (Adams, 1996, p. 201). His cartoon character Dilbert has strong (and perhaps popular) views on it, advocating, for example, that 'boredom and confusion are your allies in the budget fight' (p. 205). Atrill and McLaney (1997) take a rather more balanced view, and identify four uses of a budget (see Box 7.3). These remind us that there is more to this routine organisational process than meets the eye.

BOX 7.3 Four uses of a budget

1 It makes organisations think forward and anticipate potential problems, which enables the exploration of possible solutions. If a voluntary sector organisation wants to move into rehabilitation work that it has not provided before, using current staff, proper budget consideration will help in the planning of, and paying for, appropriate staff retraining.

2 It helps in co-ordinating the various parts of the organisation. In the above example it would involve the personnel/training parts and the finance section.

3 It can motivate managers to improve performance. Being specific about goals, including budget management, is a more effective motivator than simply an exhortation to perform well. Along with this, budgets are one potential means of helping managers link their responsibilities to the broader organisational goals.

4 It gives the organisation a means of control. The ability to compare the actual rate of expenditure with the planned means that performance can be more easily and objectively evaluated.

(Source: adapted from Atrill and McLaney, 1997, pp. 235–6)

Dilbert might take issue with the contents of Box 7.3 for, as with most management frameworks, these advantages can sometimes go too far and become problems.

- Managers may stick rigidly to plans when circumstances indicate that a change is needed. For example, a training manager refused to recognise the significance of major new legislation: 'There is no provision for it in the Training Section business plan, so there is no budget for it.'
- Where there is a 'blame culture' in the organisation, managers may be more concerned with finding someone to blame than with solving a budget problem. They may also take steps to hide problems for fear of being blamed.

- Unrealistic budgets can demotivate. A manager of a residential service for young people was asked to make savings by trying to reduce staff sickness in the coming year, as part of the budget plan. No one had thought out whether this could really work and the manager did not challenge the request. The budget then became a major source of unresolved anxiety, separated from the unpredictable world of service delivery.

- Appropriate control can shade into oppressive control, creating a senior management style that is unhealthily defensive and a frontline management style that mirrors this. It can also mean that budgets (the 'numbers') gain a higher profile than quality.

Managing and monitoring budgets

Budgets have a fundamental place in organisational life. The overall budget process was discussed earlier, locating it within the business planning cycle. Next, the middle stage of budget management concerned with monitoring is discussed. All managers, whatever their organisation and whatever form of planning their employers adopt, are expected to monitor expenditure and play a part in dealing with problems that emerge. This contributes to budgetary control. Typically, managers get budget reports against pre-set codes and are asked to check for accuracy and problems. Coombs and Jenkins (1991) suggest three basic principles for this: timely, relevant and accurate information; keep responsibility clear; ensure consistency.

Timely, relevant and accurate information

Frontline managers need to be active in identifying what information (and in what form) they need to enable effective monitoring. For example, information that clearly identifies variations from budget allocation is much more usable than information that lacks this. Equally, it should be in a form that makes variation easy to spot and on a timescale that enables action to be taken.

Keeping responsibility clear

Budget responsibility may be vague, which militates against effective monitoring. The clearest scenario is one in which managers are only held responsible for expenditure that they certified. Deviating from this, one manager enabled other people to spend from a budget for which she was responsible and had difficulty later in explaining overspends; this suggests a need for clear protocols in such situations.

Angela, the voluntary sector manager, argued that clarity about budget authorisation was a necessary part of the organisation's approach to budget management.

Ensuring consistency

Consistency is difficult to achieve when budgets are managed both centrally and locally. One manager reported that she and her co-managers were bewildered by apparent overspend on a budget, only to discover that a central finance officer had decreased it when budgets were revised (to bolster another budget) without informing her or changing the figures on the budget print-out. Therefore, the two figures were inconsistent, meaning that she saw herself as within budget but the finance section reported that she was overspent.

Exploring variation

Monitoring is only of use when managers can act on the basis of their findings. Geneen and Moscow (1985, p. 140) offer a helpful warning about this: 'Numbers serve as a sort of thermometer, which measures the health and well-being of the enterprise.' They continue, you should 'insist that management must manage. You don't want to manage the numbers. That is like treating the thermometer instead of the patient' (p. 141). So, budget reports alert managers to possible problems which they investigate, using the 'numbers' as prompts. At this stage there are two issues: first, who might helpfully be involved and, second, what might explain the variation.

Who is involved depends partly on a manager's style. Managers who believe in participative ways of managing involve anyone who has something to offer. Where this is practicable in terms of time, it invariably assists: several heads are better than two, which are better than one! It is at least worthwhile to involve a financial specialist if possible. Sandy, a senior manager, argued the virtues of developing an 'us' culture between the operational and finance parts of organisations, rather than one based on 'us and them' divisions.

Explanations for variation can fit into only two broad categories. First, the report might be wrong – some expenditure might have been wrongly coded. Second, actual expenditure might be at variance from that expected. It is important to check the first. Budget reports are not self-evidently correct. Indeed, a common first response to a report saying that a budget has been overspent is 'The figures are wrong!' Among the other common reasons for reports being wrong are:

- human error – a figure has been entered wrongly
- someone has spent money that is not recorded – for example, stamps have been bought but not entered in the petty cash book
- expenditure has been placed against the wrong code.

These are reassuring reasons for frontline managers in that they explain apparent discrepancies; but what if the figures are apparently correct? Clearly, variation then needs investigation and, again, there are common reasons for this.

- Some expenditure does not flow evenly through a year. Commissioning managers know that they need to spend more money in the winter than at other times of the year. Therefore, they expect to find an underspend for the first half of the financial year.

- There is an important distinction between 'actual' reports and reports on commitments. 'Actuals' tell you what you have spent that has been paid for; a commitment report tells you what you need to pay for in future. An actual may suggest underspend; a report on commitments usually gives a more accurate picture.

- The budget may represent an unrealistic view of what is necessary. A manager required to make a staffing allocation budget balance by significantly reducing staff sickness, while desirable, may find it impossible, as staff sickness is unpredictable.

- Price changes are reflected in budget variations. It is not always possible to forecast accurately the cost of supplies throughout a year.

- Managers have consciously not followed the budget set for them. There may be good reasons for this: someone's needs may have increased; the number of people needing services may have risen beyond that anticipated; and so on. It is important to identify reasons here; after all, it is possible that managers have simply been inefficient.

Behind the search for explanations lies the need to understand. Such understanding is necessary to ensure that subsequent corrective action makes sense. This action may involve a decision about where to decrease expenditure in order to bring the budget back into line; or it may involve the organisation finding money from somewhere else to cover the variation. As discussed earlier, these decisions are made in the context of Best Value requirements. Costs and quality exist in a balance. How decisions are made depends in part on the approach of the people who are responsible. Therefore, this consideration of budget issues concludes with that dimension in the next section.

Key points

- A budget is a financial picture of the service.

- Attracting funding depends on showing Best Value.

- Budgets are central in the business-planning process.

- Involving frontline managers, staff and service users in budget allocation is best practice.

- The manager's role is to link budgeting theory with the realities of the service.

7.4 Personal style and budget management

Managing budgets is not just a technical activity: the way managers manage budgets is partly determined by their style or approach. Whatever model you use to analyse your management styles, it will tell you something about your way of handling budgets, the advantages and possible problems. Hay (1993) offers a framework for understanding the relationship between management style and handling budgets. She works from a Transactional Analysis model (TA), popular in the 1960s in psychotherapy, as a way of understanding how relationships work. TA provides a description of ego states such as parent, child and adult. Hay's book is an accessible introduction if you want to investigate TA at work further.

Applying TA to the work environment, Hay identifies five working styles, driven by past experiences (see Box 7.4).

BOX 7.4 Hay's five working styles

1 **Hurry up** people like to pull out all the stops, and so like it when urgent work comes up. They move into action very quickly.

2 **Be perfect** people take pride in accuracy. They are well organised and forever want to do things better.

3 **Please people** people make getting on with people a priority. They are good team members, always willing to help others.

4 **Try hard** people enjoy the challenge of the new. They are less conscientious in following things up.

5 **Be strong** people take pride in their ability to cope and keep calm in crises. They seldom if ever complain.

(Source: adapted from Hay, 1993, pp. 91–2)

These are types and you should not expect to meet anyone who fits one of them exactly. However, as Hay suggests, people are probably more like one than the others and this is often accentuated when they are under stress. A feeling of stress is very common for managers who are new to managing budgets, prompted by such internal dialogues as 'What if I get it wrong?' Pause for a moment to see whether the five working styles sound familiar to you. Each has its clear strengths: for example, it feels reassuring in a crisis to have someone around who always seems to be calm. Equally, people with a concern for others are important in any team. Most strengths, however, have downsides, and this is certainly true of working styles. The way this may operate with budgets is shown in Table 7.3.

Table 7.3 **Potential problems of working styles for budget management**

Working style	Problems
Hurry up	Lack of focus on small but important details. Lack of patience for broader, strategic thinking that links budget with business plans
Be perfect	Constant concern for 100% accuracy. Too much time allocated to task at expense of more important work. The excellent drives out the good
Please people	Avoidance of difficult decisions about resources that may affect people. Inability to make unpopular decisions. Lack of interest in non-people-related issues. May end up overspending because cannot say 'no'
Try hard	Initially keen to manage budget but soon become bored with routine of budget monitoring. May start well but fail to do necessary routine checking over a long period
Be strong	Unwilling to seek help from own manager when there are problems and may resort to bluff. Less willing to get ideas from staff, so unable to maximise use of group's creativity in resolving budget problems

Now consider the relationship between your own working style and that of a manager you know. Hay (1993) argues that people feel most comfortable with those whose working styles are similar to their own. It may not always be the most effective combination, as shown in Table 7.4, which describes the impact when both managers have the same working style.

Table 7.4 **The interplay between the same working styles**

My and my manager's working style	The impact
Hurry up	Both managers skim information and there is a danger something important may be missed. Neither has time for careful thinking through of future requirements
Be perfect	There is no voice for the 'good enough' approach that busy managers sometimes need. Deadlines are missed because both are focused on perfection
Please people	Budgets take inappropriately low priority
Try hard	Both may start well but then find the pursuit of detail boring. There is a danger that the budget will not be monitored and no one will spot problems until too late, when preventive action becomes very difficult
Be strong	Strong managers may give out the message that, even if someone says they are struggling, it is seen as a sign of weakness and noted accordingly

It is not difficult to think about the impact on budget management of having a *different* style from your manager. What would happen if you are a 'be perfect' person managed by someone who is more of the 'hurry up' type?

Lessons for budget management and service development

The realisation that budget management at any level involves a series of activities and is more than a technical exercise suggests some basic principles, as described in Box 7.5.

BOX 7.5 Lessons for budget management

1 Understanding yourself is a key aspect of effective management, including budget management. The working styles described all have strengths and potential problems. Recognising your style is the necessary first step to using your strengths and dealing with any problems that may result.

2 There must be clarity about:

- what budgets a manager is responsible for, in the sense of being held to account for performance

- the manager's room for manœuvre in dealing with budget variations

- whether a budget is held for convenience at local level but is really part of a larger, corporate budget, or whether it really 'belongs' to the local manager.

3 It is sensible to view budget and service development as a collaborative exercise wherever possible. This makes potential for the manager to harness the creative ideas of a range of people, including staff and service users.

4 Efficient and simple-to-administer monitoring systems are necessary to keep control over budgets. The more unpredictable the use of money, the more such systems become essential, and the more frequently monitoring is needed.

5 Managers are responsible for actively managing budgets: burying their heads in the sand is not an option. Organisations expect managers to take responsibility.

6 Operational managers are not accountants. Rather than seeking to become financial specialists, they should focus on developing good working relationships, so that collaboration over budget management becomes possible. Finance sections should be partners in

---

effective budget management. The combined creativity of financial specialists and operational managers can enable service development to progress more effectively.

7   Accountants are not responsible for managers' budgets; their task in most organisations is to offer their expertise to help managers manage. If operational managers specify to financial specialists what information they need, in what form, and how often, the relationship will work better to the strengths of each partner.

8   Numbers, in Geneen and Moscow's (1985) use of the word, are symbols. Budgetary management and monitoring is one means to the end of effective and efficient management, not a replacement for it.

Revisiting the big picture

These ideas about budget and service management have echoes in some of the wider debates about management. They are represented by three central questions:

1   Will measurement become more important than management?
2   Will frontline managers become increasingly involved in the whole business-planning and therefore budget-planning process?
3   Will care organisations develop budget-management systems that take into account the fact that care is a people-intensive business?

As computer programs become more sophisticated, organisations will inevitably find better management information systems almost yearly. There is a danger that organisations could fall into the trap of believing that the measurement these systems offer can replace the manager's judgement in the context of an uncertain environment. One of the features of Best Value – the setting of targets expressed numerically – exemplifies this. Rogers (1999) reminds us that an organisation's performance can be measured in several ways, one of which is using statistics, as shown in Example 7.2.

EXAMPLE 7.2 A statistical review of a play

Play 'x' was performed by 'y' theatre company at 'z' theatre last night. 12 actors were employed to play 19 roles (representing efficient use of thespian resources) on a stage measuring 'b' metres. It was performed in front of 'c' customers (64% capacity utilisation) with production costs of £d and box office income of £e. The play was performed as fully specified in the programme with the exception of its overrunning by three minutes and 25 seconds (a 2% overrun on stated completion target). The performance was followed by 2.47 minutes of applause.

(Source: Rogers, 1999, p. 61)

However, you might ask 'But what was the play like?' Similar questions emerge if you think that numbers alone can tell the story of any care service.

The trend towards devolving responsibility for decision making down organisational hierarchies is well established. However, there is much variation in the extent to which frontline managers are involved in the whole budget process, an important aspect of organisational responsibility. There are many reasons for this, not least of which is time. None the less, concepts such as consultation, empowerment and partnership with service users cannot be logically embraced without also applying them to frontline managers and frontline staff. As *People Need People* (Joint Reviews, 2000) argues, the approach to service delivery must be mirrored by the approach to management.

One feature that distinguishes service organisations from manufacturing companies is the role of frontline employees. In service organisations, production and consumption are simultaneous. A residential worker's care for a resident coincides with the resident's receipt of it. In a review of early Best Value practice, Lewis examines the implications of this:

> The more interactive the role of the client (introducing uncertainty) in a service process, the more significant the role of the employee becomes in managing quality. This significance in both defining and managing quality implies that particular attention should be given to role definition and staff selection, training and supervision.
>
> (Lewis, 1998, p. 16)

Despite this important realisation, many organisations still view training and development as a cost, not an investment, and an obvious target for cost cutting. Armstrong (1995) argues that this attitude towards training and development stems from the basic principles of traditional accountancy practice. The significance that he places on this comes from his view that accountancy has grown very influential in business practice. If this is correct, much thought is needed in care agencies about Lewis's statement. As the saying goes, 'If you think education is expensive, how much does ignorance cost?'

Key points

- Managing budgets does not just involve numbers: your management style determines your approach.

- Understanding yourself is key to understanding the way you approach budgets.

- Budgeting and service development are closely linked.

- Wider management issues affect how budgets work in agencies.

7.5   Conclusion

This chapter focused on the frontline manager's role in managing budgets and giving Best Value. It has grown from a role that was relatively tightly prescribed to one that is more flexible, yet critical in service delivery. As customer care practice has grown, and with the advent of more intense competition, the belief in devolving responsibility as far as possible down organisational hierarchies has become an orthodoxy.

The introduction of Best Value has added impetus to thinking about how to achieve a balance between quality and cost. It has probably also brought the concerns of managers in the private, voluntary and public sectors closer together. This chapter sought, therefore, to increase your understanding of Best Value and its messages for budget management. Central to this was the proposal that budget planning and management are integral aspects of business planning, and that frontline managers should be key players throughout. The main lessons are summarised in Box 7.5.

This chapter ended by raising some questions about the bigger organisational picture. Behind these questions lies a simple reality: care is a set of services from people to people. Organisations that grasp the meaning of this in their business planning, budget management and quality assurance processes are likely to fare well in an increasingly competitive world.

Chapter 8
Managing information and using new technologies

Martin Ousley, John Rowlands and Janet Seden

8.1 Introduction

Managers sometimes say they suffer from 'information bombardment'. You may identify with that comment and have experienced information overload yourself. Perhaps you have had too many leaflets pushed through your letterbox or too many people telling you too much, too fast. An important aspect of management concerns the flow of information in the organisation, so managers have always needed to process organisational and personal information sensitively, and to use data to inform evaluation and planning. Perhaps now they receive more information, more quickly and in more detail. A senior manager in children's services, talking about frontline managers, put it this way:

> The team managers pass information upwards, downwards, and with a wider range of media than ever before, with more different purposes, and different timescales ... what matters is that they manage information in ways that are linked to the expectations of the work.
>
> (Manager consultations)

A frontline manager recorded her experience of handling information as follows.

> I met with my managers and the team to discuss our recent review. It went well and positive comments were received, but more and more I realise how much in the middle I am. Several times the team were asked if I had passed on organisational information which in most cases I had, but some things had got 'lost' or are in my pile waiting for dissemination. I am the conduit from the team to the managers, and it is only what I choose or remember to say that is passed on, and I do wonder what sort of a slanted picture I may unintentionally create. By necessity, it can only be subjective and not as objective as I would like. There should be more cross-over between team members and senior managers to avoid this but I am not clear if that is ever possible unless the team become more involved in organisational matters, for which they do not have a fondness!
>
> (Manager consultations)

There is power in holding, withholding or deciding to share information. Perhaps the art of managing information well is gathering it and using it ethically for service objectives. After all, data is information only when it is 'accessible and useful to both staff and consumers' (Darvill, 1992, p. 106). Information is probably only useful to managers if they select the right kind at the right time. For service users, lack of access to information, clarity about what happens to information, and informed consent are important matters. A practice-led approach to managing information is to view it as part of providing the service in care environments, where practice values underpin managers' actions.

Mintzberg (1975) describes managers as spending much of their time on informational tasks, which, he suggests, fall into three categories:

1 *monitoring* – collecting information through networking and contacts
2 *disseminating* – passing information to the team
3 *speaking* – informing people outside the organisation.

New technologies have added another dimension to these activities by providing a way to process large amounts of data quickly. These developments in information collection and processing do not take away the manager's role in communicating on paper, by word of mouth or in meetings. They do bring their own benefits and dilemmas with which managers have to grapple. Management information systems have to be managed and understood by someone before they can be useful.

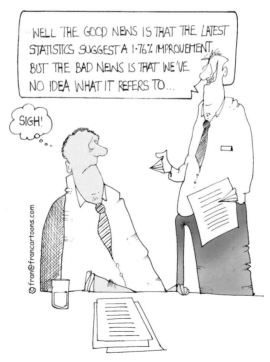

Someone has to manage information for it to be useful

In this chapter we explore some of the opportunities and concerns that managers meet when using new technologies for recording and processing information. First, we consider the debate about whether technologies control activities in care – for example, by monitoring practitioner activities and increasing workloads – with the result that users' views may be overlooked. By contrast, we also argue that the effective use of data-based information can help managers do a better job. They can evaluate more precisely the outputs (numbers of participating people, rates of attendance, meals delivered) and the outcomes (the result and intended improvement to a person's wellbeing). We then consider some aspects of integrating the use of management information systems with practice agendas. Finally, because much information that comes to care managers is sensitive, there is a summary of the Data Protection Act 1998 and a discussion of some issues about sharing information.

The aims of this chapter are to:

- explore how current practices are affected by using new technology and examine some challenges and dilemmas
- argue that the use of management information is an integral part of a frontline manager's role
- consider some ways to make sense of the potentially vast amount of readily available information and how using new technologies for data collection affects practice
- examine the requirements of the Data Protection Act 1998 and discuss some issues of confidentiality, conflicts of interest and data sharing.

8.2   Someone to watch over you?

We referred above to some managers' feelings about the amounts of information they routinely handle. New technologies enable local and central government to use management information systems for data collection in new ways. This use is linked to outcome measures and performance indicators, which are employed to assess the performance of teams and agencies against centrally selected objectives.

Harris (1998) provides an analysis of these changes which suggests that central control is eroding local flexibility and professional autonomy. He comments that in the 1970s and 1980s, despite arguments to the contrary, practitioners maintained much individual freedom in their practice as 'bureau-professionals'. In other words, there was a rational bureaucratic employment structure within which professional expertise controlled the content of services. Frontline managers made local decisions, and practitioners could also make and influence decisions through 'permissive supervision' (Harris, 1998, p. 849). This discretion was eroded in the 1990s, as the state redefined its role in social welfare and the relationships between central government, local government, middle and frontline managers changed. According to Harris, these changes were, first, operational managers had to become 'businesslike'; second, rationing and gatekeeping became major social work activities; and third:

> In order to monitor social workers' rationing of resources, the discretion of social workers has been curtailed by information technology systems which prioritize budgetary considerations in the allocation of services.
>
> (Harris, 1998, p. 857)

Fourth, information technology systems were coupled with close supervisory control; and fifth:

> Human information technology surveillance can be combined with workload measurement integrated into the worker's routine on-line recording. The amount of time needed to manage a caseload can then be determined and managerial attention can be given to 'slow workers'. Supervision sessions can focus on the social worker's 'productivity'.
>
> (p. 858)

Speaking of the future, Harris concludes, 'the likelihood is that social work as an occupation will remain a more heavily constrained part of the state's welfare apparatus than it was in the 1970s/early 1980s' (p. 859). Harris's analysis is of fieldwork in social services departments, but other care workers may have experienced similar changes. This link between information technology and the use of performance indicators to monitor local authorities has persisted. *Community Care* (2001a) reported on a keynote address given to the National Social Services Conference in 2001, in which the Health Secretary described how performance indicator results, produced from data requested by central government, would affect local councils' future development opportunities. Some of the responses are shown in Box 8.1 (opposite).

The debates about whether performance indicators improve or control practice are likely to continue. Perspectives vary and the view will differ according to your situation, whether in government, in a hospital waiting-room, at a frontline manager's desk or at home waiting for a care worker. New technologies have created new ways of collecting and collating data, and contribute to the ability of managers to evaluate outcomes. The questions are about the uses such data are put to and whether measurement becomes an end in itself, eroding the energy of practitioners to improve services for everyone.

BOX 8.1 Performance indicators and league tables

'If naming and shaming actually helped the public, it could perhaps be justified. Do let's be clear. It doesn't. The performance assessment framework only benefits the service users if they can be shown how it works, and what complex tasks are being measured. Simply telling people they live in a "poor performance area" isn't much use to them. It makes the relationship between the public and local services more difficult, and exacerbates the public's disengagement from local democracy. And if the complex performance assessment framework is of little benefit to service users, it's hard to see how the even cruder "star rating" system ... will improve matters.'

(Editor)

'Staff are slogging their guts out to turn that council around ... we are improving.'

(Lambeth councillor)

'Raising standards is part of the solution, not an extra burden.'
(Chair of the National Care Standards Commission)

(Source: *Community Care*, 2001a, pp. 5, 11)

You probably have views on these matters based on personal or workplace experience. Everybody has an investment in knowing that the information held about them is accurate and will not be shared without consent, and what kind of service monitoring and information gathering might lead to improvements for all. As Lyon (2001) identifies, there are relationships between cyberspace and citizenship. On the one hand, more access to information makes citizens into consumers, and seems open and democratic; on the other, the possibility of government surveillance of the individual increases. Lyon argues that engagement by citizens with these two modes of 'virtual citizenship' may bring a 'moral' dimension to the uses to which this technology is put.

Key points

- Data collection is now closely linked to performance indicators and measuring outcomes. Local services lose resources if they do not perform well.

- There is a tension between collecting information to monitor and improve services, and using information to control professional activity.

- Both service users and citizens have an interest in the use of information about themselves and others.

8.3   The information environment

The use of new technology in the workplace has developed alongside a focus on evaluation, outputs and outcomes. There is also a concern to ensure that services are achieving what service users and others expect (Smith, 1996; Utting *et al.*, 2001; Pinnock and Dimmock, 2003). It has been suggested that some professional activity, far from benefiting people, has disadvantaged them. For example, work on equal opportunities has shown the disadvantages experienced by several groups on the basis of ethnic origin, gender and disability (Fawcett Society, 2000; Osler and Morrison, 2000). These unhelpful experiences were not intended, so everyone involved in the delivery of services needs to consider how to find out whether they really are useful. Do they achieve the objectives with outcomes that stakeholders find satisfactory?

Manager and practitioner investment in good information

The overall performance of any care system is built up from the collective activities of many individual practitioners, usually guided by a frontline manager. Aggregated information can be useful to evaluate outcomes across a unit or an agency, or nationally, so the impact of these actions can be considered as a discernible trend. Evidence of unintended outcomes suggests the need to have agendas for clear standards of practice. Systems have been introduced for assessments in local authorities, where both the contents of assessments and the time-frames within which they should take place are specified. Managers need to know whether staff are meeting these targets, which are based on what is considered to be good practice.

Statutory returns are sent to central government to contribute to the creation of a national picture, so that managers can evaluate local outcomes against it. The measurement of service delivery against such prescribed outcomes is now an embedded feature of care activity (Smith, 1996; Pinnock and Dimmock, 2003). Smith suggests that, while there are difficulties and complexities to be overcome in gaining useful measures, it is important to continue because:

> Without information about the broad impact of public services on society, there is a grave danger that resources are misdirected and that – in the process – the usefulness of the public sector is discredited.
>
> (Smith, 1996, p. 18)

There may be differing views about what is an outcome and how it can be measured but, Smith suggests, 'there are two fundamental reasons' to persist in efforts to conceptualise and measure outcomes:

> The first is to identify effective modes of delivering public services; the second to identify the competence with which those services are delivered.
>
> (p. 196)

As Gallop argues in Chapter 7, initiatives such as Best Value (Audit Commission, 1999a, b) require authorities and their partners to be clear about the quality and cost of their services. Social services departments use information to show they are providing value for money, and this involves the voluntary and private agencies they have service agreements with. Central initiatives usually link the allocation of future resources to outcomes inferred from information that has been collected. This means that managers, and practitioners too in some settings, have no option but to invest time and energy in data collection. Integrated systems for children's and adults' services are in place, as are mechanisms for information sharing between health and social care (Department of Health, 2001c, d). Managers need to make sure that, with respect to information, the link between practice activity and the allocation of resources for service users is understood and acted on by the team.

Pressures on managers and practitioners

The requirement to collect data for central government, as well keeping up with other kinds of local information, exists in a climate where managers are already working under pressure. The monitoring of effectiveness against performance measures means that units identified as performing poorly are singled out, which is discouraging, as this adults' services manager comments:

> I think it's very difficult because, as a manager, on the one side of the coin, there's the expectation that you meet these targets. If you're not achieving, you don't get a genuine crack of the whip at why you're not ... and I think that puts you in a very difficult scenario.
>
> (Manager consultations)

Practitioners find that league tables give the impression they are not working hard for service users when, in fact, they are:

> I've often wondered why departments are now starting to put out these tables. You've got the management information that comes down and the way you feel when you realise your team has actually come down the table, rather than gone up the table. It makes you feel so bad, and it makes the team feel bad as well, that they're not producing the work they should. They probably are, but the fact is that it isn't being measured correctly: they're not measuring the correct qualitative aspects of the work.
>
> (Manager consultations)

Managers usually know why their teams cannot achieve certain standards; for example, they may be short of staff. Monitoring activity can provide managers with evidence to demonstrate their wider concerns about their unit or to support bids for resources, or with the means to share innovative ways of responding to the requests of service users. The collation of information becomes difficult, if not impossible, without the tools and time for the job. Staff may need to set aside time to learn new skills, such as how to record what is needed in a new, standardised format. The Looked After Children records (Ward, 1995) provide a standardised way of recording, designed to ensure that children in foster care and children's homes receive services such as education and health care and that their wellbeing is properly considered. However, it has been difficult to implement the records in computerised form. Kerslake notes:

> At first sight, computerisation would seem to be a natural extension to implementation of the paper-based forms. There are some obvious advantages; it offers easier aggregation of data, it aids legibility, it is a useful way to reproduce the documents and avoids repetition of data entry. Some 18 months later, although 12 authorities have taken up the system, progress in achieving wider implementation is slow. Why have such difficulties been encountered and how might they be overcome?
>
> (Kerslake, 1998, p. 236)

He suggests:

> The overall message is that child care, like other public welfare sectors (see Aldridge, 1995) lacks an information-driven culture. Trying to implement a computer system in such an environment is further hampered by the variety of computer implementations that have developed in SSDs in the absence of any strategic direction from central government.
>
> (p. 237)

Kerslake concludes that cultural and policy changes are needed, and that wider debate on how information is managed can only be beneficial for social care practice and service users. He makes some strong arguments for the benefits of computerising records, while accepting that there are difficulties with implementing a synchronised system. You may well have experienced some of the frustrations of using computers and computerised records, while trying to gain the advantages of structured recording for your agency.

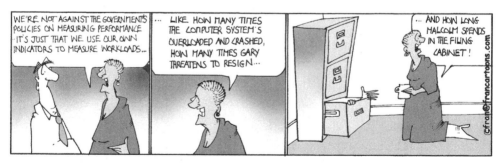

There can be difficulties implementing a synchronised system

The culture of the organisation

Kerslake suggests a shift in culture to balance the tension between the requirement to gather good information and the pressures managers and their staff experience in day-to-day implementation. A culture of blame or avoidance does not help but is hard to prevent when people know that information may be used to criticise their work. However, if information gathered can be used to enhance team learning and planning, its value becomes apparent (Bates, 2003).

Managers have responsibility for giving a lead and promoting a learning approach to information among their staff. The culture of the organisation may be determined by the senior managers but frontline managers can both add to or subtract from that culture. They can encourage staff to take responsibility for their areas of work and to implement changes. Managers' ability to understand and use information in meaningful ways makes all the difference to their staff's experience. A crucial factor is a feeling of confidence that the data collected are useful for the agency's tasks.

Ways of gathering information

Managers and teams may feel more confident about data used to inform practice if they are involved in deciding what is collected and how it is collated and analysed. The most useful information for frontline managers and their teams relates closely to their practice experience. This is an argument for data to be collected routinely which, when reviewed, are more useful than reviews driven by the need to tighten budgets or respond to a critical audit (Ousley and Barnwell, 1993). It is better still if frontline managers and staff are actively involved together in the development of information-collection systems (Darvill, 1992; Department of Health, 2001c, d).

Collecting statistics that measure only part of a unit's activity can put frontline managers in the position of highlighting areas where standards of performance may be declining but missing out information that shows the reasons. In adult fieldwork services there is a requirement to measure whether assessments are completed on time. Managers are expected to record how many reviews for adults receiving services are held later than the specified date. Analysing the information recorded may not be straightforward, as Example 8.1 shows.

EXAMPLE 8.1 Measuring performance

Authority A conducted 70% of reviews within the required timescale, but the other 30% were conducted within one week of the required date. Authority B conducted 80% of reviews within the required timescale, but the other 20% were conducted within one month of the required date. According to a simple measure of the percentage of late reviews, Authority B is better. However, the effectiveness of Authority A in dealing with those that were late is significantly better than Authority B.

This example suggests that knowing what can be measured, how to measure it, and how to analyse the information is as important as the sophistication of the system for data collection.

Information is only as useful as the way it is managed and understood in context. Manufacturing processes can be monitored easily from hard information about production targets. Care organisations are more complex because of less measurable elements, such as the quality of practitioner interventions with service users. Numerical information, taken out of context, can be misleading. The debate about league tables in education and health focuses on the fact that it is impossible to reduce the activity of a school or hospital to a single measure, or even combinations of such measures.

Factors that contribute to patient wellbeing may be interactive rather than static. They can depend on a range of unpredictable factors, making it difficult to know exactly what is being measured. Ranking schools by examination results alone says nothing about the pastoral care offered to students, or their other significant achievements. Essential 'soft' information, such as service users' views, needs to be considered together with numerical information in order to give a comprehensive view of any situation.

A review of how effective a home care service is might measure the number of people who received a service (output). It could be brought to life with other information from a survey of users saying how the service helped them (outcomes). A senior manager explained how she always tried to consider what kind of picture was being formed of her child care agency through information gathering. Increasingly, she thought it best to gather information in several ways: through statistical data collection, as required by central government; through the internal review system; by reading case files; and, not least, by talking to people.

I also look at process, timescales and the quality of the intervention ... and unless that feeds into future planning it is meaningless ... it is a thermometer, it gives me an idea of how things are going. I use complaints information, the outcomes of inspections and joint review, but I go out and look at case files. I also contact users and try to get some softer feedback, and ask things like 'Do you think you see your social worker often enough?' ... I personally make a point of seeing the worker and getting their view on the case. What you hear from people is very different from what you read, and you get a rounder picture ... it is important to collect personal feedback, so they don't think they are just inspected and monitored.

(Manager consultations)

The area this manager was speaking about was listed in the government's top ten best performing authorities in 2001 and 2002.

Key points

- Managers, service users and practitioners all benefit if they have good information to evaluate services.

- The measurement of services against centrally defined indicators is now expected. This is another source of pressure for managers.

- Computerised records can help with the tasks of recording and monitoring services but using computer systems is not always straightforward.

- Managers need the ability to understand and use information in context to evaluate services.

- Numbers alone give only a partial picture of the service; other sources of information such as local networks and service user groups remain essential.

8.4   The management information system

The information agenda

Since the 1990s managers in health, education and care may have experienced requests for information as a 'top-down' process. In all the countries of the UK the government has driven developments in gathering information. However, the system only works well if it is fed regular, careful, routine recording of information by workers. The returns that are sent via managers to the government are simply an aggregation of information that is routinely recorded. Its accuracy depends on frontline managers and practitioners seeing the meaning and purpose of doing it. If this recording is inaccurate or omitted, the information given to central government and senior managers will be wrong. The system therefore only works well if it is as much 'bottom-up' as it is 'top-down'.

The Referrals, Assessments and Packages of Care (RAP return) is an example from adults' care services (Department of Health, 1999a). This information is collected and sent to central government (returned) by local authorities in England. A similar system exists in Scotland and Northern Ireland and is being developed in Wales. The information required is the numbers of adults who make contact with social services and receive advice, a basic service or referral for assessment. It is a way of collecting statistics to measure how teams and authorities are working. It is based on practice activity and can also be used for collecting an agency's own statistics.

This method of gathering information depends on a duty worker receiving and recording the referral. If a modern database is used, the referral can be recorded directly on to the system, so that if the person is referred again, data can be found directly on the system without repeatedly inputting facts such as name, address and date of birth. Frontline managers can use the data input to look at the amounts of work coming in. They can check how many urgent referrals have been taken on a particular morning or print out more detailed information about all referrals in the previous week. This instant monitoring of workload can assist managers' operational planning although, as discussed earlier, it can easily become a tool for management surveillance.

Middle managers receive information about relative workloads across their department and see regular weekly or monthly updates. Planners and senior managers receive the same information about requests for assistance and compare this with measures of need across the authority. Some groups of similar authorities have formed benchmarking groups to compare data between themselves. Senior managers should make the outcomes available to frontline managers, who can then see more clearly whether activities in their agency are part of a wider trend. The benefits are that resource allocation can become more strategic across an area.

While there are benefits from management information systems, they are far from unproblematic for frontline managers. Apart from the additional workload involved in making sure staff can operate the system, and are using it, managers have questioned the categories by which service users are assessed, arguing that people do not neatly fit the given descriptions, and may perhaps fit several. For some managers, categorising individuals by age or service received does not accord with the values of putting people first that permeate the care services. For example, one manager commented during an online discussion:

> While I appreciate the need for records to be kept, there is a degree to which individual people are constructed as 'service users' by the use of these labels. This destroys the individuality of their need and makes a mockery of the value intentions of a 'needs-led' service for community care.

Frontline managers may find that data give them evidence to argue for resources to meet a particular local need. The performance indicator that asks social workers to record the educational attainments of care leavers draws a national picture of the educational attainment of care leavers. It also draws attention to the needs of individuals for support in education, and it can be used to provide evidence of need by managers seeking educational resources for young people.

The management information system, used well, can be a tool for providing information relevant to the roles of staff in different layers of large organisations such as health and social services. If the information for RAP returns, for example, is entered as a routine part of recording new referrals, by the time it becomes necessary to produce the figures for central government, all that is required is a higher-level aggregation of the data. The information has already been useful for evaluation and planning by operational and strategic managers in the organisation.

Integrating case information and data collection

In the past it was mostly administrators who used computer systems in care organisations. Information was entered on paper case files and data were entered into the computer later. Now that practitioners can enter data directly, a middle stage of work is removed. The computer system itself becomes the source of case information, as Figure 8.1 illustrates.

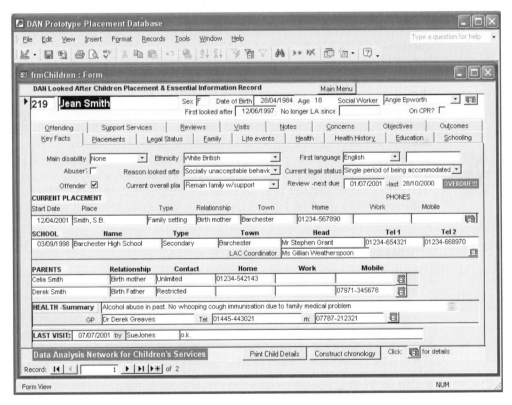

Figure 8.1   **Screenshot of Data Analysis Model for Children's Services (Wales)**
(Source: Gatehouse, 2001, p. 42)

If paper copies are needed, they can be printed out. If other information needs recording, it can be added and repetitive recording is avoided. The development of systems that allow the database to be the casework record means the amount of data stored electronically is growing. Once stored in this way, information becomes immediately available for further analysis. At the heart of practice in care services there is a narrative, and the recording system needs to be capable of reflecting this.

The use of computer systems as the main case-recording tool need not leave practitioners feeling they are simply data processors because the system relies heavily on their professional skills of accuracy in recording to be useful. Breaking down a referral into several key issues, with a brief narrative associated, develops it into a better tool for storing both commentary and decisions. Practitioners may find the task of inputting data more relevant to their work if more attention is paid to giving them feedback via outputs from the system. The tendency to see databases as 'information sinks' (Gatehouse, 2001), where data are entered but the outcome is not fed back (disaggregated) to teams, means practitioners may lack the incentive to put valuable information into the system.

In the past, service users have suffered because information recorded about them has been irrelevant and inaccurate or because their life stories have not been carefully recorded and stored. When workers seeking information about individuals' histories have access to paper records, they are often incomplete and unreliable. Sometimes workers have moved on and information carried in their heads has not been recorded. A computerised system alone cannot remove human error or poor practice. Used well, programs that provide workers with prompts and frameworks to structure information and remind them of what to record can benefit service user, practitioner and manager alike. Records built up over the years from many small entries can become very significant later. This is particularly relevant for individuals who require information about their origins. Example 8.2 illustrates that systems need to take account of this need.

EXAMPLE 8.2 Seeking information

Many people who were in care, but not adopted, know little of their past or how to find out about it ... there are few services to cater for them ...

While it might take an hour for some adopted people to go through their records, someone in care may be presented with the accumulated evidence of 18 years: school reports, parents' letters, and correspondence between the agency and the various homes where the person lived ...

Adopted people want to search for their birth families and the discovery of information is secondary; people who have been in care primarily seek information.

(Source: adapted from Philpot, 2002, pp. 32–3)

People who want information about themselves from years ago need it to be accurate and accessible. The use of technology for recording cannot be just an 'add-on' to the care task. Practitioners and service users already have easier access to information technology, and electronic records are likely to become the most usual form of recording. The introduction of remote devices, linked to an agency's database, could enable assessment information to be recorded while meeting service users in their homes. This would make the process more open and transparent for the service user, as they could check the accuracy of the record immediately.

There is a power issue here, concerning who has access to computers and electronic records, and who is excluded. Arguably, if service users have electronic access to information about themselves, this has the potential for improving equality and accessibility. Developments designed to improve people's access to their records, by providing access to computers, are happening in some areas. This is an essential advance, without which there will not be equality of access. Stoke-on-Trent Links is a project to provide access to internet services for the poorest people in the community (Department of Health, 2001c). More councils will need to take steps like this to counteract the 'digital divide' through the provision of technology to improve access for service users.

Outputs from information systems

Information can be produced from modern databases in a variety of ways; the detail varies depending on the particular software. Standard letters and forms can usually be produced from a system, which can make it seem more manager- and practitioner-friendly. When a request for a service is received by an agency, and the practitioner receiving it records it on the information system, a letter of acknowledgement can be produced at the touch of a button. Further, a standard letter offering an appointment can be sent out and a referral form produced. Of course, standard letters are not substitutes for personal responses where needed, or careful, detailed replies to complaints. If an assessment of need has to be considered by an allocation panel, requests to the panel can be made electronically, or as a print-out, very quickly. No additional forms need to be completed by the practitioner. Also, the effectiveness of the panel's decisions can be monitored from information input after meetings. In the past, reports were produced centrally by administrative staff.

Modern software enables frontline managers to retrieve information directly from the system to gain a current picture of activity in specific areas of work. For example, a manager could check that information is being consistently recorded about the ethnic origin of looked-after children by producing a list of cases where this had not been done. This information could be produced on a regular basis and sent to each of the practitioners concerned. The manager could easily check later whether practitioners had responded to the request to record the data.

Timeliness of information

A computer database can increase the regularity of feedback on what is happening in practice. Central returns are usually produced annually. By the time information is collected locally, sent to the central agency, collated again, analysed and published, it might already be six months old. It is then not updated for another year. As a result, the published information could be anything between six and 18 months old, and so possibly less useful to practitioners, especially if the situation has changed significantly in the meantime. Large retail organisations with many outlets download sales information for the day, analyse it overnight, and make comparisons early the next day. This kind of immediacy may not be relevant to care but it is an interesting example of what can be done.

There is no technical reason why central government departments could not increase the frequency with which they collect and share information. If they did, local authorities could receive comparative information to act on in their daily management of services. The effects of policy changes would also be apparent more quickly. The importance of more timely information is that, first, it provides the opportunity to refine the models for collecting data. Second, if information is analysed quickly, the feedback given to practitioners is more relevant to current practice. As suggested earlier, regular useful feedback about practice would help practitioners to see the usefulness of inputting data. Shifts in patterns of service delivery, changing patterns of need and the increasing failure to meet standards are examples where, at a unit or an authority level, timely reporting can give managers an opportunity to respond. It may be no good knowing what happened 18 months ago!

Standardisation of practice

Standardisation is a central government concern and a local issue too, authorities being keen to avoid wide local variations in the experiences of service users. Frontline managers may experience a tension between equity and sensitivity to local need. Standard processes perhaps can only be established against a backdrop of how tasks are done on a day-to-day basis, and of professional values and practices. Legal requirements may drive developments in certain directions. When the NHS and Community Care Act was implemented in 1991, social services departments were reorganised into purchaser and provider arrangements because of the way the legislation had been drafted. It required local authorities to make a distinction between the assessment of people's needs and the provision of services to meet those needs.

For provider agencies, the standardisation agenda has created dilemmas. For example, projects have been set up and funded with value bases and service objectives that may differ from those of commissioning agencies. Current innovative projects may not be entirely in tune with centrally defined performance measures. If providers want to attract the funding of commissioning agencies, which have to meet central government agendas, they may have to adapt and change.

Voluntary organisations may find it difficult to maintain their campaigning activities. Community development work with politically active groups may have a campaigning element. Such work will not meet the funding objectives of statutory providers of money, who exclude all campaigning and prioritise high levels of dependency. The same is true of charitable trusts, so the only possible source of funding may be individual donations and sponsorship in order to maintain existing services and continue the campaigning. Standardisation through management information systems can offer commissioning agencies some benefits. However, if the criteria for allocating resources are too standardised, it can stifle local innovation and take support away from some voluntary sector and service user-led projects.

Key points

- Once information is stored on a central database, the potential for extracting useful information quickly and cheaply is increased.

- Information from computer systems can help frontline managers and their staff better if it fits with the ways practitioners work and what managers need to know.

- If frontline managers can use such information to argue for increased resources, it will benefit service users and workers.

- While standardisation might disempower small agencies, direct access to records could empower service users.

8.5   Joined-up thinking

The introduction of separate assemblies for Scotland, Wales and Northern Ireland means the traditional links between some of the central government returns have been broken. Scotland has always had its own legal system and different styles of service and methods of central returns. Wales has had its own central reporting system, but in many respects this has followed the line of the Department of Health. Central reporting in England has been primarily via the Department of Health, although increasingly there are reporting requirements from the Audit Commission

and other central government bodies. The Audit Commission has also
been the lead agency in developing the method of joint review in England
and Wales. Scotland and Northern Ireland have their own Audit Offices.

Attempts have been made to develop common performance indicators
for the same areas of work, but as yet there is no consistency and there
have been variations in the definitions used. From a single authority
perspective this involves duplication of effort; at a central agency level it
leads to incompatibility of data. There are also issues concerning the
sharing of specific information about individuals. The Youth Offending
Teams in England and Wales have representatives from existing agencies –
social services, education, police, health and others – all working together
to reduce how often young people offend. If information from each
organisation is pooled, there are implications. For example, should a
police officer have access to health information about the service users
attending a unit for drug users? Similarly, the development of care plan
approaches in mental health involves medical staff and care practitioners
working jointly.

Winchester (2001, p. 20) raises some concerns about confidentiality,
saying 'it's always difficult to balance the service user's right to privacy and
an agency's right to access confidential information to do its job.' She
wonders whether the Health and Social Care Act 2001 tips the balance too
far against service users in that it allows information held by GPs to be
accessed by the Secretary of State for Health and by any organisation he or
she sees fit. Most people would expect what they told a GP to go no further
than the consulting room. Changes in legislation, and the move to close
collaborative working between care agencies, require careful thought
about what kind of information exchange is permissible, and have led to
the development of protocols and policies. In practice this can be complex
for managers. In Example 8.3 a manager outlines some of his experience of
sharing information between agencies.

EXAMPLE 8.3 Information sharing in adults' services

Sharing information between agencies is potentially one of the most
complex issues we've faced and I don't think anyone has all the answers.

You can spend years and years devising policy documents about
information sharing.

The whole concept of partnership is about improving the service to the
service user. If we ask service users, when we are carrying out an assessment,
something like 'Would you be happy for me to share this information with a
colleague who works for whatever organisation, so that they can help you
get access to X?', I think the majority of people will say yes, rather than be
assessed again by that other person.

We're making it a bit more complicated by trying to devise an all-singing,
all-dancing agreement between the agencies at the outset.

Shared information systems have probably been my biggest nightmare. We can get people working together, we can get them into buildings, we can hopefully devise single assessments, we can hopefully devise a way that the person can get the service they need through this partnership, but can we heck as like get a joint system?

We've got three health trusts on our patch and one social services department. All use completely different systems of recording information, all of whom put large investment into it, none of whom want to give up their system. How do you resolve that? In one authority they've got dual entry. They're putting all the information on to the social services system, and then putting it all on to the health system, and the workers are getting really fed up because they have to do it twice.

What you really need is one system that everyone's signed up to. But they've invested – you think of Social Services Information Database. We all think it's brilliant, don't we? And I guess the health people feel the same about their system ... so I don't know!

(Source: manager consultations)

This example shows some of the complexities for a manager who is committed to working towards the best for his service users and staff. He may be right that the most straightforward action is to put decisions about 'who is to know' in the hands of service users. Even that becomes more complex when decisions about risk and safety are involved, and managers have to consider 'who needs to know'. In Example 8.4 a children's services manager explains some complex issues which arose from new procedures to safeguard children. These were in response to the requirement to work together with other agencies.

EXAMPLE 8.4 Information sharing in children's services

What is evident is that if you formally say this is a child protection issue to another agency, they need to disclose information. If what you are doing is contacting another agency about anything else, they are not supposed to give you information without the user's consent. That is a particular issue, especially at a time when all our assessments are supposed to start with the assessment of the child as in need of support. So you don't always start out thinking this is an inquiry about significant harm [the Children Act 1989, section 47]. Halfway through the work it might change, then agencies have a duty to disclose information with or without parental consent.

We would always want parental consent, and if agencies ring up we say 'Have you talked to the parent? You need to go and get permission from the parent before you refer this child.'

There are some instances, and I think these are the easier ones (in information terms), such as sexual abuse, where you may want information without parents being told.

The Data Protection Act and the Human Rights Act impinge on some of our work here; it's complex.

Individuals may use the Human Rights Act to take action against local authorities to argue things weren't done well, and it is possible to feel incapacitated by that.

We have had to write a range of protocols to accompany the new procedures and one is about information sharing. Another one is about having shared understandings about what is a section 47 inquiry under the Children Act 1989 [possible significant harm] rather than work under section 17 [support for a child in need]. That's the first time we have put those kinds of things down on paper. They are multi-agency and it's about sharing and good practice.

Increasingly, we define what people do, and the protocols are an example, as is our guidance. Never before have we put down on paper how social workers prioritise, but in some ways the more you define it the harder it gets. The question then is how much do you erode social work judgement as you define more and more on what basis people make assessments? Managers need to communicate these things through supervision and team meetings, and help staff through phenomenal changes in the role.

(Source: manager consultations)

Another issue in obtaining consent is making sure that people have the opportunity to express their views. Involving a person with learning difficulties effectively in a decision necessitates using a variety of ways of communicating (Edge, 2001). People need both good support and the right opportunities to make informed decisions. Practitioners have to be sure that communication is happening, and to understand people's worlds so as to create more opportunity for choices.

Key points

- Working in partnership presents new issues about information sharing.

- Protocols alone will not resolve the issues if they are not accompanied by sensitive practice in relation to complex matters such as informed consent.

8.6 Data protection

Data held in single agencies and across disciplines have to be relevant and accurate. The early implementation of data protection principles often removed opinion from case records, but opinion may be recorded if it is identified and evidenced. If the implementation of data protection principles has driven unsubstantiated opinion from the record, it has achieved a significant benefit for service users. An increasing reliance on electronic records means as much attention must be paid to the accuracy, completeness and relevance of electronic records as there was for paper records. The Data Protection Act 1998 consolidates the legal regulation of the storage and transmission of data held in three ways:

1 in electronic form, for example, in word-processing or database files
2 in paper filing systems in which specific information about individuals is readily accessible
3 manual data on an accessible public record, which includes manual social work case records.

There can no longer be distinctions between information held in these ways. Manual information can be transferred to an electronic format and, with the increased use of direct input by workers, records that were created manually will in future more often be created electronically. The principles of the Data Protection Act 1998 and their detailed implementation in legal and ethical practice in care work are complex, involving the interplay of social intervention and the rights of the individual. The key ideas and principles for lawful data processing are outlined in Box 8.2 (overleaf).

Two individual rights are paramount with respect to social care information held by public authorities and their voluntary and private associates.

1 *The right of access:* the right to know what is written about you in a record held by a social care authority. The right to check that it is accurate and fair.
2 *The right to confidentiality:* the right to expect that other people do not have unwarranted access to information held about you.

BOX 8.2 Principles of data protection

The rules

Anyone processing personal data must comply with the eight enforce-able principles of good practice. They say that data must be:

- fairly and lawfully processed

- processed for limited purposes

- adequate, relevant and not excessive

- accurate

- not kept longer than necessary

- processed in accordance with the data subject's rights

- secure

- not transferred to countries without adequate protection.

Personal data covers both facts and opinions about the individual. It also includes information regarding the intentions of the data controller towards the individual, although in some limited circumstances exemptions will apply. With processing, the definition is far wider than before. For example, it incorporates the concepts of 'obtaining', 'holding' and 'disclosing'.

(The full explanation of the principles can be found on the Information Commission website.)

(Source: Information Commission, 2002)

The right of access

With certain exemptions, discussed below, any living person about whom information is held by a social care authority has the right of access to that information. This includes facts, opinions and the intentions of the authority in relation to that person. With care information, there may be the complication that information about people other than the subject of the record is held on the file. This reflects the complexity of care situations. Generally, a person cannot see what is written about someone else without that person's consent. However, if consent is withheld, the 'controller' of the record must make it possible for the subject to see as much information as they are seeking without revealing the third person's identity. This restriction is not absolute. The Data Protection Act 1998 recognises that occasions may arise when it is 'reasonable in all the circumstances' to reveal information about a third person, particularly if they are a source of recorded information about the subject of the record. These are fine, sensitive judgements that must be made about individual cases. Other information in case records is exempt from disclosure and may be withheld when someone requests access to their record. These exemptions are quite tightly prescribed and cover the following circumstances:

- when the information is being used to prevent or detect crime
- when disclosure of information to the subject would prejudice social work by causing harm to the physical or mental health of the subject or another person
- when the information concerns the subject's physical or mental health and an appropriate health professional has not consented to disclosure
- when other legislation prevents disclosure, for example that associated with adoption.

Each of these circumstances is dealt with in the Act or an associated statutory order.

A consequence of developments in another technology – embryology – has produced some very complex ethical dilemmas about access to information and confidentiality, as Example 8.5 indicates.

EXAMPLE 8.5 A conflict of interests?

The rights of individuals to find out about their origins is one that has begun to establish itself slowly. The legal right of adopted people to trace their birth relatives has existed since 1975, but other groups, such as those who have been in local authority care, have no parallel right in law to find out about their pasts.

Another group on whom the spotlight has recently fallen comprises children born through donor-assisted conception, for whom there is actually a legal prohibition on access to information about their origins. Speakers at a conference on donor conception ... argued that children conceived by this method should be told as early as possible ... the identity of the sperm donor concerned. Even Baroness Warnock, whose 1984 report led to the Human Fertilisation and Embryology Act 1990 which protects the anonymity of sperm donors, admitted that she had changed her mind.

(Source: *Community Care*, 2002a, p. 5)

One person's right to access information has to be balanced with the right of another – the sperm donor – to confidentiality about their identity. The 1990 legislation to protect donors conflicts with the right of a child to know their biological origins. The issues of protected data also go beyond recording systems to professional judgements about balancing one person's right of access with another's right to confidentiality.

The right of confidentiality

Electronic systems can hold detailed information about individuals which can be extracted to compile lists of people who share characteristics. These can be anonymised but unique identifiers may remain. Aggregated data may be extracted for analytical purposes so that only numbers and characteristics appear without any individual data being revealed. This may be beneficial if, for example, information obtained about ethnicity shows that a particular group is not receiving an equitable service and action follows to provide this. However, the opportunity to misuse information still exists, and some people argue that the routine collection of sensitive data is not good practice.

The Data Protection Act 1998 is there primarily to ensure that the confidentiality of information is respected with regard to the purpose for which it was collected and that it is not misused. It is sometimes represented as prohibiting data-sharing generally. There are many statutory prohibitions to the disclosure of information – for example, the confidentiality associated with adoption – but limitations on data sharing are as much about a cultural unwillingness to share across departmental boundaries as they are about statutory restrictions. There is indeed a sense that information is power and that, if you share it, you lose some of your power.

Key points

- Databases are a crucial tool for modern managers. However, the rights of the individual to confidentiality must be considered paramount.

- The Data Protection Act 1998 is not a barrier to transmitting data for legitimate social care goals, but it does impose a discipline in the matter of individual privacy and dignity.

8.7 Conclusion

New technologies in health and social care services are having an impact on frontline managers' activities in all sectors. The key questions for managers are:

- What do I need to know to be able to do my job better?
- What kind of working systems will enable this?
- What are the practice implications of using data to inform our service, our service users and our other partners?

When information systems are implemented well, ready access to useful, relevant, timely information can assist frontline managers greatly in their day-to-day jobs. Data collection depends on practitioners being confident and competent about recording the required data on the system. The relationship between manager and staff, levels of trust, and an ability to discuss tasks openly affect whether the use of information and new technology is viewed as a creative practice and learning tool or, as Harris (1998) and Lyon (2001) suggest, as a means of managerial surveillance of workers and citizens.

Returns to central government also depend on accurate practice information. While the data collection agenda is driven from the top down by central government, its success and relevance to practice depend on a bottom-up response, where practitioners engage with a systems approach to recording. Practice by care agencies can have unintended consequences and without detailed information this cannot be easily identified. A practice-led approach to information recording and use means practitioners and their managers can work to ensure that the information produced assists the tasks they have to achieve.

For service users this may be a mixed blessing. While immediate access to records can be empowering, it is easy for the interests of service users to be secondary to the requirements to respond to central government requests for data.

The power of modern technology, and its use in organisations, means that the risk of getting lost in a welter of information is high. On a positive note, there is now a potential to develop sophisticated and comprehensive models of data collection which give an accurate picture of the workings of an organisation.

However, it is important that:

- the information obtained fits the practice environment
- the information gathered supports service development for service users
- there are safeguards to ensure that service users' rights under the Data Protection Act 1998 are protected.

With these requirements met, managers and their staff can perhaps use new technologies to benefit service users.

Chapter 9
Managing to protect

Hilary Brown with Janet Seden

9.1 Introduction

In this chapter we explore the role of managers in protecting children and adults who may be vulnerable to abuse. The manager's role in these circumstances is a complex one because it involves managing at the interface between the interests of many agencies and considering the competing interests of a diverse range of people. Therefore, the approach taken here is to explore some issues and principles of legal mandates and practice situations and the underlying themes and concerns in a way that marks out the territory and maps the areas of responsibility managers have to engage with. In this contested space, which managers occupy because of their position in the agency, there are no simple rights and wrongs. The legal mandate may be clear but the actual interpretation and practice processes that managers oversee are as varied and diverse as the situations of the people with whom they are concerned.

A differentiating feature of being a manager rather than a practitioner or a key worker is the level of responsibility. In some settings managers are at a distance from the main events, relying on what they are told by other people and assessing the accuracy and usefulness of that information. Managers in residential and day care settings are at the centre of both the practice activity and the management responsibility. Most managers have the task of gaining an overview, weighing the information they have, making decisions about the nature and level of interventions with service users, and considering their own ability to be objective, ethical and accountable.

Decision making in social care is practice-led and not simply driven by procedures. Therefore, this chapter cannot offer a set of rules and guidelines about decisions (see Chapter 1). Moreover, if you are a manager, you want to work in a disciplined way, with proper grounds based on knowledge and using evidence to back up your professional judgements. It takes courage to make your best decisions and stick to them.

Managers have a vital part to play, whether that part is small or large. Managing particular inputs to the process of protecting people is as important as it is difficult: as many actors say, it is the 'bit parts' that often demand the most skill and the best sense of timing. Some managers have to support the person who is centre stage without getting in their way or treading on their toes. It is also tough when *the manager* is centre stage and co-ordinating others to make a decision that can have very far-reaching consequences in the lives of service users.

This aims of this chapter are to:

- consider the complex role of managers in protecting both children and adults
- explore how issues of abuse and vulnerability interact
- discuss the role of the manager in working with several agencies in protection cases.

9.2   The manager's responsibilities

The responsibilities of managers depend on the setting: whether it is commissioning or providing, in the statutory or voluntary sector, with adults and/or children. In 2000 the Department of Health introduced a statutory framework for vulnerable adults called *No Secrets*, in which local authorities are directed to co-ordinate work across all relevant agencies. One requirement is that they must clarify the 'role, responsibility, authority and accountability' of everyone involved in the protection of vulnerable adults. This parallels the requirements of *Working Together to Safeguard Children* (Department of Health *et al.*, 1999).

The mandate managers hold on behalf of children is arguably less ambiguous than that for adults. The state has a duty to protect all citizens and, as part of that, to intervene when any child is at risk of significant harm. The powers and duties of local authorities in England and Wales are prescribed in the Children Act 1989, where the twin aims of meeting children's needs and safeguarding them from harm are seen as two sides of the same coin. 'Safeguarding and promoting children's welfare' are intertwined principles that underpin the structure and philosophy of the Act (Department of Health, 2001a, p. 41). This is a mandate to act positively to intervene where any child has an identified need for support, to attain reasonable health and development and to protect them from any significant harm. The Children (Scotland) Act 1995 and the Children (Northern Ireland) Order 1995 embrace similar philosophies for safeguarding and meeting need.

For most adults, however, action is retrospective, through the criminal justice system and a mixture of mainstream legislation. The guidance, which requires local authorities to protect adults, refers only to people who are deemed to be particularly 'vulnerable' on account of older age and mental or physical impairment. While children are deemed 'vulnerable' because of the failure of the environment or care givers to provide for their proper development to adulthood, adults often view the label 'vulnerable adult' as a mixed blessing, fearing it may undermine the more positive attitudes and identities they have carved out for themselves. Children and young people who are caring for their parents and contribute to supporting their families would also see themselves as having strengths. They may not wish to be labelled as 'vulnerable'.

Although social services are responsible for co-ordination, protection is a multi-agency responsibility. Managers in different agencies therefore have different roles. They may be responsible at different stages and for different components of the process. Taking a chronological view, managers from a range of agencies play a part in:

- promoting good practice as a way of preventing abuse or neglect
- picking up early signs that all is not well and passing them on to appropriate agencies
- investigating concerns and assessing the needs of individuals who have been abused or whose care is not meeting their needs adequately
- acting on these assessments to provide services or treatment to people who have been harmed
- taking action against a service or an individual if the investigation has uncovered a criminal offence, breach of professional standards or culpably negligent service.

A diagram showing the numbers of staff involved at each stage looks top-heavy (see Figure 9.1 overleaf). It is wide at the top to show that all social care staff have a responsibility for prevention and channelling concerns into appropriate referrals. These pass through a narrow neck where more specialist staff take on the role of assessment and then investigation. The diagram widens out again to include different professional groups who take action to put things right or apply sanctions where these are thought necessary. At the widest point, where most people are involved, there is the greatest scope for ambiguity. This is the point at which managers pick up concerns from the review of case files, or because they witness glimpses of poor parenting or negligent practice, or sift through worrying impressions and information presented to them in supervision sessions.

Within this framework managers have different functions across a wide spectrum of activity. Their role may be to run high-quality services that promote good practice and avoid insensitive or institutionalised regimes (stages 1, 2 and 3 in Figure 9.1). They may be in charge of a team responsible for assessment and investigation (stage 4). They could be responsible for legal actions and/or prosecutions (stage 5) or for post-assessment services (stage 6). Managers might be involved at several or all of these stages.

Some managers may have responsibilities towards one particular party in a situation. The police deal more closely with a potential perpetrator, while social workers or care managers take a direct interest in assessing the needs of a vulnerable person. Others manage overall services rather than individual situations, for example through commissioning, policy

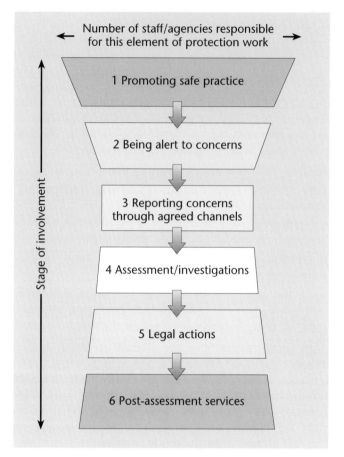

Figure 9.1   **A model for responsibilities to protect**

development or regulatory activity. All of these elements need to fit together; therefore, all managers have to be aware of the point at which they need to hand over to someone else whose job it is to take action or bring relevant agencies together.

Pressures on managers

Managing these tasks is no different from other forms of partnership working. It can feel more pressured because any newspaper on a particular day is likely to report the fall-out from complex cases and difficult decisions. At the heart of managers' efforts to protect are fundamental dilemmas. In relation to children, there are complementary duties to intervene to prevent harm to a child, while at the same time trying to respect the integrity of the family and support the parents (Department of Health, 2001a). In relation to vulnerable adults, there is a tension between respecting autonomy and acting to promote welfare (Preston-Shoot, 2001). Most managers have concerns and anxieties about balancing factors in complex situations.

These responsibilities go with the territory of managing, where the context can be one of raised emotions, difficult judgements, complex communication across family and agency boundaries and the risk of media scrutiny if things go wrong (Ayre, 2003). The resulting heightened anxiety is very understandable but may be counterproductive, leading to paralysis and prevarication rather than prompt consultation and decision making:

> In a number of instances, when professionals visited the home to assess a parent who was displaying evidence of irrational thought process and unpredictable behaviour, concerns about the child's safety became obscured by their primary focus on the parent's psychiatric diagnosis. It was as though their capacity to think about the safety of the child had become paralysed as a result of preoccupations about the parent.
>
> (Reder and Duncan, 1999, p. 97)

Also, not everyone has the same stake in bringing issues of protection out into the open. In a commercial market of social care there are powerful interests which sometimes work against openness.

Clarifying principles

In this chapter we take the view that to be a confident manager in this arena you need to be *sure of your ground*. This means knowing the principles you use to arrive at difficult decisions and being prepared to share and stand by them. If contributing to child or adult protection processes were a mathematical equation, it would mean 'showing your workings' in the margin, so that you could justify the route you took and the answer you arrived at. Your ability to make decisions (and manage) will depend on your grasp of the issues and the needs of participants. In the next section we explore some terms and the different ways of understanding them. You cannot assume that another person will necessarily share your particular concerns and understandings.

Words such as 'vulnerable', 'risk' and 'abuse' do not have fixed or uncontested meanings. Child abuse is defined by different societies in different ways (Seden, 1995). Not long ago in the UK the physical chastisement of a child was seen as an adult's right to discipline rather than an act of physical abuse. Being sure of your ground means taking account of a range of views, understanding the reasons for different ways of seeing things, and having the ability to make professional judgements in the light of the agency's legal responsibilities and partnership obligations. It means being able to give a clear account of the reasons for taking actions within this framework of responsibilities.

> **Key points**
>
> • Responsibilities for protection are an integral part of a manager's role in health and social care.
>
> • Being sure of their ground can enable managers to feel more confident about complex actions and decisions.

9.3   The interaction between abuse and vulnerability

The term 'abuse' is controversial and so is the concept of 'vulnerability'. They are both used very loosely in conversation, while they are cited in official documents to mean something very specific. Not all 'vulnerable' people are at risk of 'abuse' and not all 'abused' people are 'vulnerable'. It helps to start by being clear about how these words are used both informally and formally, and how the two concepts interact. Managers in agencies involved with children, young people and vulnerable adults are all concerned about service users' safety and the need to pass on their concerns in a timely way. They need a broad understanding of the roots of bad practice and abusive relationships, and to be clear about when their concerns should be acted on.

Abuse and the risk of downplaying harm

The term 'abuse' is used to cover many kinds of harmful actions and failures to act in a range of circumstances: it is used to refer to abuse *by* an individual or an agency. It includes abuse *of* a person's human rights, and abuse of a *position of trust* when a relationship that is supposed to work in a vulnerable person's interests is corrupted. The word 'abuse' tends to be applied only to people who are seen as disadvantaged and, perhaps because of that, it can seem to disguise the severity of violent or criminal acts perpetrated against them: for example, when the term 'sexual abuse' is used instead of 'rape' or 'financial abuse' instead of 'theft'. This may have the effect of minimising the *impact* of any harmful acts and thereby undermines a person's right to support and redress. This is the case when the criminal justice system does not allow evidence to be heard from vulnerable witnesses, or when children or adults who cannot make their feelings heard are assumed to be untouched by acts that would horrify other people.

Shared risks

Different terminology can obscure the fact that vulnerable people are at risk in the same ways as all citizens. Everyone is a potential victim of personal and sexual violence in their home and community. There is an argument that 'ordinary' crimes of sexual and personal violence should not be included in a systematic definition of abuse as they are not a product of the victim's vulnerability or the social care system. However, often the distinction is not clear cut and vulnerable victims of crime may have needs in common with people abused within their families or service settings. Policy frameworks (for example, Department of Health, 2000c) apply regardless of who perpetrates the abuse. Therefore, although different dynamics arise depending on the relationship between the abused person and the person responsible for the abuse, there is a common framework for shared decision making and care planning. This should augment the input of mainstream agencies and facilitate access to redress.

A mandate to protect children and vulnerable adults

A baseline provided by the Human Rights Act 1998 is shown in Box 9.1. There are rights that each citizen is entitled to have upheld: that is, *upheld*, as opposed to stepping in after damage has been caused. This is an active way of framing the responsibilities of social care agencies.

BOX 9.1 Key rights and entitlements from the Human Rights Act 1998

- Right to life
- Prohibition of torture
- Prohibition of slavery or forced labour
- Right to liberty and security
- Right to a fair trial
- No punishment (or detention) without law
- Right to respect for private and family life
- Freedom of thought, conscience and religion
- Freedom of expression
- Freedom of assembly and association
- Right to marry

- Right to an effective remedy

- Prohibition of discrimination

The prohibition of discrimination is backed up by a protocol that outlaws discrimination on the grounds of disability.

The Committee on the Prohibition of Torture and Inhuman Treatment also sets out the right to independent and equivalent health care to anyone in any form of detention, whether formal such as a prison or a psychiatric hospital, or informal such as a residential home or supported housing project.

(Source: adapted from the Human Rights Act 1998)

The mandate to intervene in relation to specific categories of abuse is set out in detailed legislation and guidance. For example, in England *No Secrets* defines abuse as it relates to vulnerable adults. Its definition of types of abuse is summarised in Box 9.2.

BOX 9.2 Types of abuse

Physical abuse, including hitting, slapping, pushing, kicking, misuse of medication, restraint, or inappropriate sanctions.

Sexual abuse, including rape and sexual assault or sexual acts to which the vulnerable adult has not consented, or could not consent or was pressured into consenting.

Psychological abuse, including emotional abuse, threats of harm or abandonment, deprivation of contact, humiliation, blaming, controlling, intimidation, coercion, harassment, verbal abuse, isolation or withdrawal from services or supportive networks.

Financial or material abuse, including theft, fraud, exploitation, pressure in connection with wills, property or inheritance or financial transactions, or the misuse or misappropriation of property, possessions or benefits.

Neglect and acts of omission, including ignoring medical or physical care needs, failure to provide access to appropriate health, social care or educational services, the withholding of the necessities of life, such as medication, adequate nutrition and heating.

Discriminatory abuse, including racist, sexist, that based on a person's disability, and other forms of harassment, slurs or similar treatment.

(Source: Department of Health, 2000c, p. 9, para. 2.7)

Looking beyond categories to dynamics

Although these 'categories' and other similar frameworks are a helpful start in describing the nature and extent of abuse, they inevitably provide a fragmented picture. Often several forms of harm occur together in one relationship or setting (Brown and Stein, 1998). Many situations cannot be represented accurately as single incidents or one-off lapses or outbursts, even though this is how they seem in statistics gathered from reports to care agencies. These accounts may obscure the process by which abuse is recognised, often through a gradual accumulation of concerns, with one incident or event triggering the acknowledgement that a threshold has been crossed.

The rules for intervention provide a framework for action, but it is often a matter of judgement to decide when authorities should use them and when concern should begin. Authorities have to interpret when an appropriate threshold has been overstepped. Frequently the decision has to be made before the facts are clear, which is therefore very much a matter of judgement. The criteria for assessing seriousness include the extent of the harm caused, its frequency and duration, its illegality, the intentions of the abuser, and the risk of future abuse to the person or other vulnerable persons (Brown and Stein, 1998). The particular combination will vary.

Harm arises in different contexts and because of a range of factors. Sometimes the abuse comes from an individual abuser's personal problems or learned violence. At other times it stems from ignorance or poor practice. Harm results from a failure to intervene as well as from unnecessary intrusion. It may also arise from structural issues in the way services are offered: for example, from rigid or institutionalised practice, poorly trained and underpaid staff or high staff turnover. Occasionally a person's needs may overwhelm or challenge carers or staff to the point where they cannot manage their own responses or work out what is the best way forward. Any kind of accurate assessment of risks depends on having a map of these dynamics and locating whether the propensity to abuse has arisen as a result of individual, social or structural problems.

Separating assessment of harm from assessment of culpability

Assessing and attributing blame can often draw attention away from the impact of abuse on the vulnerable person, so that serious harm committed by someone who is not seen as culpable – perhaps a stressed carer, an overworked parent or another service user who is considered 'not able to help it' – is written off, as if the harm were cancelled out. Clarity, especially by managers, in separating out issues for the abused and the abusing person is essential to avoid this kind of thinking. Managers faced with unravelling complex issues often take 'time out' to do some thinking and consulting before responding. This kind of immediate strategy is essential, as the actions professionals take immediately either add to or take away from the abuse, and they want their actions to improve service users' experiences.

More contentious forms of harm and inequality

We have argued that definitions are very selective and tend to focus on interpersonal rather than societal issues. There is a broader agenda. Piachaud (2001) focuses on the effects of child poverty and inadequate health provision. He notes that 50,000 children between the ages of eight and ten in Britain have nothing to eat or drink before they go to school. Even those children whose lives are not blighted by poverty are impoverished by advertising, junk food, television, peer pressure, lack of high-quality child care and the stressful working lives of their parents. Moss and Petrie (1996) argue for social policy strategies that support the task of parenting. Given the dominance of commercial pressures and the failure to address poor parenting, physical and cultural environments, Piachaud remarks ruefully that 'it is sad that a real strategy for childhood is thought too difficult or dangerous to merit serious discussion' (2001, p. 451).

The European Disability Forum (1999) emphasises the links between abuse and discrimination for adults with disabilities, including the oppressive attitudes expressed in selective abortion, underemployment of disabled people, lack of access and social exclusion. In relation to vulnerable adults, abuse is tackled outside the mainstream agendas of funding, professional or service regulation and charging for care services. Prioritising different forms of abuse is a political and, some might argue, an expedient way of focusing on a manageable cluster of hazards.

A strategy for safeguarding requires a social policy infrastructure that supports it, as argued by Hardiker *et al.* (2001), who analysed the role of the state in services for children. They mapped involvement at different stages and at different levels and show how authorities which regard their role as residual become involved at a later stage, and only with individuals who have already been damaged. Conversely, authorities that embrace a broader commitment become involved before harm has been done and attempt to influence attitudes across the whole population, to prevent abuse from occurring in the first place.

Vulnerability, frailty or susceptibility?

Managers find that, in practice, abuse and by implication strategies for prevention are usually located at the interface between the harmful act and the vulnerability of the individual. It is important to analyse how this interaction works. In conversation, 'vulnerability' is used to express two separate ideas:

- frailty and liability to be more easily hurt or harmed
- heightened susceptibility to risk and/or harmful events.

Children or adults may be seen as inherently vulnerable and thus more exposed to certain kinds of risk. The association of vulnerability with frailty means that individuals who challenge are often overlooked when it comes to protection, as there is a tendency to operate with a binary view that someone is either dangerous or vulnerable but not both. Hence the protection needs of young people who are homeless or who have been caught up in the criminal justice system, or people whose mental health problems or challenging behaviour present risks to others, may be downplayed or overlooked.

Social factors leading to vulnerability

Vulnerability can also be used as a pretext for paternalistic or patronising interventions. In official documents 'vulnerability' is often a label attached to individuals who fall within particular 'client groups', but not as an indicator of the circumstances which combine to make them vulnerable. It is easy to assume that inexperience, an impairment or frailty in older age lead automatically to vulnerability, without questioning how social inequalities and service structures combine to make people vulnerable in ways that have nothing to do with their individual needs or competence.

Like the social model of disability (Drake, 1999), a 'social' model of vulnerability draws attention away from a person's impairments or difficulties and focuses on the impact of discriminatory responses to their needs. This takes into account the way certain groups are *more* exposed to risk and may be *less* well protected than others. Individuals may only be *vulnerable* to the extent that their rights are not upheld or because they are excluded from, or cannot gain access to, mainstream mechanisms for protection and redress.

This model often underpins the activity of campaigners. Organisations advocating changes in the law about the physical punishment of children point to the inconsistency in allowing more powerful adults to legally assault small children when they would be prosecuted for hitting another adult in a public place. Campaigners for changes in practice relating to domestic violence point out that physical harm inflicted by men on women within the home is less likely to lead to prosecution than corresponding violence between men, say, at a football match. The law is designed to protect public order and not police private relationships even though this leaves more vulnerable people less protected.

Until recently (Home Office, 1998 and 1999) the criminal justice system and arcane courtroom procedures effectively excluded people with learning disabilities, so that crimes against them were less likely to lead to any sanctions or redress. These forms of discrimination *create* vulnerability and reinforce disadvantage.

Double jeopardy and multiple causes of vulnerability

Labelling certain groups as 'vulnerable' may be counterproductive in that it implies risks arise out of their own impairments or difficulties. It also takes the spotlight off the agencies that are supposed to protect them as equal citizens and obscures the extent to which abuse takes place against the backdrop of broader, and often multiple, forms of oppression, exploitation, social injustice and conflict. Girls and women who fall into particular 'client groups' share the disadvantages of all girls and women and they are also disproportionately victims of sexual violence and sexual harassment (Sorheim, 1998). Tilley argues that women with disabilities are doubly affected by stereotypes relating to disability *and* gender so that as women they are 'represented ... as victims, stereotypes of dependence, which reinforces the "sick" role often ascribed to people with disabilities' (1998, p. 89). Women with disabilities who are victims of domestic violence may have fewer avenues for leaving violent relationships, entering refuges or seeking appropriate redress.

Children, elders and adults with disabilities from ethnic minorities can be doubly disadvantaged in their dealings with social and welfare institutions through vulnerability to racially motivated abuse and discrimination. Refugees and asylum seekers also experience these 'extra' disadvantages which, running in parallel, act as multipliers of difficulty (Roberts, 2000; Hermansson *et al.*, 1996). They create a unique identity for individuals with impairments, who may be resisting hostile attitudes within their communities at the same time as struggling with the effects of social and economic discrimination because of racism from the dominant community.

While children can be represented generically as a 'vulnerable' group, they are also disproportionately victims of poverty, affected by violence within and outside the home, exploited as cheap labour and as naïve consumers, and sexualised through pornography. The accumulation of the impact of a range of factors can lead to children needing the safeguarding actions of social care agencies (Bebbington and Miles, 1989). Similar factors can apply to disabled people and older people.

Individual impairment and lack of capacity as contributing factors

None the less, there are individual characteristics that produce particular vulnerabilities: physical illness and frailty, challenging needs and behaviours, and loss all play a part. 'Capacity' is a term for the legally recognised ability of people to make their own decisions, but the law also treats *mental capacity* solely as a characteristic of the individual rather than a product of their circumstances. Psychological assessments focus on the extent of a person's understanding of the issues germane to any specific decision and their ability to make a choice and express their wishes. However, a broader assessment also needs to address the extent to which the person may be pressured or intimidated, or to have been manipulated and exploited, especially by those in familial, authority, care-giving or professional relationships.

The law is a blunt instrument and less able to incorporate these issues. Proposals to change the legal framework in England, Northern Ireland and Wales (there has already been reform in Scotland) focus on removing the idea of a blanket 'capacity' and adopting a more graduated approach. This recognises and supports individuals in taking those decisions they can manage while authorising someone else to act in their best interests over matters that are too complex. Within all jurisdictions, a person's ability to make a reasoned judgement is critical to determining whether some actions or transactions (especially sexual or financial transactions) are abusive or not and therefore central to the assessment process. Such assessments are more challenging in situations where the person's capacity is eroded gradually or fluctuates.

Cumulative factors leading to vulnerability

Hence vulnerability is not usually caused by a single factor such as youth, frailty, disability or mental illness; it is much more likely to occur at the intersection of these factors with other forms of social disadvantage and to be complicated by insensitive or discriminatory service provision. This places 'protection' very much at the same end of the spectrum as other strategies for social inclusion and empowerment: not at the other end, since vulnerability is theorised as a product of discrimination and exclusion and not a personal characteristic. Practice-led managers have to balance this broad understanding with narrower definitions in official documents used to govern when agencies are required or empowered to intervene.

Managers are helped by an awareness of the complexity of concepts such as abuse and vulnerability when monitoring practitioner actions and agreeing service provision. Thinking about risk as a multifaceted concept, based not on single incidents alone but on clusters of factors, is important when managers make decisions about referrals and instigate protective action.

> **Key points**
>
> - Care agencies have a legal mandate to protect certain people. The Human Rights Act 1998 is a positive baseline for intervention.
>
> - Terms such as 'abuse' and 'vulnerability' cover a range of harmful actions and are interactive.
>
> - Harm is a dynamic event: it is the result of both social factors and individual characteristics.

9.4   Managing heightened risks

Vulnerability can lead to a greater risk of abuse (see Chapter 10) and an increased risk of harm from that abuse. In addition to the risk of 'ordinary' crimes (which may not be taken as seriously when the person concerned is in a group without social status), children and vulnerable adults are at risk in 'extra-ordinary' ways. They may be singled out because of their perceived vulnerability or isolation and targeted as potential victims. Abusers sometimes target children; older people can fall prey to financial exploitation. People may be at increased risk as a direct consequence of their use of services or the challenges presented by their impairments. They are also at risk of their needs being ignored or overlooked. Taking each of these eventualities in turn, Figure 9.2 (opposite) starts to develop a map of risk on which to build preventive strategies, risk assessment and multi-agency responses.

Neglect and failure to uphold human rights

Vulnerable people's needs are more likely to be overlooked at an individual and a societal level. In a system that requires people to demand health care or benefits and to campaign for improved provision, those with the quietest voices, and often the most need, get the least. Disabled people are keen to link the protection agenda into the anti-discrimination policies adopted by the European Union (European Disability Forum, 1999). Failure to take up benefits probably causes as much hardship to families and older people as more deliberate forms of financial abuse and yet it might not feature in policies on abuse and vulnerability.

Accessing health care is another area where discriminatory practice can be seen to have significant and sometimes life-limiting effects, as for example in the inquiry into discriminatory decisions about heart surgery

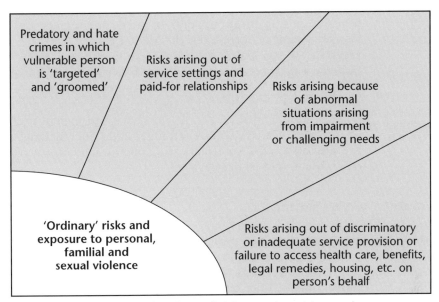

Figure 9.2 **Ordinary and heightened risks to vulnerable people**

for infants with Down's syndrome (Royal Brompton Hospital, 2001). Accessing health care for all people with learning disabilities was prioritised in the White Paper for people with learning disabilities, *Valuing People* (Department of Health, 2001b). So, at one end of the spectrum, the protection agenda merges with the need to redress discriminatory processes and structural inequalities in society. People with learning disabilities *can* make decisions: the automatic assumption that this is not the case is discriminatory.

Abuse in response to challenging needs or difficult decisions

Where rights are compromised necessarily, as for example in control and restraint or detention (under the Mental Health Act 1983), it is vital that decisions are taken transparently with proper processes for review and appeal. Where vulnerable people cannot make decisions for themselves, seek service provision or manage aspects of their affairs, they need special and formal procedures to be in place to manage on their behalf. Decisions may be complex, for example, for an older person who is gradually losing the capacity to manage her own affairs.

Where difficult decisions have to be made, it is important that they are scrutinised impartially. There is often an assumption that informality is best but, when fundamental rights are at stake, formal procedures are likely to provide additional safeguards and should not be avoided. Thus, for example, the sterilisation of girls and women with learning disabilities now triggers an automatic judicial review: far from being a sledgehammer to crack a nut, this provides essential impartiality and protection. Similarly, some actions under the Mental Health Act make it possible to access a second opinion for medical treatment and/or a review of important decisions by a Mental Health Act Review Tribunal.

In England the Care Programme Approach (Department of Health, 1999b) ensures that both risk assessments are carried out and aftercare services are provided for people who have had mental health problems. It provides for systematic arrangements for making assessments, the formation of a care plan, the appointment of a care co-ordinator (key worker) and regular reviews.

Abuse in service settings

There are also very specific risks arising in educational and service provision: for example, bullying at school and institutionalised care practices. Everyone is vulnerable when they surrender themselves to the care of others. A person having an operation would routinely expect that the person operating is capable, has been appropriately trained and supervised, and is regulated and managed. When these systems do not work, it causes a justifiable outcry. Where less formal practices cross social boundaries, as for example when personal and intimate care is involved, it is important that managers of the services create strong cultural norms, through supervision, guidelines and leadership to protect individual dignity. *No Secrets* (Department of Health, 2000c, p. 35, para 7.5) specifically recommends written guidance for staff on:

- challenging behaviour
- personal and intimate care
- physical interventions (control and restraint)
- sexuality
- medication
- handling service users' money
- risk assessment and management.

Guidance may not be enough to prevent poor practice but it creates a benchmark against which standards can be audited and training designed.

Predatory or 'targeted' crime

Even if the criminal justice system develops more robust ways of addressing ordinary crime against children or vulnerable adults, some crimes are *deliberately* targeted at them and require a more rigorous approach. The sexual abuse of children and vulnerable adults (especially adults with learning disabilities) tends to follow a pattern in which the victims are 'targeted' and 'groomed'. They are made to believe that they are 'special' and that the relationship is one of choice. Sexual abuse tends to be serial and gendered (the vast majority of perpetrators are men). The financial abuse of older people may also follow this route, with the perpetrator infiltrating an older person's network and ingratiating him- or herself in order to exploit or defraud them. It is often very difficult to obtain evidence for these crimes or to get successful convictions.

Contested definitions

Managers responding to heightened risks to vulnerable people need to consider all the possible elements arising from the framework in Figure 9.2. Often a provisional decision about whether the risk justifies intervention has to be made on the basis of very limited initial information, before the facts are made known as a result of an investigation. This is often a very delicate judgement for the frontline manager to make.

The definition of abuse may be contested by either the alleged perpetrator and/or the person thought to have been victimised, especially when the definition depends on an assessment of capacity or consent, or when the best interests of the person seem to conflict with their expressed or implied wishes. When the person who is supposed to be the victim contests abuse, it is important to switch the focus to the perpetrator's intent. Helen's situation in Example 9.1 shows this dilemma. Her relationship can be construed as a consenting relationship or as an exploitative one, depending on whether the emphasis is placed on consent or intent.

EXAMPLE 9.1 Helen

Helen is a young woman with moderate learning disabilities living in a sheltered housing project, and receiving some help from staff with shopping and cooking. She became involved in a sexual relationship with a man she met in a local pub who is ten years older than her. After three months the staff were increasingly concerned about his motives and about her welfare within this relationship.

Although the relationship seemed to proceed with her agreement, he gradually took over the management of her bank book and benefits. On several occasions she appeared to have bruises on her arm and he urged her to stop taking her contraceptives. He regularly stole food from the fridges of other residents and, whenever challenged, he had a line of plausible defences, including the fact that the staff were treating Helen like a child just because she has been labelled as having learning disabilities.

On several occasions he took Helen away for a few days. During this time she did not seem to eat any proper meals or have access to a bath or shower. She did not take her medication for epilepsy either. She appeared withdrawn and depressed, despite saying she loved him and did not want anyone to say anything to him.

Much later, as a result of inter-agency consultation, it was discovered that the man was a registered sex offender and that he had targeted other women with learning disabilities in this way before. This accounted for his sophisticated rebuttal of challenges using the jargon of normalisation. The service staff had been very unsure whether they were justified in seeking out additional information at an earlier stage.

A decision to intervene further here would hinge on the seriousness of the risks the staff believed Helen was exposed to. For example, if the man has a history of serious violence towards his previous partners, they might act more forcefully than if they were primarily concerned that he would leave Helen and hurt her emotionally. Any intervention would be considered according to the principle of *proportionality*. Care would be taken not to cause further harm through the processes of intervening. So, as a manager, you might not agree to a serious action over a small risk, but over a significant risk it would be necessary to consider a definitive action; for example in Helen's case, taking out an injunction to keep the man away.

Assessing capacity in context

No Secrets warns that a simple assessment of mental capacity is not enough in such circumstances, and that:

> Assessment of the environment, or context, is relevant, because exploitation, deception, misuse of authority, intimidation or coercion may render a vulnerable adult incapable of making his or her own decisions. Thus, it may be important for the vulnerable adult to be away from the sphere of influence of the abusive person or the setting in order to be able to make a free choice about how to proceed. An initial rejection of help should not always be taken at face value.
>
> (Department of Health, 2000c, p. 11, para 2.16)

Similar dynamics emerge with older people and their finances. For example, an older person might be seriously overcharged for some simple building work, and at face value the transaction may seem to be freely made. Even where formal processes are in place to protect an older person's assets, this cannot rule out the corruption of those systems by individuals who target vulnerable, isolated people and pretend to offer assistance when their agenda is to ingratiate or exploit. As *No Secrets* points out, an initial rejection of help by a person should not always be taken at face value.

McCarthy and Thompson (1994) illustrate how these perspectives should be analysed in the context of the sexual abuse of adults with learning disabilities (Table 9.1), an approach which can also be applied to other situations.

Table 9.1   **Analysing the intention to abuse**

	Intention to abuse	**No intention to abuse**
Experienced as abusive	Abuse	Abuse
Not experienced as abusive	Abuse	Not abuse

(Source: adapted from McCarthy and Thompson, 1994, p. 45)

This model suggests that an act should be construed as abusive if it is *either* intended *or* experienced as such. Therefore, managers have to weigh up the factors carefully before sanctioning protective action.

The key elements to consider when assessing abuse and deciding to intervene are shown in Box 9.3.

BOX 9.3 Factors to consider when protecting people from abuse

- The seriousness of the act

- The person's level of vulnerability

- The person's ability to consent

- The person's rights

- The level of pressure or intimidation

- The likelihood of abuse re-occurring

- The mandate to intervene

Key points

- Risks occur from a cluster of factors, including perpetrators, poor service settings, individual vulnerabilities, and the cumulative impact of disadvantage and discrimination.

- When the person concerned contests the definition of abuse, another layer of complexity is added to the manager's decision about intervention.

- Managers need to weigh up the complex factors carefully when deciding on intervention to protect people from abuse.

9.5 Using theory in practice

So far, the term 'abuse' has been used to refer to a range of different types of harm: harm that is rooted in, and arises out of, different contexts, relationships and structures. Therefore, it is unsurprising that models of prevention are built on different assumptions. Vettenburg (1998, p. 43) comments that 'like violence, "prevention" is a term which has many connotations and therefore needs to be described and defined clearly.'

In Figure 9.1 many managers are concerned to prevent abuse or to pass on concerns promptly to the relevant authorities. To do this they need to be alert to patterns of abuse and abusing and to the different factors that lead to increased risk and less resilience to harm.

Moreover, it is clear from Figure 9.2 that different agencies and professions are responsible for distinct aspects of prevention and that a range of theoretical models are relevant. So how do professionals with divergent orientations and backgrounds use their knowledge to make better decisions than any single person or profession could make in isolation? Do they amalgamate their knowledge, cancel each other out or 'fudge' their differences by focusing exclusively on producing pragmatic plans of action that are not based on any specific analysis of risk?

Quigley (2001, p. 6) argues that most abuse in care settings is not caused by 'bad apples' but by systemic problems in delivering high-quality care. Adherence to more simplistic individual explanations leads to an over-reliance on punitive responses such as disciplinary hearings, dismissals and tribunals. Clarity about how far, and in what circumstances, individuals are 'responsible' for abusive practice – as opposed to more general failures in management, supervision, staffing and support – is vital if protection procedures are to have the support of workers and prove effective.

Although systemic failures are implicated in many situations this does not mean that employers can overlook their responsibilities to be alert to predatory abusers and do what is reasonable to keep them out of the workforce. It means guarding against their infiltration into service and professional networks through careful recruitment and vetting (Moody, 1999). However, the threat from strangers should not be overemphasised. The murder of Sarah Payne, aged nine, in 2001 attracted unprecedented media attention, including a campaign to 'name and shame' registered sex offenders orchestrated by the *News of the World* but cases involving children who are harmed *within* their families usually occupy a much lower profile in the national psyche. While eight or nine children are killed by strangers each year, between 70 and 80 children are murdered each year by their mother or father, and 10% of all homicides are by the victim's parent (Birkett, 2001). Most violence still stems from so-called 'domestic' incidents.

Scandals and biased reporting can lead to 'procedural proliferation' rather than more targeted and evidence-based solutions. (Ayre, 2003) The adversarial culture in legal systems and academic disciplines can lead to arguments *between* theoretical approaches rather than an appropriate synthesis, undermining the whole purpose of multidisciplinary and multi-agency working. Farmer and Owen (1995) comment that, despite the presence of many well-educated professionals sitting around the table at case conferences, there is rarely any discussion about causes or patterns of abuse.

For professionals who work to safeguard children, the two major theoretical orientations are most likely to be a broad focus on socio-economic conditions and inequalities alongside a more individualised and psychodynamic picture of family and gendered relationships. Stevenson's research (1995) suggests that often *neither* are brought into the discussion, making for a very untheoretical and ungrounded assessment. Stevenson argues that this avoidance of either model may constitute the 'worst of both worlds if neither material circumstances nor family dynamics are adequately explored' (p. 230) and, in that case, Stevenson concludes, 'the conference is operating with little or no explicit content and with little discussion of "causation" of whatever kind' (p. 230).

Managers who are responsible for case conferences and support services need to be conversant with a range of theoretical models that address the different forms of abuse and the locus of concerns. Risk assessment in the absence of any understanding of where the problem lies is likely to be a 'hit or miss' affair. The 'where, why, when, how and by whom?' of intervention needs to be clarified. This is a prerequisite for effective prevention and strategic management of harm by managers. Figure 9.3 summarises the discussion of the areas to consider. The frontline manager is often the person who oversees from the centre and decides about intervention.

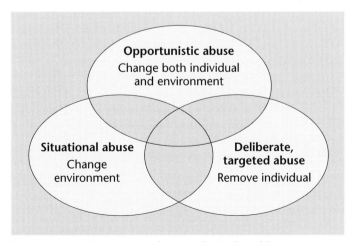

Figure 9.3 **Distinct or overlapping loci of problems**

Different approaches to intervention

Vettenburg (1998) addresses prevention in a document on the prevention of violence in schools for the Council of Europe. Her construction can equally be applied to the abuse of older people by their carers or to the misuse of control and restraint techniques in residential services for younger adults or children with challenging behaviour. She noted four distinct 'prototypes' in the range of *preventive* strategies on offer (Box 9.4).

BOX 9.4 Types of preventive strategy

- **Situational prevention**, which is attending to the environments in which abuse may take place through, for example, the design of establishments or staff supervision.

- **Punitive prevention**, where by attending to detection, prosecution and appropriately serious punishment a sufficient deterrent is established.

- **Treatment-based prevention**, which conceptualises abuse as a consequence of individual or family dysfunction or prior victimisation of the perpetrator.

- **Social prevention**, which deals with the problem in the broader social context, for example by addressing specific manifestations of abuse against a backdrop of widespread discrimination.

(Source: adapted from Vettenburg, 1998, p. 44)

This brings together initiatives that address different levels of the system, at different stages in the aetiology of the problem, and explore the *orientation* of potential strategies. A *reactive* strategy seeks to avert danger, for example through screening out unsuitable staff, whereas a *proactive* strategy tackles risks by promoting positive approaches, for example enhancing user involvement, improving key areas of practice or implementing quality assurance programmes. Mapping these orientations on to the different types of abuse outlined in Figure 9.2 shows that different responses are required to different kinds of risk, as outlined in Figure 9.4 (opposite).

Utting (1997) outlines a strategy for protecting children in local authority care from abuse (see Box 9.5). The strategy might apply equally to adults' services.

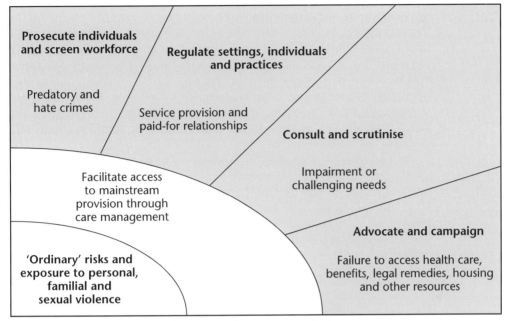

Figure 9.4   **Preventive strategies across the spectrum of abuse**

BOX 9.5 A protective strategy for looked-after children

- A threshold of entry to paid and voluntary work with children which is high enough to deter committed abusers.

- Management which pursues overall excellence and is vigilant in protecting children and exposing abuse.

- Disciplinary and criminal procedures which deal effectively with offenders.

- An approved system of communicating information about known abusers between agencies with a need to know.

(Source: Utting, 1997, p. 1)

The report *People Like Us* (Utting, 1997) also includes a range of strategies for promoting quality services for children, such as clear objectives for services, good-quality assurance systems, recording and care planning. Managers in all settings can view their role as:

- to manage systems to respond to harm that has occurred and to organise protection and support
- to manage quality services that promote safer service environments.

When agencies work together, each one has a different role and remit, so that when they address abuse issues, they come with very different responsibilities and orientations. Each of the prototypes identified by Vettenburg is claimed by a different agency. Regulatory authorities usually take responsibility for situational prevention through their inspection function. The police may focus on prosecution and other sanctions. Probation and/or mental health services address the treatment of potential offenders. Campaigning organisations work to lessen inequalities and social exclusion. These agencies are likely to be involved differently in the types of situation identified so far, and to draw on various systems and mechanisms for intervention.

All managers need to mobilise the strategy or strategies which are most appropriate: *screen*, *regulate*, *consult*, *scrutinise* and *advocate*. It is a matter of 'horses for courses'. An over-defensive approach, based exclusively on 'bad apple' assumptions, will end up cutting across important competing principles, such as fostering autonomy, improving practice, increasing openness and facilitating integration, but a naïve assumption that 'advocacy' could stop a predatory abuser could leave this and other vulnerable people exposed.

Key points

- Understanding the interplay of different theoretical approaches to harm can lead to more accurate responses and interventions.

- Managers have to be active in maintaining systems that protect people from harm.

9.6   Co-ordination and the active manager

In Chapter 6 Charlesworth argues that a lack of co-ordination and communication has serious implications for the quality of care. She also identifies that the frontline manager's role is crucial in making partnerships work effectively. The necessary work of protecting vulnerable adults and safeguarding children brings this essential activity into sharp focus.

Social services managers have two distinct roles to play when responding to allegations of abuse. They are responsible for:

- maintaining a focus on the needs of the child or vulnerable adult and for arranging service provision
- co-ordinating the infrastructure to allow different systems to work co-operatively across their geographical areas.

However, many other agencies also have an important part to play. Systems are essential and, while there are statutory frameworks (Department of Health *et al.*, 1999; Department of Health, 2000c), managers remain responsible for achieving workable multi-agency responses in practice. The complex range of possible relevant involvement, responsibility and mechanisms for response is shown in Figure 9.5 (overleaf).

The role of any manager involved in inter-agency work is to be responsible for their own agency's remit while enabling the work of others. Protocols set out agreed ways of working and sharing information, but there has to be detailed local agreement about how the agencies dovetail their contributions. In protection work, the remit to work together is mandatory: social services may have the lead role, but other agencies have a duty to respond. The way managers handle their roles and agency resources is critical to the outcome for the service users.

The first stage of any action to be managed is the clarification of concerns. The information and the evidence gathered have to serve three different ends:

1   to establish matters of fact
2   to ascertain what needs a child or vulnerable adult has for immediate and long-term protection, treatment or support (for children this may involve being formally placed on the 'at risk' register)
3   to decide what action should and can be taken against a perpetrator and/or whether that person also needs support or extra input.

These different strands will come together at strategy discussions and then case conferences. Balancing each individual's and each agency's interests requires attention to detail, skill and impartiality. In particular, however the meeting is arranged and conducted, it is very difficult to involve the child or adult who is the focus of intervention as a free 'consumer' or 'partner'. Also, there may be fundamental conflicts of interest between parents, carers or service providers. These are areas where the active manager, paying attention to detail, can make the event as positive and useful as possible.

Since the publication of *Child Protection: Messages from Research* (Department of Health, 1995), one concern raised about such procedures is their narrow focus and the consequent failure to identify a range of service provision or to co-ordinate follow-up activities. The case conference is too often seen as an end point rather than a launch pad for active safeguarding strategies. Barker (1996) comments that there is also a tendency to stipulate short-term objectives rather than long-term sustainable support for children, vulnerable adults and their families.

Farmer and Owen (1995) found that if long-term plans were made, responsibility for implementing them most usually fell to, or was left with, social services, other agencies defining their role solely in terms of the initial assessment or investigation. Looking back at Figure 9.1, this is why the diagram is top-heavy. One role of social services managers is to find

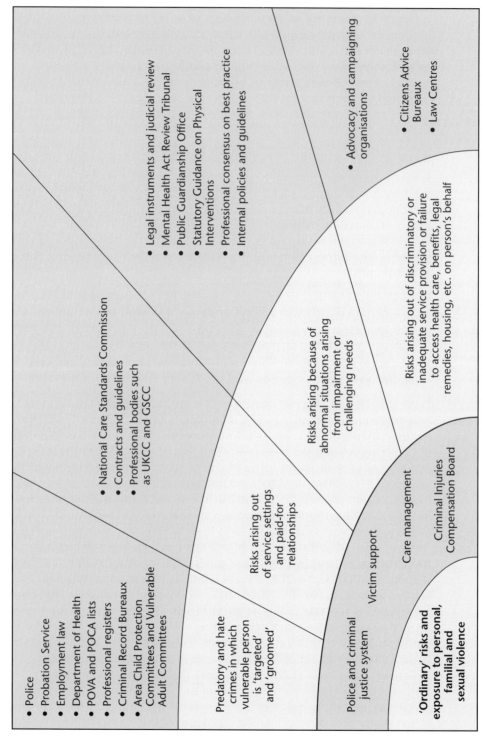

Figure 9.5 Agencies and mechanisms responsible for protection against different kinds of risk (social services have an overall co-ordinating role)

ways of maintaining post-conference support through cohesive local networks. A role for managers in other agencies is to engage actively with post-conference support plans, and to sustain their input. This involves committing resources and contributing to post-conference service provision, review and evaluation.

A critical view of multi-agency approaches to protection

In the guidance on the protection of vulnerable adults (Department of Health, 2000c), an inter-agency 'management committee' is recommended but not required, unlike the Area Child Protection Committee (ACPC). The committee's role is left less clear than the ACPC's, perhaps reflecting a lower priority accorded to adults than to children regarding protection. However, in both cases the move towards co-ordination can be undermined by a lack of resources. There is an argument that locating the responsibility for child and adult protection in the space between agencies reflects a comparatively weak mandate, which depends on maintenance by managers for its effectiveness. The protection agenda is effectively characterised as one of *co-ordination*. Weiss argues that:

> decision makers have continued to advocate coordination reforms in the face of consistently discouraging evidence because they have been seduced by the symbolic and expressive content of the co-ordination message.
>
> (Weiss, 1981, pp. 21–2)

It is easy to contrast the 'symbolic' message underlying strategies called things such as *Working Together* (Department of Health *et al.*, 1999) with systems that struggle to do just that. It is also easy to contrast the aspirations of a document entitled *No Secrets* with agencies that have complicated rules about sharing information across real, perceived and sometimes even artificially constructed boundaries, such as the wall between purchasers and providers even when they are in the same agency. Early policy documents on the abuse of vulnerable adults were considered to be largely 'symbolic' in that they enabled counsellors and managers to look good, but were unlikely ever to receive the resources and operation priority to make them 'real' on the ground (Means and Langan, 1996). Corby argues it is possible that 'co-ordinative action can be misused as a substitute for shortage of resources' (1995, p. 212).

Managing to protect is essentially about steering through complex and competing expectations in order to reach well-balanced decisions in the face of concerns about individuals.

> **Key points**
>
> - Managers are key people in creating and maintaining an inter-agency response to protection issues.
>
> - Managing to protect involves competing and complex demands that have to be understood and balanced through active management.

9.7 Conclusion

This chapter explored how protection, abuse and vulnerability are defined. We considered how children and certain groups of adults are offered formal protection, partly to compensate for the additional risks they face. The thrust of government policies has been to exhort local authorities, regulatory bodies, health and police services to work together through multi-agency committees. These locally agreed structures provide a level of co-ordination and ensure that there are agreed policies and procedures in place so that when managers encounter abuse they know how to make a referral and how to contribute to multidisciplinary investigations and case conference decisions. To be sustainable, these require active management.

Abuse is a painful topic. It confronts everyone with disturbing dilemmas. If you are a manager, you have to make difficult judgements about how the abuse has arisen, how it affects the children or adults involved and what can be done to help them in the present and protect them in future. The most important fact to hold on to is that you do not have to make these judgements on your own. You probably support your staff in working with these issues, but you can also turn to colleagues in your own and other agencies for support and expertise.

Several dilemmas arise for managers whenever protection is on the agenda. They have their value – they can make you think. They can lead you to reflect on your knowledge base and the evidence you have. They can make you check out your practice and procedures with colleagues and other professionals. You can seek second (and third) opinions. You can make sure decisions are made publicly and are open to challenge from service users and their families and from independent experts.

However, dilemmas can also cause managers to dither and prevaricate. Instead of 'act now, think later', they can cause them to 'think and think' and never do anything. While the debates are being debated, vulnerable people are not protected from crime as they should be, nor are they assertively helped to challenge exclusion and discrimination. Instead, they are put into service settings that may not be well enough resourced to resist the drag of institutionalised practice or individual cruelty. Stand back and disadvantaged and under-resourced people and their families suffer. Take a stand and perhaps they might be safeguarded from harm. That is the challenge for frontline managers.

Part 3   Managing Learning and Development in the Team

Introduction

Throughout this book, the authors argue that managers are constantly learning from the dilemmas and challenges of their jobs. The development of such practice wisdom is at the heart of the idea of a practice-led manager. Managers also have direct responsibilities for the learning, the careers and the professional development of other people. This starts from the moment a person is employed and carries on through the processes of induction, supervision and appraisal and, on occasions, disciplinary meetings and actions. Inevitably, work that is challenging and complex brings difficult and painful learning from what goes wrong, as the workplace is just as much a place to learn as it is a place for activities. A theme in *Managing Care in Practice* is that learning and development in care agencies take place in many ways and the organisation should seek to enhance a culture of development, growth and improvement. There is learning through experience, through problem solving, from training courses and from theoretical models. There is also the painful learning through recognising mistakes. The last part of this book considers what managers can learn together with their staff and organisations in several different ways.

Making a mistake and learning from it involves realising, as a result of seeing things go wrong, what might work better. All managers have an opportunity to learn from the extreme cases where the findings of inquiries provide lessons to be disseminated and digested. There are many examples of service users' needs being ignored, resulting in abuse and harm. This applies in adults' services, in children's services, in residential and social care fieldwork, and in education and medical environments. Report after report has sought to recommend improvements and much of what managers now do and expect other people to do is the result of inquiries and suggested improvements to practice. In Chapter 10 'Managing mistakes and challenges', Burton starts by accepting and acknowledging that care settings are complex and full of potential mistakes and challenges. Some mistakes are avoidable and should never happen but, Burton argues, when it does happen it is best to put it right as quickly as possible and then use this as a way of developing and improving the service.

To some extent every service user presents a challenge to services and the ability of managers and their workers to respond appropriately. Burton describes the admission of a resident to an older people's care home and discusses some of the challenges she presents to the manager. Many things can and do go wrong. He ends by considering the role of complaints procedures in putting things right and highlighting areas for the organisation's learning. Burton demonstrates how much the manager and the staff at the care home learn from the mistakes they make over this one service user and from the reactions of other residents and workers. Learning in care settings is often in the context of the relationships between managers, workers and service users as they work together.

Chapter 10 shows through an experiential narrative that managing care is fundamentally about people. In Chapter 11 'Managing significant life events', Seden and Katz develop this point and make the case for practice-led managers to learn to keep to the fore the human needs of workers and service users. They argue from a more theoretical position that the psychosocial theories of loss, transition and crisis are relevant to understanding how service users experience the problems that bring them to care services.

They suggest these theories are also relevant for understanding how workers and managers experience change and disruption, at both personal and organisational levels. Managers need to understand the underpinning theory in order to respond appropriately to the people they work with. The learning here involves taking account of employees' feelings and stress levels, and taking action to avoid or mitigate problems. Chapter 11 takes a particular psychosocial approach to understanding human need and managing care.

Peel completes this part of the book on learning and development. In Chapter 12 'Managing professional development', he considers the manager's role as an educator, both by example and by teaching 'on the job'. A part of managers' responsibilities is to improve the performance, career and professional development of the workers they supervise. Agencies have policies for such matters as induction, supervision, appraisal and disciplinary proceedings but the frontline manager is at the hub of what needs to be done. The practice-led manager makes these policies real and is active in implementing them in a creative way for the team. Peel suggests these activities are part of a whole: from the point at which a worker (qualified or not yet qualified) takes a post to the point when they leave. Managing to ensure your own professional development and that of your staff is complex. Individual experiences, qualifications and aspirations need to be balanced with the needs of service users, and the strategy and policy of the organisation. Peel argues that supervision provides the most effective tool for harmonising these competing objectives.

Supervision sessions provide an opportunity to discuss the work from the service user's perspective: to plan responses, to identify workers' training needs, and to match these with the available training and development opportunities. The practice-led manager relates the workers' training needs to the expressed needs of the service users. Often, however, managers are generous in promoting the learning needs of other people, but have difficulty taking proper time out for their own development and learning. The introduction to this book raised the issue of the urgent needs of managers for training. It is important that the valid needs of managers to keep up to date with policy development and learn new skills are not submerged by the pressures of managing daily realities and pressures. Who ensures that a manager's need for support and training is met? We hope that senior managers take seriously their responsibilities to support and provide development opportunities for frontline managers. We also hope that this book and the course *Managing Care*, which it is part of, will make a substantial contribution to meeting managers' training needs in a grounded way that relates to their practice experiences.

Chapter 10
Managing mistakes and challenges

John Burton

10.1   Introduction

Care work is full of mistakes and challenges for managers. It is a service that can itself be thought of as a product of some mistakes and challenges. People may use care services because their lives and their way of living have been disrupted, undermined or deprived, or perhaps because society has in some way failed or excluded them. They may come to the service for help and support, and they bring with them a challenging range of needs, troubles and expectations. Social care organisations exist specifically to meet those needs; without them there would be no social care managers, staff or services.

Managers generally *make mistakes* and *face challenges*. To say that they 'manage' them implies that it is possible to control all of them, and even to eliminate them. In this chapter I hope to demonstrate that some mistakes are inevitable and can lead to very positive outcomes, and that you might be making a bad mistake if you tried to avoid or eliminate all challenges, rather than welcome them as a means of developing the service. Mistakes can pile up on one another until it feels as if you are confronted by an impossible challenge. There seems to be no way out. Every move you make adds to the pile. You try to put things right and more goes wrong. No one seems to understand your point of view.

This happens to the most competent and well-motivated managers. You need determination and flexibility, the ability to accept that you will make mistakes, faith in your own good motivation, and the capacity to see other people's point of view, even if they do not see yours.

The aims of this chapter are to:

- discuss mistakes and challenges in the context of a manager's accountability
- examine some of the mistakes and challenges a manager might face, through the example of Carmen, a residential care home manager
- consider whether mistakes are inevitable or whether they are to a degree controllable
- encourage the idea that when mistakes do happen, they can become stepping-stones to move practice forward
- discuss the mistakes that should not happen and the mechanisms for complaints.

10.2 Care: a setting for mistakes and challenges?

All managers are accountable to other people. Accountability is usually most immediately to service users, a senior manager and the staff who work directly under their guidance. However, many managers also have to account for, or explain, their actions more widely. Organisations usually have several layers of accountability, such as senior managers, boards of trustees, management committees, owners, funders, elected members, the public (for example, independent visitors for looked-after children), inspection and registration officials, all the way through to central government.

Accountability and responsibility go together (Clark and Asquith, 1985). Coulshed (1990) suggests that accountability comes from the manager's organisational responsibility, the position and remit they hold. Managers of care always have to give an account, or explain their actions, with the reasons for them, to the people who might reasonably ask them to do so. Eby highlights that 'it is not easy to be accountable in contexts where practitioners feel under pressure and face diminishing resources and increasing workloads' (2000a, p. 187). She adds that there may well be 'contradictory challenges to be accountable coming from service-users, their employees and their professional bodies' (p. 187), who will have different priorities and views about what they want to happen. For frontline managers, as much as for practitioners, such accountability is multidimensional. These accountabilities are listed in Box 10.1 (opposite).

As noted in Box 10.1, managers are accountable beyond their own organisations. Heath (2000), writing about accountability in the 'New NHS', points out that accountability is a relationship between two (or more) parties. One person gives the reasons for what they have done to another. These days, because of new structures for arranging care services, managers may have to account to their employers, to networks at a local level and, as discussed in Chapter 8, through performance indicators and government returns to central agencies. Accountabilities are becoming more complex and need to be mapped. This is harder to manage, as Heath says:

> Another difficult aspect of accountability derives from the emphasis on multi-agency approaches in the new structure. This gives rise to the danger that, even if each agency accounts satisfactorily to its own stakeholders for its part in inter-agency activities, accountability for the total outcome or impact of those activities may 'slip through the net'.
>
> (Heath, 2000, p. 14)

Transparency and accountability are linked. Care services have been subject to many scandals and inquiries (Fallon, 1999; Waterhouse, 2000; Department of Health, 1991b) and they have to be open to public scrutiny. Teachers have been accused, and some found guilty, of maltreating schoolchildren; and doctors have been accused of giving inadequate or

---

BOX 10.1 The manager's accountabilities

Social

There are boundaries around what is considered acceptable behaviour in society at any point in time, and in a particular culture.

Ethical

Managers have personal values and there are standards of practice for their role and workplace.

Legal

The responsibilities of managers usually come from laws and are often stated in organisational policies and procedures.

Professional

Groups describing themselves as 'professional' have codes about how their members carry out their tasks.

Financial

Managers are usually responsible for budgets and accounts.

Public

There is an expectation that the public can subject professional activity to scrutiny and complaint.

(Source: adapted from Eby, 2000a, pp. 188–203)

---

inappropriate treatments. Subsequent inquiries have made recommenda-tions and introduced procedures designed to clarify standards and the level of service the public might expect from a particular agency. In addition, the demand for public accountability has led to new legislation, such as the Care Standards Act 2000. These are positive developments designed to produce better, more clearly examinable services but there is no doubt that they, together with the reviews, audits and inspections attached to them, put additional pressure on workers and their managers (Fletcher, 2001).

Inquiries into failures in the system usually offer recommendations for procedural change and better practice, which it is hoped will prevent the next mistake. Experience suggests that, while such recommendations may improve practice and bring about positive changes, they cannot alone prevent mistakes happening. They do not help with the unexpected or replace frontline managers' responsibilities to resolve the challenges they face. While most managers work with helpful legal and procedural guidelines about what is considered good practice, and work from their professional and ethical values, there is still much uncertainty and surprise in this highly complex, personal work.

The uncertainty that managers may feel is increased by the climate of fear, blame and mistrust that has surrounded care since the 1970s (Ayre, 2003). Frontline managers may be acutely aware that 'bad news travels faster than good' and that, when things go wrong, some senior managers and organisations focus on finding someone to blame rather than on learning the lessons for improvement. Managers might fear blame for mistakes and this can lead to actions designed to cover them up, inertia and unwillingness to take responsibility for decisions. This culture of blame and mistrust needs to be overcome if mistakes and complaints are to be acknowledged and put right as far as possible and lessons are to be learned.

It is better if managers can respond creatively and flexibly to new challenges and to use them to develop in the day-to-day experiences of managing. Lessons can be learned from past mistakes while still recognising that the present is not the past. New factors pose new challenges. The ability to recognise the potential for new mistakes and to prevent them from building into serious scandals is important. In residential settings this means creating safer environments through a culture of awareness and consistently good practice (Department of Health, 1998b; Wyre, 2000; Peace and Reynolds, 2003). These principles of awareness and consistency of practice can apply to all care settings, including the work that happens in people's own homes.

Care services aim to safeguard and promote people's wellbeing. Linked to the ideas of accountability and transparency are the values of privacy, choice, confidentiality, dignity and respect. There have been scandals precisely because a care worker has abused someone physically or sexually, or because someone's dignity and rights have been infringed. Managers of care services can work from ethical principles and consider to what extent they are enabling people to make decisions for themselves (see Chapter 9). In the case study that forms the basis of this chapter, such interwoven and even conflicting accountabilities are ones to have in mind as you read about Carmen, Irene and the others. Safeguarding and promoting welfare, managing mistakes and facing challenges are seen in the context of the daily responsibilities of Carmen, the manager of a residential home, and her staff.

As you read the story, consider your own responses: put yourself in the situation and reflect on the thoughts and feelings of Carmen. This chapter is written in a way that tries to draw out the themes and management principles which are transferable to all those settings where someone is responsible for the care of others. These could be children's homes, day centres, residential places for people with alcohol or mental health problems, fieldwork teams, education settings – wherever a service is provided.

By using a common event from a setting that is familiar to me – an 'admission' to a residential home – different sorts of mistakes and challenges can be examined. When do they occur? Who makes them?

Are some of them controllable or preventable? And what are some of the possible outcomes? The idea is to encourage you to see most mistakes and challenges as stepping-stones without which the manager, staff and residents could not move forward. Clearly, there are some mistakes that should not happen but, if and when they do, some may still lead to improving the service and moving on. Challenges may be people or events that make managers find another way of doing things and they should stimulate ideas and creative responses. Finally, there are some mistakes that should never occur and some challenges that managers should not take on.

Key points

- Managers are accountable to a range of people and organisations.

- There are conflicting accountabilities in care settings and some mistakes are inevitable.

- Mistakes and challenges can become stepping-stones to better practice.

10.3   A request for an admission

The example used here is a residential care home for older people, but the lessons could apply equally to your own setting or one you know. The home has 20 residents, more than 12 care staff, domestic and catering staff, a manager, several relatives and other visitors, all interacting. They eat together, sit and talk together, meet, visit, come and go. Some are angry and complaining, some calm and satisfied; some are ill, some full of energy and ideas; some bring in problems from home, some have problems stemming from losing their home and feeling that nobody cares for them.

The 'society' of a residential home is immensely complex, constantly changing and fraught with mistakes and challenges (Burton, 1989). Of course, this is just like a rather concentrated version of the wider society of which the home is part. The description of this home gives some clues about my picture of the staff, their backgrounds and personalities. You, the reader, can use your own experience and imagination to create your own ideas of the people, the place and the issues that a diverse group of people brings. Social care is part of the wider society it serves and so the challenge posed by an 'incontinent and drunken old woman' (Irene), swearing at passers-by on the street, steps up a gear when she ventures into the supermarket. It then becomes a set of complex and major challenges when she goes to live in a residential home. Irene's story is described in Examples 10.1, 10.2 and 10.3.

EXAMPLE 10.1 Introducing Irene

Irene has been living on the streets of her local town. She is frequently seen near local supermarkets. She is often drunk, and swears at passers-by, sometimes in a 'threatening and aggressive' way. She has been living rough for several years after being evicted from her flat for not paying the rent and for anti-social behaviour. Irene is 73.

She was admitted to hospital after an anonymous emergency call when she was found lying injured in the street. She had fallen down the stone steps of a footbridge under which she was sleeping. She was seriously injured by her fall but, after several weeks of hospital treatment and physiotherapy, is now out of a wheelchair and using a walking frame. She is still unsteady on her feet and incontinent at night.

Irene has agreed with the hospital social worker to try living in a residential home. At least she would be warm, safe and well fed. She is ready to leave hospital after several weeks of treatment for bronchitis and a broken ankle. She is discharged very quickly. The ward is under pressure to find a bed for a new admission. Carmen, the manager of the home, decides to offer Irene a place straightaway on the basis of telephone calls with the hospital social worker with whom she has a good working relationship.

So, Carmen has been approached by the hospital social worker to accept Irene as a resident. It might be a mistake to agree to this. Certainly, it would be a mistake if Carmen did not assess the risks and was later shown not to have made an informed decision about the potential for harm to other residents and staff (see Chapter 9). However, Carmen may have weighed up the risks in her own mind and, being an accepting and caring person, decided to agree to the admission. She may have spoken with staff about how to manage the challenges that Irene would undoubtedly present. She also might have thought about ways in which other residents would be consulted and prepared.

However, if there is no record of these discussions and no detailed care plan made, and if there was no formal, written 'risk assessment', Carmen will be in trouble if Irene pushes over another resident who breaks a hip in the fall and dies in hospital. Carmen has done so much that is right but she cannot produce the evidence that she planned Irene's care or took full account of the risks that she posed. With luck, support and good management, Carmen will learn from these mistakes and will not lose her confidence and commitment. Unfortunately, she could lose her job and find it very difficult to get another one. In this situation, at the very least, Carmen needs to have assessed the risks to Irene and other residents and staff and to have kept a written record.

Making decisions that could be wrong

Mistakes often occur when you have to make a decision. This can be when you have to choose between a range of alternatives, one of which may be to do nothing. There is a well-known saying that someone who has never made a mistake has never done anything. The essence of taking responsibility is using your judgement. You exercise discretion, choosing between one course of action and another. Although your decision may subsequently be considered 'wrong', it may still be acceptable, if not 'right', if you have made it in good faith and can account for it from your use of available information. As a manager, you generally use your judgement and have to make a decision in response to some kind of challenge, question, difficult or risky situation, radical idea, threat or argument. Becoming a manager means taking an increased level of responsibility. Making decisions and professional judgements go hand in hand (Dowie and Elstein, 1998). Accepting and working with uncertainty is part of the job of being a manager.

Taking responsibility and being accountable

Organisations build frameworks of rules, procedures and guidance in order to help managers and staff make decisions. Sometimes the organisation weaves such a tight and all-embracing network that there is no room for the manager's discretion. It is as if the procedure makes the decision for them. In situations governed by rules and procedures, managers face relatively few challenges and can avoid the stress and anxiety of ever making a decision if they simply follow procedure. Alternatively, in a situation where there is as yet no procedure, the manager may be expected to refer the decision upwards for someone else to take, and a new procedure will probably be invented to take the place of such decision making in the future. In these circumstances, you might wonder what managers are employed for.

In this book it has been argued that the practice-led manager's role is to engage with the issues and act on the firmest ground they can establish for their decision (see Chapter 9). If Carmen worked in an organisation that ruled out taking residents who had alcohol, mental health or incontinence problems, she would never have had to consider Irene in the first place. Alternatively, her organisation might not allow her to make any decisions about who was to be admitted, expecting the manager to accept whoever was 'sent by head office'. However, suppose that Carmen does make the decision and that the home can accept people with some of these needs, although it is registered simply for 'elderly people'. (The terms of the registration exclude residents with serious mental health problems.) Rules and procedures can reduce individual responsibility for mistakes arising from faulty decisions, but they can also result in an inflexible and unresponsive service.

The manager decides

Irene is hard to place, but the hospital social worker thought that Carmen's home might be suitable because she had arranged for someone else to go there who had a slight mental health problem and was a bit 'difficult', and it had worked out well. The social worker knows that Carmen is a warm and sympathetic person who is not likely to say 'no' just because Irene will pose some unconventional challenges to the smooth running of the home. Irene's hospital social worker telephones to ask Carmen if she would consider taking Irene immediately and briefly outlines Irene's history. The social worker feels very fortunate to have found a place and with a manager who she knows is caring and non-judgemental in her approach. She knows Carmen has worked well in the past to accommodate her 'difficult customers'.

Social workers who commission community care services have to cultivate useful informal relationships with residential managers in order to secure places in good homes. However, such comfortable, or even cosy, working relationships can lead to unjustified assumptions and ill-considered decisions. The careful use of agreed procedure helps by questioning assumptions and thereby avoiding mistakes. Even where the commissioner and the provider have a good working relationship, based on past experience, the questioning of assumptions in the present situation is still needed to avoid mistakes. A well-designed admission and assessment process requires systematic assessment of need and formal identification of why a particular admission is necessary. The regular review of admissions procedures should monitor whether they are working well (Department of Health, 2002, Standards 3, 4 and 7).

Mistakes outside the control of managers adding to those they can control

Once Carmen has accepted Irene, she anticipates that she will pose some challenges; indeed, she would be concerned if Irene posed no challenge at all. On the other hand, how should Carmen prepare staff and the other residents? She is very short of time. She may feel that too much preparation could make staff over-anxious and set up Irene to fail. However, she does not want to pre-empt Irene's quite natural reactions to arriving in a residential home after spending several years living on the streets. Yet again, Carmen rightly thinks that, without some preparation of staff and residents, Irene poses not only a challenge but also an unacceptably high level of risk.

EXAMPLE 10.2 Irene arrives at the home

There is not much time to prepare, but Carmen makes plans with a member of staff who will prepare for Irene's arrival and be responsible for her introduction to the home.

The member of staff fails to turn up on the day of Irene's arrival. Irene arrives unexpectedly early. No one is briefed to welcome her and she reacts by becoming angry and abusive.

Carmen steps in to meet Irene and then allocates responsibility for settling Irene in to other staff. This includes reassuring her and finding her some clothing and other items. She has few possessions. The hospital has provided her with an 'emergency pack' of essential items but she has little else, apart from her handbag.

Everyone is busy because the home is short-staffed. Irene does not have consistent attention from a key worker on her first day.

For anyone (of any age) the hours before, during and after the moment of walking through the front door of a home as a 'resident' are inevitably stressful. If that process has not been fully discussed and understood by staff, the manager is making a mistake. If the home has not already worked out a way of doing it well, it is about time it did. Like many other such places, Carmen's home may have 'got away with it' because previous residents, although sometimes extremely anxious and upset by the unreliable process, did not react in the same way as Irene does. Perhaps, for some, the period of depression and loss, or panic, anger and resistance, were accepted simply as a natural 'settling-in' process.

For some residents this might mean disorientation, loss of confidence and memory, and temporary incontinence, all of which have a strong chance of becoming permanent conditions. For children it may mean running away at the first opportunity, or displaying frightened, aggressive bravado with other children and staff, which sets a pattern of action and reaction that remains with the child and the staff team throughout the child's stay. The inadequate way of handling her admission is challenged by Irene. However, instead of rejecting Irene as being unsuitable, Carmen and other staff are stimulated (challenged) into thinking, 'Ah, we've made a mess of this; there must be a better way of doing it.'

There are many potential mistakes and challenges in this process. Each one could lead to a poor outcome or could result in change and progress, depending on how Carmen manages them.

> **Key points**
>
> - Comfortable working relationships can lead to assumptions and ill-considered decisions.
>
> - The careful use of agreed procedures can help to avoid mistakes.
>
> - Risks need to be assessed and communicated and a record kept of them.
>
> - Managers make judgements in an environment where uncertainty is part of the job.
>
> - Managers make decisions that influence the course of events, so taking account of the possible outcomes of judgements is essential.

10.4   Two days, a night and an incident

Many mistakes remain unnoticed because no one has challenged them. A challenge can lead to correcting long-standing faults, and to learning and making progress. However, mistakes can also accumulate and cause a crisis (see Chapter 11), and other people and organisations can be drawn in. Many different people are involved and connected with almost any event. The reverberations are seemingly unlimited. A small incident can lead to entanglement in laws, regulations, guidance and lengthy investigations, as well as involving a host of 'stakeholders' who have all been directly or indirectly affected by the event. In a children's home, a minor incident similar to the one described next, if poorly managed, could lead to a frightening and destructive breakdown of order. It can also show that well-thought-out, reliable structures help new residents to feel as safe and settled as possible.

Irene's stay has gone from bad to worse by the second day, as described in Example 10.3.

EXAMPLE 10.3 Irene's first two days and a night as a resident

For the first few hours after she arrived, Irene spent a lot of time in her room and appeared not to want to mix with other residents. The plan was for her to have lunch, but when she was taken to the dining-room she found no place set for her. Irene said she was not hungry and asked to be shown to her room. At the evening meal she remains at her table for less than five minutes and eats very little. Members of staff make an effort to talk with her but the only person she wants to see is Carmen who, by that time, has gone home.

> After her first night, Irene complains to Carmen that the night staff were 'spying' on her and had come into her room without her permission. When she left her room to look for the kitchen, the staff told her not to wander around at night. At breakfast the next morning she refuses to sit with a resident who had looked at her in a disapproving way and seemed to be making remarks about her.
>
> By afternoon teatime, Irene is still restless and upset. She helps herself from a plate of biscuits on a small table in the sitting-room and puts them in her handbag. Philippa, the resident to whom she had taken exception at breakfast, stands up from a nearby chair and tells Irene to 'leave the biscuits alone – they're ours'. Irene pushes her back into her chair and Philippa shouts 'Help! Help! She pushed me. Oh, why do they let them in here? It never used to be like this.'

In this situation, although Irene's needs have not been met or carefully assessed, she now appears to be a threat to both staff and other residents. The widespread prejudices that might be expected to operate towards someone described as a 'drunken, incontinent street person with mental health problems' have not been explored or discussed by the care team. Also, there has not been the close, careful observation that would mean a picture of Irene's needs, and the concerns of other residents, was being built up. No one noticed that Irene was very hungry. In many group care settings, it is common to lose track of what is happening to each resident over a period of time. Staff can make the mistake of reacting to residents as if what they are doing is unrelated to all that has gone before.

To understand the situation and manage it well, the staff must consider what was behind each resident's words and actions, and the way they are related. They also need to be more aware of prejudices and assumptions based on matters such as race, class and gender and, in this case, attitudes to homelessness.

Recognising mistakes and challenges, and taking action

It would be a mistake not to take the incident seriously. In many homes it would be smoothed over: Philippa would be reassured and offered another cup of tea; Irene would be encouraged to go to another room with the biscuits she wanted and, of course, a cup of tea! That might be just right at that moment for the residents themselves. However, it would be a mistake not to recognise the challenge (or whole range of challenges) that the incident encapsulated, and to ignore the accumulation of mistakes that led up to it from the time of Irene's admission. It would also be a mistake not to perceive the much more serious potential of the incident.

The situation might have escalated if a care worker had not calmly reassured Philippa and quickly, but gently, drawn Irene away from the scene and given her attention and much-needed food. This care worker was intent on reducing the tension. She was able to think clearly about what was happening to Philippa and Irene, and she helped to make the situation better for each of them. If a different care worker had intervened by loudly confronting Irene, and even gripping her arm in an attempt to 'restrain' her, while calling urgently to a colleague to come and attend because Philippa had been 'attacked', Irene might well have become 'violent'. This care worker would not be thinking clearly about the needs of either resident; rather, she would be making the serious mistake of adding her own feelings and reactions to a volatile situation.

Several other people and organisations would probably have got involved. Philippa would have insisted that her son should be called. Irene's social worker would have to be informed, along with the local inspection unit, because this would now have become a 'significant' incident affecting the welfare of residents. Carmen would also have felt that she should inform her own manager, because it would be impossible to predict just how big this small incident might become as more and more people got involved. There would be reports to write and forms to be filled in, reducing Carmen's availability to get on with the more productive parts of her job, such as finding out from the staff and residents what had gone wrong and putting it right.

So, with thoughtful planning and preparation, this event might have been avoided. Although it did happen, how it was handled was crucial to whether one set of initial mistakes was compounded by clumsy and panicky reactions. Carmen's manager, Philippa's family, the inspection unit and Carmen herself might all, with justification, be thinking, 'That should never have happened.' As a manager, that is an excellent way to think, yet you must also resign yourself to the fact that you can neither predict nor pre-empt all eventualities. Even with the best preparation and attention, Irene might still have found an opportunity to 'have a go' at Philippa or vice versa.

Also, was the pushing incident itself so bad? You may consider all that happened was a rude, prejudiced and officious old woman got what she deserved; no real harm was done; and Irene started to get the attention she needed. Or you might think that Philippa had good reason to be anxious and frightened by Irene's behaviour, and that her reaction was understandable in the circumstances. However, what led up to Irene's behaviour? Apart from anything else, she was ravenous. Of course, the incident could have been much worse. As suggested earlier, Philippa might have fallen on the floor when pushed, broken her hip and, through an all too common series of events, later died in hospital from a respiratory disease.

What could go wrong?

There is ample scope for 'mistakes' and a service user like Irene poses many challenges, even during her first few hours in a home. Table 10.1 summarises some of the potential mistakes and challenges. Each of them could lead to poor outcomes or could result in change or progress, depending on how Carmen manages them.

Table 10.1 **Irene's stay: what could go wrong?**

Challenge/event/situation	*Decision*	*Actual/potential mistakes*
Request for Irene's admission	Carmen says 'yes' in principle	Insufficient information – with more information she might have said 'no'. Carmen fails to involve staff in the decision, so all some of them see is the additional burden of a difficult resident
Handling the assessment, preparation, visit, involving staff and other residents	Carmen has to decide on a timetable and on which staff will be involved	Failure to assess, particularly a risk assessment. Irene does not have a preliminary visit. Arrangements break down: for instance, no place is set for Irene at lunch
The member of staff allocated to help Irene settle in is away sick	Carmen is very tired and decides to go home at 6 pm after a 10-hour day	No one makes it their job to give special attention to Irene
Shortage of staff on the shift when Irene actually arrives at the home. During her first day and night, she receives inconsistent and unplanned attention. Staff listen to gossip about her. Irene reacts to some critical remarks from other residents by swearing at them	Weighed down with other work, Carmen does not reallocate the work of settling Irene in and seeing her through her first few hours to one member of staff	Irene is not given enough steady attention. What she is given is intrusive. Irene and the other residents respond badly
Irene thinks the night staff 'spy' on her and enter her room without her permission. On her second day, Irene refuses to sit with a resident at breakfast	Carmen thinks Irene has a point. What to do? Move Irene to another table or move the other resident?	Carmen overdoes her criticism of the night staff or she says nothing because they could wreck Irene's placement if they chose, and Carmen cannot manage without them

Mistakes should be addressed as soon as possible

Most mistakes can be either put right or made worse. The longer they are allowed to continue, the more destructive they are likely to become. On their own, most mistakes are neither serious nor irretrievable. It is when they are not noticed, and when they are compounded by further mistakes, that they can be devastating for residents and for staff and managers. The pushing incident was handled well by the first care worker, followed by Philippa's safe (although for her slightly shocking) landing and loud outcry, which should have rung a very useful alarm bell for Carmen and her staff. Despite her welcoming and supportive attitudes, Carmen had not planned and communicated well enough, and then she was let down by the worker she originally allocated to Irene. She was preoccupied with other, equally urgent, matters; or she might have been further let down by the staff to whom she reallocated the task of managing Irene's admission.

Also Carmen guessed that insufficient information about Irene had been passed on at the handover meeting between the day and night staff. Consequently, far too little consideration had been given to meeting the challenge she presented. By failing to concentrate on these crucial first few hours of a challenging admission, and neglecting to communicate well with each other, the team had failed. The incident pointed to the absence of a useful procedure for admitting residents and to other gaps in the home's care practice. However, all was not lost by any means: out of the incident would come an honest analysis and appraisal of what went wrong, a determination to work more professionally with Irene, and a new framework for welcoming new residents into the home, including participation from existing residents.

Mistakes and messages for the organisation

Mistakes need to be put right quickly but, as well as trying to rectify the immediate mistake, other patterns and meanings, which are messages for the organisation, should be looked for and then acted on. For the manager, the choice is whether to try to manage mistakes and to accept challenges or whether to stop managing (in any meaningful sense of that term). In fact, mistakes and challenges are the very stuff of managers' everyday work, and they can expect to be involved in shaping the direction of activities, and acting on the messages they gather from what has happened, to guide future actions (Burton, 1998). From these messages they can also identify the training needs of staff and arrange for them to be met.

> **Key points**
>
> - Some mistakes result from events within managers' control. They can also be made worse by factors outside their control.
>
> - Mistakes can go unnoticed if no one challenges what is happening. Challenge can lead to helpful changes being made.
>
> - It is a mistake to react to an event without considering what led up to it.
>
> - Most mistakes can be put right quickly. The longer they are left, the worse things can become.
>
> - Mistakes have messages for organisations as well as individuals.

10.5   Carmen's next steps

If the care worker had not handled the pushing incident well, as it occurred, it could have escalated into a much more serious situation in which the series of mistakes in response to Irene's challenge would have led to some very negative and wasteful results. That daunting prospect presents Carmen with a decisive test of her managerial ability and resolve. She may take the view that whatever happens within the home is her responsibility, and she may do her best to respond to all mistakes and challenges in a positive and creative way. Alternatively, she may be tempted to argue that the lack of an effective procedure for admitting residents is a failure by the organisation for which she cannot be held accountable.

Consequently, Carmen could say she is no longer willing to be accountable for the initial assessment of potential residents and deciding whether they are suitable for the home. If she takes that view, and the organisation (whether a private or voluntary organisation or a local authority) then assumes responsibility for the 'admission process', it is unlikely to result in a better service for the residents. Although Carmen's job will perhaps be less demanding, it will also be much less satisfying. In any case, the managerial responsibility for the continuing assessment of the residents' care needs will remain hers.

The organisations and people who could get involved and take the decision making away from Carmen (if she is willing to relinquish it) include those listed in Table 10.2 (overleaf).

Table 10.2 **Influences on decision making**

Organisations with statutory responsibilities and powers	*Family and voluntary bodies that could be involved*
The 'provider' organisation and Carmen's outside management	Philippa's family
The National Care Standards Commission	The other residents' families
The Health and Safety Executive	The Relatives and Residents Association
The hospital community care management team	Counsel and Care
The social services complaints officer	Mind or local advocacy services
The local authority environmental health unit	The local Age Concern branch

If Carmen chooses to maintain her full responsibility for running the home, she might well have to accept the involvement of some of these 'outsiders'. Indeed, she would very much welcome their assistance and support in appropriate areas of her work. For instance, a good inspection unit or environmental health unit would help her to set up suitable risk assessments and admission procedures. Such units can sometimes be unreasonably demanding and officious, requiring unnecessarily lengthy written procedures and impractical levels of risk reduction that undermine residents' choice and self-determination. However, Carmen might find them a source of support in establishing better structures for practice.

Carmen would welcome the involvement of the local Relatives and Residents Association and other voluntary organisations. It would be an opportunity for wider involvement, drawing them in as partners in running the home. They could also help to work out procedures and policies and involve the residents more fully in the practices of the home. Of course, Carmen would want Philippa's family to get involved. However, if she relinquished her responsibilities as the full-time manager of the home and became more of a 'nominal' manager, these outside organisations, such as those identified in Table 10.2, could impose their own pet, but often unworkable, procedures on the home. Carmen and her staff team would then no longer be in a position to face challenges and learn from mistakes.

If the organisation running the home decides to take the overall responsibility for management away from Carmen, the development of the home by learning from mistakes and challenges would largely stop. Staff would still make mistakes, of course, but these would be regarded as breaches of official procedures rather than as opportunities for learning. The implication is that if staff follow procedures, no matter how inappropriate these are to residents' individual circumstances, they cannot make a mistake (and if staff do not follow procedures, because they are unworkable, the mistake is to get caught). Similarly, challenges will be met by the mere application of a rule or procedure. If the outcome is unsatisfactory it may be concluded that the client presenting the challenge is unsuitable for the service, rather than that the service needs to respond, change and take some considered risks to meet the client's challenge.

True management is difficult, creative and sometimes untidy. It is a developmental process. The positive use of mistakes and challenges is intrinsic to such management.

Key points

- Partnership with a wider range of organisations and more user participation in running the service can mean that some mistakes are avoided.

- Procedures can reduce individual responsibility for mistakes arising from poor decisions, but they can also result in an inflexible and unresponsive service.

10.6   Managing complaints

This 'inside' and 'outside' management response is well illustrated by what happens when a complaint is made. Suppose that Philippa's son (Paul) felt the incident had not been handled well and that, even though on this occasion his mother was unhurt, he was worried it could happen again with much more serious consequences. He may well be right, and the most obvious person to complain to is Carmen, the manager. Paul is concerned about his mother but she often complains to him about events and conditions at the home, which he thinks she has made up. Like many people who intend to complain, Paul is torn between several different pressures: worry, mixed with some guilt, about his mother; doubts about the seriousness of this particular incident; and not wanting to offend or criticise Carmen or her staff. He has a lack of confidence in himself combined with some anger and resentment about how difficult it is to be a caring relative in this situation.

Nevertheless, Paul asks to see Carmen. Usually, Carmen would be friendly, supportive and clear when dealing with a complaint. She would encourage Paul to tell her what he is worried about, both in particular and in general. Without breaking any confidences about Irene, Carmen would freely admit that she and the staff had made some mistakes with Irene's admission, which were exacerbated by staff absence. She would tell Paul what she was planning to do about it and that the complaint would help her and the staff to make the necessary changes. She would ask Paul if there was anything else he was worried about, and explain that if he wanted to take his complaint further he could contact Carmen's outside manager.

She would also give him a leaflet produced by the organisation to help complainants take matters further if still dissatisfied. Carmen would make careful notes of what Paul said, including a record in the home's complaints book. She would immediately write him a formal but friendly letter outlining the complaint, saying what she was going to do about it, and thanking Paul for his time, trouble and concern in bringing it to her attention.

In spite of the pressures on her, Carmen manages to deal with Paul's complaint just as she intended. It was difficult because she felt criticised. She had been put in the position of answering for mistakes that she could not have prevented (staffing problems) and for a situation to which Philippa herself contributed.

However, Carmen also has the professionalism, generosity and good sense to see this complaint as an important insight into faults in the home's practice and as an opportunity to make changes. Carmen knows that every complaint should be taken seriously, even those that appear to be unfounded. As with almost any event or situation in a social care setting, a particular complaint may be connected with other dissatisfactions or anxieties. It is always a mistake not to attend to a complaint, even when there seems to be little substance to it. Managers may be tempted to see a complaints procedure as yet another layer of bureaucracy but this would be a mistake too.

Listening attentively to a complaint reveals the underlying issues. A complainant who is not listened and responded to, or who is merely referred to the complaints procedure, handed a leaflet and form and told to complete it, may take it no further but is likely to make more of their

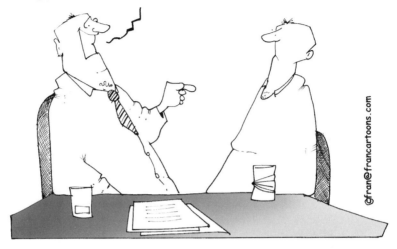

THE ANSWER TURNED OUT TO BE SIMPLE .. BY JUST CHANGING "DISSATISFIED" TO "SATISFIED" ON ALL THE FORMS WE CUT OUR COMPLAINTS BY 100%.

@fran@francartoons.com

Managing complaints and concerns does not just add another layer of bureaucracy

complaint. The complaint may then be distorted and exaggerated by their anger and resentment about their treatment. In either case, communication will break down and there will probably be a poor outcome for all concerned. A complainant may end up, after months of struggle, achieving an independent investigation or even taking their case to the ombudsman. Complaints need to be heard with care and given attention in terms of both the specific complaint and service development. Box 10.2 summarises the main points to bear in mind.

BOX 10.2 Hearing complaints

Listen to complaints with two things uppermost in your mind:

1 This person is unhappy about something and wants it put right quickly.

2 We can learn from this and improve the service – using it as a stepping-stone for development.

Be direct and open in your response.

Investigating a complaint

Some complaints from staff are more accurately called *grievances*. How did Carmen handle the complaint from Irene about night staff 'spying' on her and entering her room without her permission? You may remember that Carmen was concerned that both allegations could easily be true. Yet she was worried about challenging the night staff because, if they chose to withdraw their co-operation, she herself might be faced with the breakdown of an already difficult staffing situation.

Carmen gave the same attention to Irene's complaint as she later gave to Paul's: listening carefully, considering a course of action and telling Irene what she intended to do. In fact, having a well-recognised process for the complaints of residents and relatives and for staff grievances that is simple, fair and open helps managers to deal with the real issues and reduces the suspicion that they might have a personal agenda. If staff know that all complaints will be dealt with promptly, and that their own grievances will also be taken seriously, they are more ready to voice real grievances and less likely to make them up. For this to happen there must be a clear grievance procedure.

First, Carmen had to find out from the night staff their version of the night's events. She began by looking at the notes they had written and her heart sank as she realised how poor the notes on most of the residents were. It became all too clear that the night staff were receiving very little training, support and supervision. 'How out of touch they are with my directions', thought Carmen. The notes on most residents amounted to comments such as: 'Quiet night. No problems. All care given'; or '4 am. Incontinent of urine. Washed. Pad and sheets changed. All care given'; or, in Irene's notes, 'Restless and aggressive. Refused attention. Wandering around; swore when asked to return to room. All care given'. ('"No care given" might be more accurate,' Carmen thought ruefully.)

The night staff were not working in the way Carmen expected them to, and it was her fault for not checking that her recent guidelines for writing care notes were being followed. After a complaint the previous year that a resident had received no attention during the night and a recent inspection requirement, they had been told to write notes on every resident: so they did but not in the way Carmen had asked them to. In addition, they had reverted to an outdated routine of checking on every resident every two hours during the night.

The only exceptions were the few residents whose relatives had requested in writing that they should be left in peace! Carmen did not like this arrangement at all, but had accepted it because it appeared to comply with the requirements of the inspection unit and her own managers. She realised now it had been a mistake not to challenge it at the time. When managers make a change they always need to follow it up on the ground to check that it is working. If they accept their responsibilities as manager, and then object when changes they disagree with are imposed from outside, they may be doing the right thing but at the wrong time.

Now, because Irene had, in effect, challenged the arrangement, Carmen wanted to get back to the roots of the problem and put it right. She had in mind some training for the night staff combined with doing some shifts with them, so that she could discuss issues as they arose. They would also need regular supervision and appraisal, but when would she get time? She needed to prevent the mistakes of the first night being made on Irene's second night. She was annoyed with herself that she had gone home at 6 pm the evening before. She decided she would have to meet the night staff in person. She resolved to stay until 10.30 pm so that she could both discuss Irene's complaint and start talking with them about ways of improving care practice. This brings Carmen into conflict with Margaret, a night care worker, as described in Example 10.4.

EXAMPLE 10.4 Margaret's grievance

Margaret, who clashed with Irene on her first night, has worked at the home for 15 years. Carmen has been manager for two years. Margaret is one of the staff against whom a complaint was made about lack of attention a year ago, when Carmen tried to stop routine two-hourly checks being made on residents. She told night staff to check only those residents who needed attention or were at particular risk during the night. Margaret was very upset by the implication that she was at fault, first for checking all the residents and then for not checking them, when, as she said, she was only doing what she had been told. Now Carmen was bringing a complaint from Irene, a new and troublesome resident, who is 'difficult and violent', according to the gossip Margaret had heard. Carmen even had the cheek to criticise her recording all of a sudden, when she had been writing the same way for the last year without attracting comment, ever since Carmen had asked the night staff to make a record for each resident. It was all so unfair.

Margaret knows she is the most reliable person on the staff; she is never off sick like the others and she is always willing to fill in. Most of the residents like Margaret; they are used to her and can rely on her. She is kind, skilful and very experienced. She was only doing her best when she went into Irene's room because there was no answer when she knocked. She was genuinely worried about Irene.

Carmen knows very well what Margaret is thinking, and consequently she approaches the meeting with great sensitivity, doing her best to get a true discussion going so that they can talk about the real issues. However, Carmen is 'running on empty': her reserves of patience and energy have been used up. In spite of Carmen's best efforts, Margaret is angry, resentful and immovable. She keeps saying she just wants to be told clearly what to do and she will do it, adding that 'things have really gone downhill since the old matron left'.

> Carmen, who arrived at work at 8 am and is now in her fifteenth hour of
> consecutive work, knows in her heart that she is just too tired and stressed
> to deal with Margaret's intransigence.

Carmen made a mistake by staying late. She felt helpless and resentful. She
loses her temper and leaves the meeting saying, 'I am sick of this. I came to
discuss this issue, not to be insulted. I am not satisfied with your recording
and I can see that Irene's complaint is justified. I will put my instructions
in writing.' Margaret is very upset and that night writes out a grievance
against Carmen. Many management decisions are about when to
intervene and when not to. 'A stitch in time saves nine' is often true for
social care managers. However, they must also avoid putting themselves in
stressful and demanding positions when they have insufficient reserves of
energy and patience.

Carmen goes home feeling that everything is falling apart, and
questioning her capacity to manage all these things that keep going
wrong. She finds herself thinking, 'I am giving up. I'll just hand it all over
to my manager. I am tired of struggling with it.' She wants to say to her
manager the sort of thing Margaret said to her: 'Just tell me what to do.'
She has a sleepless night but forces herself to get up and go into work at
8 am the next day. She is confronted by Margaret's letter stating her
grievances: 'unfounded and repeated criticism; giving contradictory
instructions; finding a resident's complaint justified without proper
investigation; and being spoken to in an angry, rude and unreasonable
way.' Carmen is alone in the office and bursts into tears. When she stops
crying, she has to decide what to do next.

Learning from mistakes to improve practice

This example ended at a low point for Carmen. However, later, when she
reviewed the lessons with her own manager and received some support
herself, it was the launch pad for some excellent developments in the
home. Carmen's handling of Margaret's grievance led to a new understanding and respect between them. Margaret became Irene's key worker
(the first occasion a night care worker had taken on key work) and, with
her support, Irene flourished. Carmen held regular meetings and training
sessions with the night staff, starting by helping them with a handover
meeting once a week. The home created a clear and comprehensive
checklist for admissions.

From this point onwards, no resident was admitted without an
allocated worker to support them through their first few hours in the
home. Philippa's son, Paul, with Carmen's encouragement, started a
Relatives and Residents Association affiliated to the national organisation.
In managing these changes, Carmen had to renegotiate and reposition

herself with her manager and the outside organisation. She gained authority and her responsibilities grew. Of course, mistakes still happened, challenges arose, and further advances came out of them. The culture of the home had been changed by the series of events. Carmen's underlying faith in herself and her principles enabled her to respond creatively.

Key points

- Management is difficult, creative and sometimes untidy.

- The positive use of mistakes and challenges is integral to managing care.

- When a change is introduced, it should always be followed up to make sure it is working.

- Managers should avoid dealing with stressful situations when they are tired and lack reserves of energy and patience.

10.7   The lessons summarised

When Carmen reflected on this experience with her supervisor some time later, she could draw out for herself what she had learned for her future practice. She took this to a training event to share with other managers, as summarised in the following diary extract.

CARMEN'S DIARY: SUMMARY OF LESSONS LEARNED

It really matters to assess risks, to communicate them to my staff, to keep a record and regularly assess them.

Taking responsibility means accepting and working with uncertainty.

Rules and procedures can reduce individual responsibility for mistakes arising from faulty decisions, but they can also result in an inflexible and unresponsive service. I am trying to get a balance.

Comfortable working relationships can lead to unjustified assumptions and ill-considered decisions.

The careful use of agreed procedures helps by questioning assumptions and thereby avoiding mistakes. I need to talk each admission through better with commissioning social workers. We also must have a full needs assessment before someone joins the home.

Many mistakes go unnoticed because no one has challenged them. A challenge can lead to putting right long-standing mistakes, and to learning and making progress. I would not feel so bad if I could use challenge to change things for the better.

It is easy to lose track of what is happening to each resident over a period of time. Staff can make the mistake of relating to residents as if what they are doing is unconnected to all that has gone before. Thanks to the incident with Irene and Philippa, we picked up a major flaw in our practice.

Most mistakes can be put right or made worse. The longer they are allowed to 'run', the more destructive they are likely to become. The trouble is you do not always have the time and energy to take action immediately.

As well as trying to rectify the immediate mistake, I could look for patterns and meanings, messages for the organisation, and then act on them. It's not all down to me. My senior manager has a responsibility here too. We do need to keep more detailed records though.

Management is a difficult, creative and developmental process. Part of it is the positive use of mistakes and challenges. I can be right in there working towards change, even though I get tired!

Next time I make a change, I will follow it up to check that it is working in practice. Without follow-up, changes do not take root.

If I accept my responsibilities as manager, I will not accept without objection changes with which I disagree being imposed from outside, although this might be difficult.

I will try not to put myself in stressful and demanding positions when I have insufficient reserves of energy and patience.

10.8   Conclusion

This chapter began by describing how managers in all care settings are accountable to a range of people, from service users through to government. It was suggested that it can be difficult to manage mistakes and challenges creatively if managers are concerned about being blamed when something goes wrong. However, mistakes cannot be avoided in care, and they are better managed openly, as stepping-stones to individual learning and organisational growth. The story of Irene, Carmen and the others is a way of illustrating this in practice. The learning from the mistakes that Carmen experienced is summarised in the extract from her diary. You can compare her experiences and learning with your own.

Finally, it is impossible for a manager to do everything and not to make mistakes. There are choices to be made and decisions to be taken. If there is no room for error, there is nothing to make a choice or decision about. In the same way as there is no such person as the perfect parent (and who would want one?), there is no such person as the perfect manager. Just occasionally managers achieve what seems like perfection for a few hours or even days, and then something goes wrong, mistakes start happening, and more challenges are posed, and so they move on. As a manager, you respond to complex and ever-changing pressures and events. You keep balance; you move; you correct and overcorrect; you lean one way and then the other. If you try to stay still, you lose balance.

Chapter 11
Managing significant life events

Janet Seden and Jeanne Samson Katz

11.1   Introduction

Managers in care services have a variety of responsibilities. Some of those which superficially appear to be routine and not unduly stressful concern organising workloads and shifts, meeting departmental deadlines and processing paperwork. However, much of managing care is involvement in the life events of other people. Some of these situations were explored in Chapters 9 and 10, where some complex human dilemmas are discussed in the contexts of the protection agenda and learning from mistakes and challenges. This chapter focuses on the emotional impact of such demanding social care work on managers, their staff and their service users.

Researchers and observers alike have noted the enormity of the emotional burden faced by practitioners and managers in many care environments. For example, Dr Margaret Tonnesman, speaking at a conference in 1989, suggested that, 'the human encounter in the helping professions is inherently stressful'. However, she went on to say:

> By contrast, if we can maintain contact with the emotional reality of our service users and ourselves then the human encounter can facilitate not only a healing experience, but also an enriching experience for them and for us.
>
> (Tonnesman quoted in Hawkins and Shohet, 1989, p. 157)

Frontline managers' day-to-day work brings them into contact with the emotions, feelings and reactions of both staff and service users towards all kinds of life events. This is demanding, challenging and often stressful. For managers, interactions with their workers and senior managers are often as significant and stressful as those with their service users. Dealing with unexpected events is also part of the character of managing in health and social care. These events can impact on many facets of managers' work and on the whole spectrum of their service user and staff groups as well as on them personally and the way in which they carry out their work. These events might include death, impairment, injury and other kinds of trauma, or sometimes all of these at once.

The aims of this chapter are to:

- argue that management approaches in social care are better when made sensitively
- consider the relationship between management style, agency structure and stress and wellbeing
- explore some ideas that help managers to understand and manage agency responses to their own and other people's experiences of loss, transition and crisis.

11.2   Management with a human face?

You might wonder whether, in the regulated market which is the context for most care services, management can have a human face. Some of the stereotypes of managers in cartoons and encountered in daily life might lead you to think otherwise.

Have you ever experienced an unhelpful 'macho' management style operating in a social care environment? Some writers on social care management have suggested that this happens and also that the styles women bring to management lead to a more enabling and caring approach (Grimwood and Popplestone, 1993; James, 1994). It remains true that, in general, entry to management at senior levels is more difficult for women (Davidson and Cooper, 1992). There are still more women managers in social care at frontline level than at more senior levels. According to Davidson and Burke (2000), there has been a gradual increase in the percentage of women in the workforce, and a slight increase in the numbers entering management. However, 'the average profile of the female manager has changed little'. Further, 'the glass ceiling still exists, with the majority of women concentrated in the lower levels of management' (p. 3).

Organisational research suggests there is still a long way to go before men and women of all ethnic backgrounds experience equality of opportunity at work. In 2002 a survey by the Social Services Inspectorate

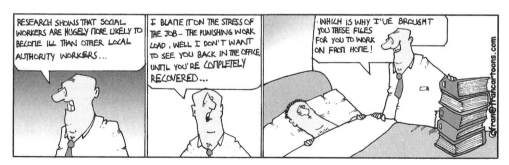

Management with a human face?

in England reported on 2633 posts, of which 1266 (48%) were held by women (see also Chapter 3, pp. 77–8). Although there were more women in management posts than in the 1997 survey, the shape of the situation remains a pyramid, with more women at the base tier than at the first or second tier in their organisations. However, women in the survey held 34% of director posts. There is still much to do to improve the numbers and achievement levels of women in the top tiers of management, and also of black managers (male and female) in council-based management of care in England, but the number of such managers is increasing, especially in the front line.

This chapter draws examples from the practice experience of Surrinder and other managers. You have seen extracts from her diary in earlier chapters. She is a black woman, born in Yorkshire, who describes her identity as Indian and Hindu. She is a frontline manager of a social services family centre in an inner city area with a multi-ethnic population. She manages a deputy, several nursery officers, a cook, a person who repairs the building and equipment, and transport and other support staff. She is one of a team of six frontline managers responsible to a senior manager. She manages the day-to-day running of the service, including the allocation of places, recruitment and appraisal of staff, the building and the budget. She has a view of managing which includes her experiences as a black woman, parent and practitioner as well as her management practice. She works to develop a management identity consistent with her own, with all the dilemmas and challenges this undoubtedly brings.

Accounts written by professionals in the social work press (*Community Care*, 2000) sometimes describe management behaviours that are neither professional nor acceptable when viewed through the lens of what is considered good social care practice as exemplified in professional codes of conduct. If senior and frontline managers treat their workers with a lack of respect this inevitably leads to such practices being passed on to service users. It has been frequently pointed out that frontline managers are in a pivotal position between senior and frontline staff. They face the dilemma of upholding what they see as good practice among their own staff, while perhaps receiving little assistance to maintain these standards from the layer above them. The kind of practice-led management we argue for in this book advocates that those values and actions which practitioners bring to best practice are the same values and actions that inform best management.

The low staff morale that can result from feeling alienated from the manager can lead to a lack of motivation, disillusion and unwillingness to work. While recruitment shortages are the outcome of many complex factors, it has been suggested that 'the quality of management may be the key factor to health in the workplace' (*Community Care*, 2001b, p. 29). In conversation, practitioners often say that when managers minimise or ignore the demands and pressures on them, it contributes significantly to the levels of stress they experience. In this chapter we argue that practice-led managers aim for a style of management that enables and supports practitioners with difficult and complex tasks and acknowledges their humanity and possible vulnerability to strong feelings. This kind of awareness on the part of managers may play an important part in retaining staff, keeping morale high and enabling people to deal with the inevitable pressures of care work.

The challenges faced by managers are often a combination of personal and emotional issues compounded by pressures imposed by the organisation and higher authorities. Henderson and Seden (2003) found that frontline managers are often acutely aware of the need to balance meeting strategic departmental deadlines, achieving operational objectives and managing the professional and developmental needs of staff in a positive way. Surrinder was interviewed during the research (referred to in Appendix 1) in 2000 and 2001. She said her professional and personal values meant that she tried to achieve a balance between good operational service processes, good outcomes for children and their families, and valuing her staff. She wanted to achieve the goal of ensuring that agency responsibilities to service users and staff needs were all met. She also asserted that, in her view, competent management could have a human face and take account of workers' feelings as well as the demands of the organisational structure and service delivery:

> I say to staff that I am not a mind reader, but if things are happening in your life, you need to value yourself enough to come and speak to me.

> I have always said to them that if you feel you have stress or something is bothering you, or something a child or family says stirs up emotions for you, you can come in here and let me know that you need some time out or a break. You need to come and tell me so that we have an understanding and awareness of what is happening.

> I have a job to do and that is to manage and see that the staff are effective for the children, but I try to be human in the process. I think that's the thing I try to bring home to the staff, that you are still human, but there is a level of professionalism within that which they have to maintain, so that's my drive.

>   (Manager consultations)

Surrinder's personal views reflected those of several other managers, male and female, interviewed by Henderson and Seden (2003). These managers believed that, in order to manage staff, they needed to find the balance between awareness of the emotional impact of the work on staff and maintenance of the clear and firm boundaries that make the care environment caring and fair. They said this made heavy demands on them personally; for example, a manager of a children's home commented:

> The staff need support over problems that arise. In a home or establishment you are there to raise staff morale, keep it as high as you

can, so you have to know each member of staff personally. That is very time-consuming, so you've got to hold meetings, make sure staff are informed, so personal issues and personal skills are part of the job, definitely ... a very time-consuming part of the job, I find.

(Manager consultations)

Managing care processes

There is a theoretical model for this kind of managing. Brown and Clough (1989) suggest that managers of residential care in particular work with differing constants. In other words, the certainty of managing in care is that situations will vary and individual needs will differ, but the task of the manager is to recognise and work with that reality. The manager's central objective is to 'establish a facilitative culture and climate based on a clear purpose and value-base, creating an atmosphere and way of doing things which permeates everything in the centre' (Brown and Clough, 1989, p. 193). Acknowledging the feelings and experiences of the individuals involved in service provision is integral to managing in a humane way. This is because 'we are all different people with different experiences, work-styles and strengths; and this needs to be recognised and taken into account in making the most of the different resources of individual users and staff' (pp. x–xi).

Surrinder recognises this in her work and aims to manage the culture, climate and environment in the unit to meet the needs of the individual children and their families, managing the staff so they can play their part in doing this. This responsiveness to a complex process is practice-led. Fieldwork managers also experience their work as managing different constants. The same situations occur (for example, children needing safeguarding from harm) but the factors to consider are different each time (for example, this unique child in her particular environment). This is what makes managing care a practice-led matter and thus different from managing, for instance, car production lines.

Brown and Clough also argue that:

The real test of the 'grand' objectives of social agencies is to be found in the daily life of the people who live and work in the centres about which we have been writing. If those people are to have more say in what happens within the centre, the inevitable consequence is that there will be less control from management. However, the gains are startling: users are reassured when staff are able to share their own struggles to adapt and cope with all the different demands.

(Brown and Clough, 1989, p. 213)

This is a style of management where being sensitive, listening to what people say and working openly with constant change and complexity is the approach taken, whatever the manager's formal role. Therefore, in this chapter we view the manager as a human being first, whose management activity is guided by protocols, but who actively responds to contain and support the life crises, losses, transitions and uncertainties that are part of other people's life events.

With the exception of the work on group care that we just considered (Brown and Clough, 1989), it is arguable that, perhaps in the past, writing on management in care tended to neglect the relationship between the core skills, knowledge and values of care work and effective management practice. The human relations school has helpfully sought to apply psychological theories to management (Obholzer, 2003). More recently, an identifiable management literature has emerged that recognises the links between understandings of psychological theories of behaviour and management style (Glastonbury *et al.*, 1987; Hersey and Blanchard, 1993; Arnold *et al.*, 1998). However, it is perhaps not always as widely drawn on in practice as some other, more instrumental or 'hands-on', models of management.

This issue of integrating management activity with professional values has also been explored by Bilson and Ross (1999), who attempt to link the methods of social work management to the practice activities of the agencies, and by Exworthy and Halford (1999), who argue for a synthesis of managing and professionalism. Most social care managers appear to learn on the job by adding management experience to practitioner qualifications (Lawler and Hearn, 1997). This means that a public sector management based on the purposes, conditions and tasks of the agency has developed in practice. This kind of practice-led management has grown incrementally with the increase in management roles available under the current arrangements for organising social care. Exworthy and Halford (1999) also argue that understanding the professional–manager link, and what it means, is a key issue for the delivery of services. The participatory model, which involves workers in making decisions (Pine *et al.*, 2003) shows how this kind of practice + professional + management coalition can be effective.

Key points

- There is an opportunity to be sensitive when managing.
- There is a theoretical basis for a practice-led model of managing care.

11.3   Stress and wellbeing in the workplace

The ways of considering the management task discussed so far underpin the argument that psychosocial theories of stress, loss, transition and handling unexpected events can be useful to managers. Everyone involved in helping other people will at some time experience:

- *loss* – perhaps of a job, a person close to them, a possession or a hope
- *transition* – response to a life change involving emotional adjustments, for example when moving home, moving into care or forming a new relationship
- *crisis* – a sudden unexpected event, such as an accident or a disaster, the shock of which temporarily makes the usual ways of managing both personally and professionally feel inadequate, and for which new coping strategies are needed.

You may be familiar with ideas about loss, transition and crisis from your own experiences or practitioner training. They are also relevant concepts for managers since they interact with staff and make decisions about how services are organised. It is precisely this need to manage complex events that makes managing care a potentially stressful occupation. The failure to manage transitions, losses and changes well, taking account of their emotional impact on individuals, can lead to an accumulation of unacknowledged pressure, which may lead to stress. Consequently, this chapter first considers stress, stress management and the maintenance of wellbeing for managers and the people with whom they work, before returning to some key ideas about loss, transition, crisis and their effects on people.

Arnold *et al.* (1998) describe workplace stress as a force that pushes people psychologically and physically beyond the ability to adapt. Each of us has our own individual coping mechanisms, which have personal and cultural origins. As already suggested, stress is inherent in social care work and it is helpful to be open about it. The manager of a children's home put it this way:

> I have taken a different approach. I say 'This is going to be stressful – let's see if, as a team, we can manage it together.' We also have our own risk assessments, so that when a child comes here we check if that child self-harms or is known to attack staff. This helps us identify issues early. Staff know that their concerns are heard and we are able to bring in the right staff on rota, and perhaps specialist services that might help. We try to have a proactive approach. The stress is still there but people are enabled to manage it. We had a very threatening young person here recently and we managed that without staff going off sick, as they might have previously.
>
> (Manager consultations)

All managers, whatever the setting, need to find ways of adapting to the pressures created by the demands of other people. Surrinder described some of hers as follows.

> There are times when I need to get certain things done, and they are constantly asking for stats and things. Sometimes I would have to close my door and set some clear boundaries around myself and say, 'I have to have an hour to do this and can I not be disturbed? Any messages can be redirected or taken down.'

> I have recently appointed a deputy to cover maternity leave, because my deputy left. So when the senior and we two get together we have a management meeting and look at all the management tasks and delegate from that who will have responsibility for what. I have to be clear and say what I can and can't do. When I first actually started I felt like I had to be superwoman and do everything.

> Also, being a black woman and being in a peer group where the majority were white, I think I had to succeed better and put in a lot more. I was being really hard on myself and have had to really lower my expectations and be realistic.

> (Manager consultations)

Surrinder has developed strategies to help her to manage. Stress occurs when habitual psychological ways of coping with pressure fail or physical illness develops as a result of psychological pressures. The cost of stress to individuals and their families is high, and so are the costs to society, as employees become sick or leave their jobs. Arnold *et al.* (1998) have shown that certain occupations seem to entail particularly high stress levels, for example medicine and nursing. Social care workers are also high on the list of those whose jobs make them prone to sickness and absenteeism because of stress. According to the authors, 'stress costs industrialised economies around 10 per cent of Gross National Product, through sickness absence, ill health and labour turnover' (p. 422). They identify five factors (pp. 430–8) that in varying degrees have been linked to work-induced stress (see Box 11.1 opposite).

Walsh (1987) suggests that the stresses social care professionals experience in their work make them vulnerable to *burn-out*: a state of physical, emotional and mental exhaustion. It has also been described as a 'feeling of helplessness, hopelessness' and 'the development of a negative self-concept and negative attitude toward work, life and other people' (Walsh, 1987, p. 280). Many people have some of these feelings, some of the time, but what characterises burn-out is its chronic and overwhelming nature. Walsh also suggests that the gap between the expectations workers may have of their roles and the realities of agency life may contribute to the stress they feel, in which case a management style that enables workers to sustain professional values and derive satisfaction from their work will contribute to their wellbeing. It will also contribute to improved staff retention, a key issue in all care settings.

BOX 11.1 Factors linked to work-based stress

1 Factors intrinsic to the job

These include poor physical working conditions, shift work, long hours, elements of risk and danger, the introduction of new technologies, work that is too much or too difficult, long periods of inertia coupled with the possibility of needing to respond swiftly to crises.

2 Role in the organisation

Three critical factors are major sources of stress: role ambiguity (not being sure what you are supposed to do); role conflict (having contradictory expectations to meet or personal reservations about your remit); and responsibility for others.

3 Relationships at work

Other people are sources of stress and support at work. Lack of trust, poor communication and poor problem solving between people can cause stress. The three key relationships are with superiors, subordinates and peers.

4 Career development

Job security, progression and rewards are strong motivators. The transition to retirement, or being overtaken by younger workers, may be stressors for some. Performance appraisal can be anxiety provoking both for the appraisee and for the appraiser, who may be worried about union reaction, grievance procedures or simply the responsibility of affecting the career of another person.

5 Organisational structure and climate

Participation in the shape of the organisation, and in decision making, creates a feeling of investment and belonging which gives a sense of control and wellbeing to staff. Conversely, non-participation and a feeling of powerlessness contribute to stress.

(Source: adapted from Arnold *et al.*, 1998, pp. 430–8)

Organisational responsibility for employee stress and wellbeing at work

Recently, writers have turned their attention from stress to consider what might promote a sense of wellbeing at work. Barrett (2002) argues that, while wellbeing can be seen simply as the reverse of stress, it is a more complex and positive idea. Factors which contribute to wellbeing in the workplace include genes, diet, socio-economic status, emotions, moods and past experiences. Now that organisations have a legal responsibility to protect the wellbeing of employees, they must ensure that their systems, structures and cultures all offer support to this end.

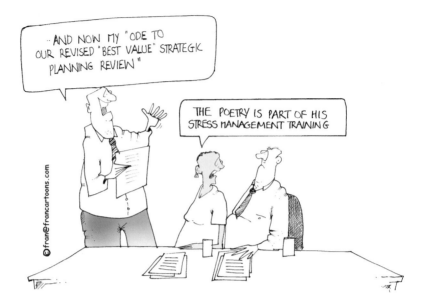

Everyone needs a way to manage stress

However much the individual takes responsibility for care of the self – for instance by jogging, eating well or attending relaxation classes – stress is best managed by tackling its source. This is where the frontline manager has a key role. Elkin and Rosch (1990) suggest that organisation-directed strategies are primary ways of reducing stress and promoting wellbeing at work (see Box 11.2).

BOX 11.2 Organisation-directed strategies for reducing stress

- Redesign the task

- Redesign the work environment

- Establish flexible work schedules

- Encourage participative management

- Include the employee in career development

- Analyse work roles and establish goals

- Provide social support and feedback

- Build cohesive teams

- Establish fair employment policies

- Share the rewards

  (Source: Elkin and Rosch, 1990, cited by Arnold *et al.*, 1998, p. 449)

Managers working in busy care environments such as education and health are in a position to influence some of these factors. Ultimately, such strategic decisions are the responsibility of the senior management group, but the first steps towards change often come from frontline managers identifying where to start, what to influence, and how to monitor and evaluate any changes. Managers can perhaps best reduce employee stress by creating a supportive organisational culture (Seden, 2003) with good interpersonal communication. It can be difficult for middle managers to achieve structural change in their organisation but engaging with this process step by step will be productive both for them and their workers. As one new manager said: 'You need to choose your goals and address them one by one to change the working environment for the better, otherwise too much change can be exhausting too' (manager consultations).

The organisation's responsibility to workers is brought into sharp focus by situations where individuals take employers to court, claiming compensation for work-related stress. According to the *Daily Express* (Fagge, 2002), the TUC won £321 million in compensation for workers in 2001. There has been a steady stream of reports of such cases in the media. For example, Margaret Pratley of Honiton in Devon is reported by *Community Care* (2002b, p. 7) as saying that her work for Surrey council between 1994 and 1998 became 'so overwhelming that she contemplated suicide'. She is said to have been managing between 75 and 150 cases at any one time. The council disputed her application for retirement on the grounds of ill health, saying she was fit to return to work after a long period of sick leave. In August 2002 she lost her claim for compensation. However, Thelma Conway, whose story is told in Example 11.1, won an out-of-court settlement from her employer.

EXAMPLE 11.1 Compensation awarded for stress at work

Former social worker Thelma Conway was awarded £140,000 compensation last year for stress she suffered in her job. Mrs Conway, 56, ended up running the children's home where she was deputy manager, despite her protests that she was not qualified. She retired through ill health in 1999 after pressures which were said to have left her 'withdrawn'.

Mrs Conway, a mother of four, put in 70 to 80 hours a week at the home in Redditch, Worcs., often finishing at 2 am and starting again at 7 am.

She said: 'It was the worst four years I have lived through. The money won't compensate for losing a job I enjoyed. It could have been avoided if someone had simply listened.

I kept saying I was struggling and felt I was letting people down. Normally I am a confident, bubbly person, but stress destroyed a lot of things in my life.'

Worcestershire county council admitted liability, and settled out of court.

(Source: *Daily Express*, 2002, p. 9)

Looking after yourself

While structural change to introduce worker-friendly policies might seem the best long-term goal, self-care remains essential for busy managers. West (1997) suggests managers should ask themselves the following questions to identify ways of staying psychologically intact.

- What would be physically helpful for you: for example, sports, walking, climbing, team games, massage, yoga, scented baths?
- How can your emotional needs best be met? What works best for you: sharing, talking, drawing, painting, dancing, drama, music, friends, theatre, cinema, watching football or reading?
- How might your spiritual needs be met: exploring beliefs, meditating or reading poetry, exploring complementary therapies?

If you do not know the answer to these questions already, now is a good time to think about it.

Surrinder described some of her strategies for her own wellbeing as follows.

Within work, whenever I get time, usually at lunchtimes, I try to take my break after everybody else has had theirs, because I like to have the staffroom to myself for space and time to sit in silence. Outside of work I actually do Tai Chi and meditate.

I have two very good soul mates ... one is my partner and one my best friend. And talking and writing – I do quite a lot of reflective writing now ... and just being with my children, I love it.

She also arranges both stress management sessions and informal activities for staff, which she believes contribute to team building in the workplace:

Prior to the stress management, we had a fun afternoon – we were looking at team building and we all brought food in. It was a bit social, but we had it partly because I wanted the staff to look at their own team dynamics, strengths, and weaknesses and how they pulled together.

It was very positive and did wonders for morale, but it also brought out a lot of issues that perhaps people hadn't identified among themselves and with management.

> **Key points**
>
> - Managing stress is an organisational responsibility.
>
> - Structural changes are important, and frontline managers have a key role in influencing them.
>
> - Management failure to listen to and act on workers' concerns can lead to litigation.
>
> - Self-care is an important factor in managing stress.

11.4   Some theories for understanding and managing events

Acknowledging issues as they arise

So far, we have argued that managers in care settings can manage in a humane way, but that this takes time and attention and can be inherently stressful. Surrinder's view is that it is best to deal with issues in an honest and open way as they arise because that stops pressure and tension building up. However, this is not always possible. Some events, such as the family centre's cook being off sick, can happen unexpectedly and be difficult to resolve. In this section we argue that understanding the way in which life events are experienced, and people's reactions to and ways of coping with them, can help to make them less stressful and enable people to adapt and manage them. Also, regarding life events, the simple user–professional split is artificial. The parties concerned may be in the role of service user or professional, yet each will respond at a personal level to the events and processes they share together. This is certainly true in residential settings where, as a manager of a children's home put it:

> Honesty is needed. It's a very open place to work, it's very informal at times, but you need to be formal too. You're playing dominoes and eating your tea with the young people and next thing you're in a case conference. You have to be able to change your style.
>
> (Manager consultations)

So, it is important to remember an awareness of how the professional and personal interact as you explore the relevance of psychosocial understandings of people to the management of particular events in care settings. While psychosocial theories of attachment, loss, transition and crisis may already be familiar to you, they are explored here in relation to managing. First, theories of *attachment* and *loss* (two sides of one coin in human experience) are considered and these provide an underpinning for thinking about two other key ideas – *transition* and *crisis*.

Theories of attachment and loss

Events such as a death or separation from a partner or child affect the way people behave as employees, and require sensitive responses from the manager. Surrinder had experience of this.

> There is one member of staff who has had a lot of stresses in her life. She had a loss, her sister. She is a single parent and her sister passed away last year. There was no sign – she [the sister] came down with 'flu and passed away within two days.

> We maintained contact by ringing up and asking how she was, and she had compassionate leave for a while before going off sick. I think she attempted to come in, for me, but she was very upset and emotional, very tearful and we said, 'You need to take some time off for yourself and come to terms with things, and understand what is going on for you.'

> We stayed in contact so she felt she had that support, but also that work wasn't something miles away. One of the other managers visited and I made phone contact. When she came back, what we looked at was 'therapeutic hours' and set that up so she only came in a couple of hours each morning. She was breaking the ice but didn't feel pressurised to get things done ... and then increased her hours gradually over a period of two months until she returned to work fully.

Surrinder was very clear about the need for sensitive personal support for this staff member, but also about her responsibility, as manager to the agency, for paperwork and for making formal agreements about working arrangements through the occupational health department. She had to balance her responsibilities to the service users with these considerations, and check that the staff member was in a fit state to provide emotional warmth, stability and consistent care for the children at the family centre when she returned to work. Surrinder thought that if the personnel department had been less flexible and supportive towards this staff member, she would not have returned to work so soon, and her valuable practice experience might have been lost. Having been supported through this difficult personal event, she was able to return to full employment. Managers are not expected to provide counselling, but they do have a personal support role. In the situation just described, counselling was offered through the occupational health department.

The theoretical material on understanding loss has developed over time, and the more recent writing places psychological issues in a social and cultural context (The Open University, 2001). Writers about loss focus on death and dying but also show how the ideas are relevant to other kinds of losses, for example having something stolen from you or losing a limb (Charmaz, 1995). In the management context it is important to be aware of the relevance of these ideas for a staff member losing a job or failing to achieve their professional goals. Managers need to recognise the impact of personal life events on workers in order to offer the right support, to encourage them to take leave when necessary, or seek more intensive help outside the workplace. Managers have a role in recognising staff's and service users' reactions to loss; being alert to the implications in their actions and decisions is crucial. As one manager said:

> Good practice in dealing with underperforming staff is, I feel, to use policies and procedures as a support mechanism. In terms of M. having a problem and going off sick because of it ... I would have advised her [manager] to use that as a support, not a disciplinary, and if as a manager you keep in your head that you're there to support the person, to try and help them get through the problem they're having, it becomes a far easier meeting than thinking about going into a meeting as a disciplinary.
>
> (Manager consultations)

Loss of whatever kind causes pain in two ways: first, the actual pain of being without something or someone and, second, the pain of adapting to the absence and the changes that this adjustment involves. Next we consider three theoretical explanations for the experience of loss. John Bowlby uses an individual approach, Colin Murray Parkes a psychiatric one, and Peter Marris's approach is a sociological one. These ideas, which were developed during the 20th century, still provide a basis for understanding people.

John Bowlby and attachment theory

Bowlby (1969, 1973, 1980) was the first to argue that what he calls 'separation anxiety' is the price people pay for being attached to someone or something. Bowlby, and those who have adapted his ideas, present the force of attachment to the mother, other early care givers and significant people in our lives as a powerful and universal force. Since the early 1950s Bowlby's theories about attachment have permeated studies and practice in care work, and have been critiqued, developed and refined to include attachment to culture and place (Rashid, 1996; Daniel et al., 1999). Bowlby's idea that attachment is a characteristic of human beings 'from cradle to grave' has been developed and attachment viewed as a significant factor in adult life as well as in childhood (Parkes et al., 1991). Howe (1995, 1996) makes applications to current social work practice.

Colin Murray Parkes and psychosocial transitions

Colin Murray Parkes (1986) considers the social dimensions that explain losses and their psychological effects. He points out that people are generally good at adapting to change but suggests that some life events are more difficult and so potentially more dangerous than others. He identifies three distinguishing criteria for these most difficult changes, which he calls 'psychosocial transitions', which he says:

1 require people to undertake a major revision of their assumptions of the world
2 are lasting in their implications rather than transient
3 take place over a relatively short time, so there is little opportunity for preparation.

He argues that, as individuals, we all inhabit an 'assumptive world', that is, a world that contains what we consider to be true based on our previous experience. When new experiences challenge this truth, revising the assumptive world is not easy. Thoughts and behaviour can no longer be taken for granted. The familiar world becomes unfamiliar: we have to think before we act and this takes time and energy. We no longer have confidence in our assumptive world to keep us safe and the process of adaptation can be painful.

Peter Marris and sociological perspectives

Peter Marris (1974, 1986) offers a sociological explanation of loss, using three key concepts to explain the link between loss and change.

1 The conservative impulse

We are surrounded by change much of which we neither notice nor absorb. Marris suggests that everyone has an in-built bias towards predictability, a resistance to change. He calls this 'the conservative impulse', which is a drive towards finding ways of feeling familiar with our environment, or at least most of it, and of reducing uncertainty.

2 Structures of meaning

Marris suggests that individuals relate to social and physical environments by recognising familiar patterns. He calls these 'patterns of attachment' and 'structures of meaning', which he defines as 'the organised structures of understanding and emotional attachments by which grown people interpret and assimilate their environment' (1974, p. 4). Marris's structures of meaning are similar to what Parkes describes as 'assumptive worlds'. Marris understands structures of meaning to involve both understanding and attachment. He illustrates this by the commonly used expression 'that means a lot to me'. He suggests that people attach meaning to objects and people from early childhood and carry that meaning from one situation to another.

3 Grieving

By grieving Marris means the psychological process of adjustment to loss. It involves feeling bereft not only of the lost object but also of part of our understanding of, and adaptation to, our environment. There are many useful studies of different aspects of bereavement and grieving (Worden, 1991; Lendrum and Syme, 1992; Kubler-Ross, 1970).

The message that emerges for care professionals is to be cautious about seeing grief as occurring in stages and to avoid being prescriptive about what they might feel or experience (The Open University, 2001). Reactions to loss can include many emotions, some of which are listed in Box 11.3.

BOX 11.3 Feelings associated with loss

Tearful	Guilty	Hurt
Sad	Angry	Helpless
Numb	Panic	Worthless
Insecure	Tired	Relieved
Apprehensive	Disoriented	Vengeful
Dazed	Burdened	Distressed
Misunderstood	Alienated	Grief
Bewildered	Unhappy	Restless
Pain	Unwanted	Anxious
Shocked	Lonely	Afraid
Liberated	Vulnerable	Unloved
Unburdened	Powerless	Self-pity
Release	Disbelief	Denial

(Source: adapted from Ward and Associates, 1992, p. 109)

Managing and understanding the impact of loss is an important part of a manager's role, be it deaths in the families of either staff or service users. Other losses could be someone losing a home, losing a foster placement, their liberty, job or promotion. Losses of all kinds trigger a range of strong feelings and reactions, all of which are best acknowledged and managed openly and as part of the process in the workplace. Most of the situations that bring people into contact with social care professionals and their managers involve elements of separation, transition and loss.

Caution is required in all studies of human development in relation to gender, culture and race. In general, theories of human growth and development do not always take enough account of the diverse experiences of different ethnic groups and of women. There are many accounts which re-evaluate theory and examine bias and prejudice (Gilligan, 1982; Pederson, 1994; Burck and Speed, 1995; Lago and Thompson, 1996). However, it can be argued that psychosocial theories, subject to reinterpretation and careful checking against the lived realities of people's experiences, remain a powerful way of understanding some of the personal processes which are part of the daily work of managing care.

Life changes and events

Transition remains a powerful and persuasive concept in social care because it describes the impact of the change and adjustment which happen in various human experiences such as being made redundant, retiring, changing partner, experiencing terminal illness and bereavement, or moving house or country. Transition has immediate relevance, too, to the lives of service users (for example, entering and leaving care) and how this is managed, as well as to workers faced with organisational change, such as becoming a manager or having some other new role in the organisation.

Different events affect people in different ways. Researchers have looked at the kinds of life event and how they may make an emotional and/or a psychological impact. Scales developed over the years indicate the different impacts of certain kinds of event. One example is the scale compiled by Holmes and Rahe (1967) (see Table 11.1).

Table 11.1 **Holmes–Rahe social readjustment scale**

Life event	Score*
Death of spouse	100
Divorce	73
Marital separation from mate	65
Detention in jail, other institution	63
Death of a close family member	63
Major personal injury or illness	53
Marriage	50
Fired from work	45
Marital reconciliation	45

Life event	Score*
Retirement	45
Major change in the health or behaviour of a family member	44
Pregnancy	40
Sexual difficulties	39
Gaining a new family member (e.g. through birth, adoption, [person] moving)	39
Major business readjustment (e.g. merger, reorganisation, bankruptcy)	39
Major change in financial status	38
Death of a close friend	37
Change to different line of work	36
Major change in the number of arguments with spouse	35
Taking out a mortgage or loan for a major purchase	31
Foreclosure on a mortgage or loan	30
Major change in responsibilities at work	29
Son or daughter leaving home (e.g. marriage, attending college)	29
Trouble with in-laws	29
Outstanding personal achievement	28
Spouse beginning or ceasing to work outside the home	26
Beginning or ceasing formal schooling	26
Major change in living conditions	25
Revision of personal habits (dress, manners, associations, etc.)	24
Trouble with boss	23
Major change in working hours or conditions	20
Change in residence	20
Change to a new school	20
Major change in usual type and/or amount of recreation	19
Major change in church activities (a lot more or less than usual)	19
Major change in social activities (clubs, dancing, movies, visiting)	18
Taking out a mortgage or loan for a lesser purchase (e.g. for a car, TV, freezer)	17

(continued)

Life event	Score*
Major change in sleeping habits	16
Major change in the number of family get-togethers	15
Major change in eating habits	15
Vacation	13
Christmas season	12
Minor violations of the law (e.g. traffic tickets)	11

*Less than 150 life change units = 30% chance of developing a stress-related illness
 150–299 life change units = 50% chance of illness
 Over 300 life change units = 80% chance of illness

(Source: Holmes and Rahe, 1967, pp. 213–8)

This scale orders life events according to the responses of a group of subjects, and has changed over time, as individual responses to change have varied with changing social contexts. Change, even when chosen and possibly positive (e.g. marriage) appears to be stressful and can lead to illness. Work-related events are included too, appearing nine times as high-scoring stressful life events. Trouble with the boss, included in Table 11.1, is usually higher in research focused on work-based stressors only. This implies that, as a manager, you might be a 'stressful life event' for one of your staff, and you might view your manager as a source of pressure or stress. Such scales cannot identify what might be a troublesome change for a particular person, but they give an idea of the kinds of event that might require time for adjustment. Individuals may need practical support, or time off for preparation or afterwards to make the necessary adjustments in their lives when faced with a significant loss or change.

Managing life events in care environments

Managers can use their understanding and awareness of the impact of life events on people when they plan and provide services. They can also use their understanding to minimise disruption to individuals during times of change to the service, which can be frequent. Service users may experience many more transitions when they are recipients of care than they might have done otherwise. For example, someone may choose a residential care home carefully, sell their house and move in expecting to stay permanently, only to find the care home is to close through unforeseen financial difficulties.

Patients admitted to one hospital for treatment may be transferred to another with little notice. Such disruption adds to the stress and adjustment the person is already experiencing. Events like these require an adjustment of thinking, perhaps for meeting new workers or changing carer or treatment. People who go into hospital or residential care well prepared for what might happen, with some of their own clothes and belongings, are likely to feel more at ease.

Some transitions result from unavoidable circumstances such as becoming ill or reaching the age for changing school. Others come from making choices such as finding a new partner or changing job or location. While change is a common experience, and transitions are part of most people's life experience, factors such as the challenges to a person's assumptive world and structures of meaning, together with the amount of support available, will affect how the transition is experienced.

Parents often spend a lot of time preparing their children to start school. Strategies such as explaining what is expected, reading stories about children starting school, making sure clothes and equipment are ready, visiting in advance and practising walking the route to school beforehand all help. Teachers find those children whose parents have prepared them for beginning school or nursery, and have friends who help them to adapt, are the ones who make the transition from home best.

In contrast, children looked after in local authority care may experience many moves from foster home to residential unit, back to foster home, and often without there being much preparation or purposeful arrangements about schooling (Shaw, 2003). This can be very disruptive and upsetting. Likewise, moves made by older people from home to hospital, to nursing care, to home, can leave them feeling they have no control of their circumstances and choices. The way such moves are managed makes all the difference to how they are experienced.

Changes can be policy-driven and managers and care staff are often preoccupied by keeping up with developments. The changes in the organisation of social work and social care which have been experienced since the 1980s have affected managers and practitioners alike as well as influencing the experience of users. Managers need to have oversight of how changes are managed for service users at practical as well as procedural levels. When under pressure to follow procedures conscientiously, it is easy to overlook some basic human elements that may be the aspects of most significance to the person whose life is changing. For instance, it is more important for a two-year-old, coming into a foster placement and leaving familiar carers, to have her favourite toy, cup or food with her than whether the new admission forms have been completed properly, important though that is.

> **Key points**
>
> - Theories about attachment, loss and transition are helpful in managing care.
>
> - Managers can use these theories to understand what changes might mean for individuals.
>
> - Managers can be instrumental in guiding practitioners to help people manage change more successfully.
>
> - Managers can use their understanding of the impact of life events on their staff, for example by arranging compassionate leave.

11.5   Managing unexpected events

Adjustment to loss and change makes heavy emotional demands on everyone, even when things go relatively smoothly. Pressure on people is greater when they are in situations of deprivation and hardship, with limited access to those financial and other material resources that might make adjustment to change or loss easier to manage. Such pressures may tip transition into crisis. Individuals may have different thresholds for managing transitions and crises depending on their previous experience and background. Marris (1974, 1986) suggests four sets of conditions that may help or hinder people to adjust when faced with loss, transition and change.

1   Childhood experiences of attachment affect our general world view and resilience in the face of loss.

2   The more there are conflicting emotions or the more doubtful or unresolved the meaning of what has been lost, the harder the process.

3   The less opportunity to prepare for the loss, and the less predictable and meaningful the event itself, the more traumatic the experience.

4   Events after the loss itself may support or frustrate the recovery process.

Social factors are also significant: for example, experiences of discrimination such as racism and sexism. If a manager understands more about the dimensions of change for individuals (including dimensions related to cultural values), this can make the implementation of care plans or changes in workplace practices go more smoothly. Often, clumsily managed changes become a crisis. Some events overwhelm people because they are too big and are outside their experience. Those who write about crisis (for example, Seden, 2001) often describe it as a temporary period of upset and disequilibrium, sometimes brought on by the impact of change, shock or a traumatic event, when the person's usual abilities to cope are temporarily suspended, while they find new ways of adjusting.

Some crises, such as the events of 11 September 2001 in New York, when two passenger aircraft were flown into the twin towers of the World Trade Centre, causing them to collapse, are defined by their unexpectedness and the scale of the disaster. Coping with unexpected serious events at work adds another dimension to the manager's support task and to the emotional load on the practitioner. Even the most experienced practitioners can struggle to cope with an unexpectedly demanding situation. There are immediate challenges to resources and to management practice.

However well prepared they are, any manager may have to deal with unanticipated situations. Examples are the King's Cross fire (1987), the Hillsborough disaster (1989), the Omagh bombing (1998) and the Dunblane shootings (1999), all of which required supportive work from local health and care organisations. In Northern Ireland health and care managers operate in the context of political tension and associated violence (Pinkerton, 1998). Events such as the abduction of children or rail accidents in their area require managers to respond quickly, often with little or no preparation. The death of a service user may lead to an inquiry. Managing sudden and unpredictable events such as those mentioned, and their aftermath, is a challenge.

Social care workers were involved in many ways after the bodies of several missing girls were found buried in Fred and Rosemary West's home in Gloucester in the 1990s. They helped the Wests' other children to talk through the awful events they had experienced and found them new places to live. One of the workers wrote:

> Eventually, the children were found permanent placements and the care team's task came to an end ...

> The personal cost was high. All of us felt we would never be the same again. We had gone round for so long with all this information locked in our heads and we were unable to let it out. You felt you could never be normal again ...

> We were all offered counselling and many of us are still receiving it. We have group sessions where it is a real relief to be able to say anything you want and know that no one will be shocked or upset by it.
>
> (Social worker quoted in *Professional Social Work*, 1996, p. 10)

It was not just the social workers who found themselves exceptionally emotionally affected. All those close to such events, such as the person who keeps the records, can find themselves emotionally changed and involved. The management response to the workers makes all the difference to their coping and recovery mechanisms. Managers can never be fully prepared for the unexpected, but the following conclusions were drawn after the Hillsborough football stadium disaster about the impact of such events on the professionals involved (The Open University, 2001).

1 They are likely to feel overwhelmed by the sheer size of the problem and feel helpless. The chaos at Hillsborough made the doctors' tasks much more difficult.

2 They need to recognise that trained professionals are as traumatised as everyone else by such experiences.

3 They will need help and support in the aftermath of a disaster such as Hillsborough.

Expertise has developed among emergency services personnel, who recognise the need to train and support other staff in the event of such unexpected tragedies. Psychological support may take the form of debriefing immediately afterwards or long-term counselling. Managers and their teams of staff are unlikely to have any useful experience to draw on in such situations, which puts them in a vulnerable position. Managers are no more protected than their staff when dealing with traumatic events. Therefore, it is important to ensure they also are offered or seek appropriate help.

Key points

- Transitions are changes in people's lives that may become crises if unsupported or mismanaged in care situations.

- Social factors are very significant in supporting or disadvantaging those experiencing changes in their lives.

- Managers may have to support staff through unexpected traumatic events. They will do this better if they understand the possible reactions of staff and themselves and seek resources for support.

11.6 Conclusion

In this chapter we argued for an approach to managing care that takes account of the humanity and psychological make-up of managers, staff and service users within their cultural contexts. Ignoring these elements can contribute to the build-up of stress and reduce any sense of wellbeing at work. It was suggested that managers do a better job if they take into account the psychological, social and practical impact of changes, life crisis and loss on themselves, the people they manage and the service users, as they go along.

Several practitioners quoted in this chapter indicated that it is essential for managers to listen carefully to service users' and workers' concerns and to respond actively to them. Through recognising the impact of the work on people's feelings, and by heeding service users' and workers' needs and concerns, managers are more likely to oversee the provision of services in ways that make service users' situations better rather than worse. Furthermore, there is a relationship between the way managers approach their staff, and the demands on them, and staff sickness and staff retention.

Managers ignored Thelma (Example 11.1) when she raised concerns about her ability to cope with the increasing demands on her in a new role, which led to her experience of stress and her claim for compensation.

Workload management has to include a consideration of the emotional impact of caring work on those who do it. Managing a service can only be done well if account is taken of the consequences of loss, change, transition and crisis for the people using the service and those who are working with them in a professional role.

Chapter 12
Managing professional development

Mark Peel

12.1   Introduction

At one level, professional development simply 'reflects a personal commitment on the part of individuals to seek out the answers to questions that continually arise in the context of practice' (Eby, 2000b, p. 48). Motivated individuals look for answers to the challenges and dilemmas they face through a range of activities, discussions with colleagues, professional journals, training courses, research reports, taking advice and seeking supervision from managers. In this chapter the emphasis is on managers' responsibilities for enabling the professional development of their staff, while also managing performance. This means considering the processes of induction, supervision, appraisal, managing poor performance, delegation and disciplinary procedures as linked together. Managing professional development includes overseeing the career development of both qualified and non-qualified workers.

Managers want their own professional development to be taken seriously within their organisation. This is because the frontline manager's role in the professional development of other people, with the linked responsibilities for ensuring the quality of professional practice within their area of influence, is such that support for the manager in carrying out this task is essential. Active attention to the learning needs of others is a demanding practice-led activity, whereby the individual development and performance of staff are enhanced to meet the needs of service users, the organisation, employers, professional bodies and policy makers. Practice-led managers, who take service users' satisfaction seriously, will want to make sure that workers are well equipped to work with people and provide services.

Professional development and career progression are linked concepts in nursing, teaching and social work (Eby, 2000b). While managers supervising in the 1970s and 1980s might have emphasised emotional and professional support, by the late 1980s and 1990s they were increasingly concerned with assessing performance, managing workload and measuring competence in ways that feed into appraisal systems and promotions. Supervision has become an activity where all these parts of practice are managed (Pritchard, 1995; Horwath and Morrison, 1999). In this chapter professional development is considered as a concern of service users, individual practitioners, frontline managers, senior managers and organisations. It draws on examples from colleagues who were interviewed as part of the preparation of this book.

The aims of this chapter are to:

- explore the idea of professional development
- identify the frontline manager's role and responsibilities in the organisation for the processes that contribute to staff development
- discuss the processes through the use of examples.

12.2   Managing the professional development of other people

In terms of professional development managers provide a personal point of contact for their staff within the organisation and they mediate between the requirements of individuals and those of others in the work group or team. However, what does development mean? Marsh and Triselotis (1996) observe, from their research study into the experiences of newly qualified practitioners and their managers, that different managers or supervisors rarely define development explicitly. They found that, 'the meaning they [the supervisors] attributed to "development" was seldom explained, but, like support, it was seen to take different forms' (p. 159). Usually two related concepts were involved: the identification of existing strengths and the identification of areas where further training or experience was needed.

Also development probably means different things to workers at different times in their careers. For example, when Barbara, a newly qualified social worker, was first appointed she felt a need to gain more confidence in her basic professional skills and establish herself as part of the team. A few months later she felt more confident in her skills; she also felt better integrated as a team member. Barbara was then able to identify more specific and advanced development needs, such as improving her assessment skills. This had not been apparent to her or her manager at the earlier stage.

In an educational context, O'Neill (1994, p. 87) defines professional development as 'meeting the needs of professional role responsibilities at various career stages' and 'improving professional performance and capability'. Middlewood (1997) puts professional development in context, describing two contrasting, and potentially conflicting, explanations of the objectives of professional development either as being 'for organisational improvement' or as a means of 'harmonising the needs of individuals and the organisation' (p. 187).

These definitions suggest that, far from managers and practitioners simply agreeing on their professional and personal ideas, professional development has an agency function: improving individual performance improves the agency's services. Individuals are assimilated into the culture of the organisation, by developing the skills and abilities they need to do their jobs. There is a further element in that professional development will also continue to be influenced by wider changes to the professional landscape, such as the impact of new legislation, changes in the expectations and needs of service users, developments in the field of post-qualification training and awards, and organisational restructuring.

In summary, professional development is driven by:

- the individual aspirations of individual workers, specific to both their current job and, more generally, to their future career development
- organisational requirements for workers' development to reflect the remit of the organisation, enabling them to be as efficient and effective as possible in the context of their present job and future opportunities within the organisation
- external circumstances such as changes to professional qualifications or legislative mandates.

It might be argued that a more standardised approach to professional development is preferable to the less formal, implicitly highly variable system often negotiated between individual workers, their managers and their organisations. Individually agreed arrangements may be unregulated and out of step with the modern emphasis on evaluation and consistent quality standards. A standardised approach helps to ensure that all workers gained fair access to scarce resources, and regional and national standards could be developed to ensure the highest possible quality. The development work done by the General Social Care Council (GSCC) in England and similar organisations in the devolved countries of the UK, together with National Occupational Standards for social care and health workers being developed in the early 21st century, are designed to create more consistency in qualifying courses and subsequent career development.

Is supervision mainly concerned with regulating working practices and ensuring quality? Kitchener *et al.* (2003) examined the extent to which the new public management approach in social care has permeated the management practices of children's homes in 12 local authorities. They found that while a series of abuse scandals had led to a concern for tighter management control over practitioners and more emphasis on monitoring and procedures, the extent to which this was implemented in practice was uneven. Managers preferred to use supervision to discuss what they saw as professional practice issues.

Workers thought that managers promoted from within residential child care practice understood their concerns better. Managers without such practice experience needed to work at demonstrating their ability to listen to, empathise with and advocate for staff. Supervision had not changed radically – it still encompassed professional development matters – yet managers were also responding to the requirement to engage in formal monitoring and inspection. There was still continuity with past supervisory practices of support and modelling. Most importantly, Kitchener *et al.* found that in most cases departments continued to be orientated towards maintaining collegial relationships and respecting practitioner autonomy.

Thus it appears that the more managerial functions of supervision are being grafted on to established models of supportive, educative and practice-led professional activity. Some tensions remain in practice. Thompson (1999, p. 18) says 'social workers want supervision to provide them with emotional and professional support. Managers increasingly see it as a way of measuring performance and results.' In this chapter professional development, and the place of supervision within it, is presented as a holistic process encompassing both elements.

The manager's role in promoting workers' development accords with the role of individuals in taking responsibility for their own learning together with recognition by organisations that facilitating individual professional development offers benefits both for the organisation and, most crucially, for its service users. Individual responsibility for career and professional development is very important. Workers have a responsibility to keep up to date with new publications and research into other professional developments and to assess the usefulness of research-based findings for practice. Managers have responsibility for stimulating and supporting this (see Chapter 5).

Organisations have a responsibility to ensure that they embody and promote a culture in which learning and development can take place, and where career development is acknowledged and appropriately rewarded. When many organisations in health and social care are finding it increasingly difficult to recruit and retain qualified people, the maintenance or development of an organisational culture in which personal development is actively supported may be especially important. Kydd argues that:

> Although individual development may not necessarily have tangible outcomes for the organization, a developing individual is likely to make a richer contribution to it. Conversely, organizational development will only happen if the individuals within it are developing. Professional development and organizational effectiveness are then inextricably linked.
>
> (Kydd, 1997, pp. 1–2)

Managers at all levels need to consider whether they are creating and developing a learning organisation and how it might become a reality (see Chapter 1). There is a useful literature about learning organisations (for example, Senge *et al.*, 1994; Mabey and Salaman, 1995; Pearn *et al.*, 1995) where the key features and elements can be found. There are also some studies of and applications to care (Gould, 2003). Perhaps more familiar to care practitioners and managers is the notion of creating the environment in which individuals, groups and agencies can truly be said to learn, grow and change. David Behan, writing on training as Director of Social Services for the London Borough of Greenwich, considers this in Box 12.1.

BOX 12.1 Learning in the organisation

How do we create an appropriate environment for this individual and organisational learning to occur? When I reflect on my own development as a worker and a manager, I recall the people I have worked with who have helped me to learn, grow and change. As a Director of Social Services I hold a responsibility for a large number of staff from a variety of backgrounds, disciplines, experiences and cultures. One of my responsibilities is to establish a culture within the organisation which values learning at both an individual level, a team level and at an organisational level. My task is to create what Peter Senge refers to as a 'learning organisation'. I would argue that every senior manager has a duty to 'make a difference' to their organisation by the creation of a culture which values learning.

However, the commitment of senior managers alone will be insufficient to deliver effective change within organisations. It is dependent on a range of individual managers who will work together. It is therefore crucial that all managers within organisations are able to answer the question 'How do individuals learn and how do organisations learn?'

(Source: Horwath and Morrison, 1999, pp. x–xi)

This is a strategic vision for a learning organisation from a senior manager, and many organisations have training and development strategies. There are no prizes for recognising that it is the frontline manager who will implement the strategy in practice. To do this, they will need to analyse the blocks and barriers to embedding learning in the workplace and engage others in learning processes. The frontline manager is the communicator of agency strategy as designed by senior management, the mediator of training resources to the team, the educator through supervision, and also the troubleshooter when things go wrong. It is the frontline manager who amid the daily realities of other functions reviews with staff who should be learning what, why and when. Many managers are now S/NVQ assessors and mentors for staff on post-qualifying and other in-service training. 'Educator' is another of the 'add-ons' to the frontline management role as it has developed in care settings (Henderson and Seden, 2003).

> **Key points**
>
> - Professional development involves individuals, organisations and the wider context.
>
> - Managers need to balance strategic, operational and team objectives with individual needs.

12.3   The manager at the centre

So far, some factors that influence professional development have been considered. Next, some elements that appear to be integral to the managerial role are discussed. Frontline managers are usually responsible for organising the team's learning opportunities, often making decisions about who will have training opportunities. Some years ago, when I was working as a team manager in a busy social services office, my line manager and I discussed who from my team might attend a two-week training course. Only one person could go, and we could not agree who to select. I was surprised that my manager nominated the person I considered would gain least from the course. I argued that another worker had more interest in the subject, would bring more back from the course to the team as a whole, and had not been on any training events that year, whereas the person she suggested had already been on several courses.

My manager agreed that from my perspective my nomination was valid, but she thought that her nominee was close to 'burn-out' and, in the wider context of a forthcoming external inspection of services, we should give him some time out or we might lose this experienced worker altogether. From her perspective, nominating this person offered maximum benefit to the whole organisation, which she felt should supersede individual or team considerations. Thus audit and staff retention were prioritised over the strictly educational needs of individuals. This is the kind of dilemma frontline managers engage with when allocating scarce training resources. No doubt the team members would have been vocal in their responses to this questionable decision. The same complexities might apply when managers themselves seek training.

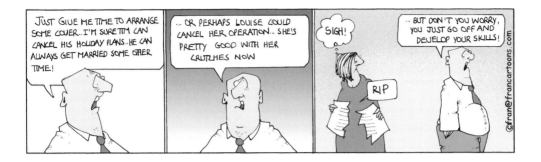

The frontline manager's role and responsibilities

It is useful to model the relationships between an individual, a team and an organisation, and to clarify the manager's position and responsibilities in such a system.

In Figure 12.1 the manager is at the centre of a system that balances the requirements of an individual team member (circle 1), with the combined requirements of a team (circle 2) and the overall requirements of the organisation (circle 3). Intersections between one circle and another illustrate circumstances in which the requirements of one part of the system impact on those of another. This pattern of managerial relationships with the individual, team and organisation can be applied to the majority of social care settings in the voluntary and statutory sectors, and also in many commercial, health and educational settings. Ainscow *et al.* (1994), describing a project to improve the quality of education, use a similar model to describe the management of the professional development environment they found in schools they studied.

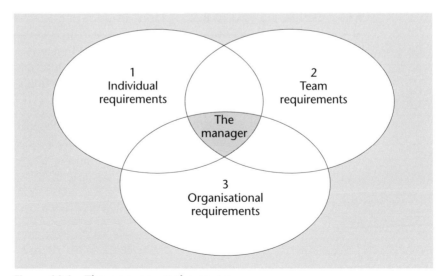

Figure 12.1 **The manager at the centre**

The pattern shown in Figure 12.1 can now be applied to the work in a typical social services access (or intake) team. This is a team responsible for the initial telephone calls and office visits from the public. Their task is to respond immediately to requests for services, often dealing with complex and urgent issues. Also, when appropriate, they put service users in touch with other service providers or teams within their own organisation who can offer the relevant service.

Barbara, the recently appointed social worker referred to earlier, has worked for Southshire Social Services access (intake) team for a few months. Her manager, Manju, has worked there for seven years. The team has six other members and two vacancies. Betty, the most experienced person, has been with the team for 11 years, and Chris and Bupen joined just before Barbara. Looking at Figure 12.1, Barbara is in circle 1 (individual requirements), while Betty, Chris, Bupen and the other social workers in the team are in circle 2 (team requirements). The wider organisation of Southshire Social Services, including staff training officers, the personnel section, other social work teams, multi-agency teams and senior managers, are in circle 3 (organisational requirements).

Manju, the team manager, is responsible for considering where the circles overlap, and balancing the needs and requirements of all three elements of the figure. Individual, team and organisational requirements are related. Manju has responsibility for managing Barbara's professional development, but this is not a one-way process. As her development progresses, Barbara will have responsibility for putting the confidence and skills she gains into practice in her day-to-day work and into her responses to service users' views. As Barbara gains experience, her ability to offer as well as receive support within the team should grow. This picture shows the complexities of the frontline manager's role in balancing competing requirements.

Key points

- The manager balances the training needs of individuals, the team and the agency.

- The pattern of needs and opportunities is complex and changing.

12.4   Induction

The shortage of suitably qualified social workers and other care staff has been a concern for managers since the late 1990s. In circumstances where demand (the need to recruit) exceeds supply (the pool of potential applicants), it is increasingly important for managers to ensure that the induction process addresses the fears and anxieties that new staff often feel. This may also go some way towards retaining staff, who, even if they have relevant paper qualifications, may still feel unready to practise, especially if their training period was short.

Marsh and Triselotis (1996) found that about half of the newly qualified social workers and probation officers they interviewed felt less than fully prepared for the demands of the workplace. They reported that the early period of employment was a testing and anxious time:

> Only about five per cent of the respondents indicated that they had no anxieties about starting work. The rest mentioned at least one specific area which was causing them concern, either in relation to their own degree of readiness or to agency related factors and not infrequently to both. Having to be 'accountable' or 'responsible' for their actions frightened many of them. As students, a large part of this responsibility had been carried by their supervisors.
>
> (Marsh and Triselotis, 1996, p. 133)

This anxiety about inadequate preparation may be common. Proper induction makes all the difference to the quality of the experience of staff joining a new team (see Chapter 2 for a discussion of induction into the team). Active managers see induction as the first experience of training and development, when new employees have time to match the abilities they bring from their past experiences and learning to the requirements of the post. Some of the potential concerns are described in Example 12.1.

EXAMPLE 12.1 Steve joins a new team

Steve is a newly qualified social worker who started work with a local authority fostering and adoption team three months ago. Steve has limited pre-qualification experience of social work, but completed a very successful student placement with the team he has now joined. He is supervised by Denise, the team manager, who has been in post for only six months.

Steve said:

> I am very lucky to have got a job with this team. I know there was a lot of competition for my post. I really enjoyed my student placement here and I am sorry that my placement supervisor, Gulshen, has retired. I got on very well with her. The rest of the team have been brilliant in making me feel at home, but I have found the work much more demanding than I expected.

> I know that Denise has been frustrated that I don't know more about fostering and adoption, especially in relation to the law. I don't think that Denise understands that fostering and adoption were only a small element in my training. Gulshen and I very much worked together when I was on placement here. I sometimes don't ask Denise for help when I know I should because I don't want her to think they have made a mistake appointing me.

Denise has a management perspective:

> I've worked in fostering and adoption for the past 12 years, and recently moved to this area when my husband's company relocated him here. Fostering and adoption work needs to be done to a very high standard to ensure the best possible outcomes for very vulnerable and often damaged children. We need to be confident about our own skills so that service users and other professionals feel able to trust our assessments and work in partnership with us. I have offered to increase Steve's supervision from monthly to fortnightly and, while he was initially very keen on this idea, he now seems less convinced.

(Source: manager consultations)

The example reveals a lack of understanding about what are reasonable expectations of a newly qualified worker. Steve's anxiety to be seen as competent, and to ensure that Denise does not think that he is the wrong person for the job, increases the likelihood that he will not take advantage of the available advice and support. Denise has high expectations of the level of confidence and skill required to do the job, which may not be possible for someone newly appointed and inexperienced like Steve. The result of these two perspectives is likely to make each of them more anxious and less likely to find a positive solution.

It is a mistake for any manager responsible for a newly appointed or newly qualified person to assume that they will not need special attention to ensure that their transition through induction is as smooth as possible. It is also necessary to plan how the initial training they have received will be built on and developed. For example, what gaps does Steve identify in his learning so far in relation to his new post? Will Denise help him to identify what support he needs in the early days of practice? Her task in Steve's first year should be to:

- discuss what is competent, accountable practice at his level
- encourage his continuing professional development
- offer support through supervision, team meetings and peers
- integrate him into the organisation by keeping him informed and supported
- encourage him to listen to and learn from service users.

This means they should consider together what learning experiences Steve needs, and determine what priority should be afforded to each activity. For example, it seems more important at first for Steve to be helped to engage with his team and organisation than for undue stress to be placed on his accountable practice. The plans made and agreed at induction could be built on through supervision and appraisal as Steve becomes established in his post.

Key points

- New workers are likely to have skills gaps and anxieties when starting a new job.

- Induction is an opportunity to identify learning needs and begin the worker's professional development in the new role.

12.5 Supervision

Marsh and Triselotis (1996) identify supervision in social care as conceptually different from the more instrumental approaches common in other work settings. Social work has a stronger tradition of regular one-to-one supervision than teaching or nursing for example, so that managers responsible for multidisciplinary teams may find that staff have a range of previous experiences and ideas about what managers will expect and offer. In social work managers' supervisory responsibilities for accountability are supplemented with additional responsibilities for personal and professional development. When it is implemented well, this model has many strengths. Therefore, it is explored here as useful for professional development in all care environments. Morrison writes:

> Supervision is therefore critical to the quality of services delivered to vulnerable groups, the development and sustaining of staff and to the very life of social care organisations. It is an essential managerial and professional activity for everyone in a social care organisation. Supervision is not just for practitioners.
>
> (Morrison, 1999, p. 1)

Drawing from Richards and Payne (1990), Morrison outlines four interrelated functions of supervision:

- management (competent accountable performance/practice)
- education (continuing professional development)
- support (personal and for the task)
- mediation (engaging the individual to the organisation).

(Adapted from Morrison, 1999, p. 19)

A further function sometimes mentioned in relation to supervision is assessment. In this chapter this is included in the concept of the managerial function and performance assessment. However, work-based training includes roles for managers such as practice teacher, mentor and S/NVQ assessor. There has been some debate about whether one person can be line manager and practice assessor. Some argue that there is a clash of interests, and that there should be one supervisor responsible for evaluation, performance and compliance, and a second, independent person responsible for personal and professional development.

The argument is that the frontline manager is not the most objective person to assess competence in the workplace for S/NVQs or other work-based learning. However, it can also be argued that part of professional management practice is the ability to combine roles, negotiating differences and functions. Managers, who know what is required of the work, may be in the best position to assess competently and may also be able to balance this with a support role. This debate is a relevant one for managers to bear in mind, as they might at times want to consider the feasibility of multiple roles in relation to a particular staff member.

These four functions of supervision – management, education, support and mediation – are illustrated by an extract from a Southshire Social Services supervision record. Example 12.2 shows a record, completed by Manju, after a meeting with Barbara soon after she started her job. I have noted where each of the four functions of supervision is demonstrated.

EXAMPLE 12.2 Supervision record: Barbara J.

Completed by Manju P., 12th November

Barbara is presently holding nine cases, having built up from four at our last supervision session. I selected two cases at random, and asked Barbara to nominate a further two cases for us to discuss in supervision. [Management]

Barbara has consistently expressed an interest in improving her assessment skills, especially in relation to the completion of initial and core assessment documentation for children in need. I offered Barbara the opportunity to attend a one-day assessment course to be held soon at Southshire University. [Education]

Barbara has found the Smith case very distressing, and we spent some time discussing why this had proved so difficult for her. We talked about the level of support on offer to Barbara within the team as a newly qualified and appointed social worker and how she might more easily find such support for herself. [Support]

It has become clear that Barbara has a much better grasp of the new computerised record system than anyone else in the team, including myself. Barbara has agreed to make a brief 'hands-on' style presentation during the next team meeting to help us all get to grips with the system. [Mediation]

Supervision in most agencies remains the place where different agendas meet, establishing the worker's accountability to the organisation and promoting professional development. Sometimes these agendas can seem to be in tension rather than interwoven. In relation to the managing, teaching and support roles of supervision, Sawdon and Sawdon write:

> The challenge has been to work creatively with that tension, and to recognise that each of the three core functions of 'managing', 'teaching' and 'supporting' require a place on the stage as part of the whole, rather than to give one purpose assumed or explicit priority over the other.
>
> (Sawdon and Sawdon, 1995, p. 4)

Mediation as described by Richards and Payne (1990) is part of the whole, too.

Morrison, in an interview with Thompson (1999, p. 19) for *Community Care*, says 'the task is not about ensuring that managers understand social work, but that they understand exactly what is entailed in being a supervisor.' He speaks of managers who have supervised for ten years and yet received no training for their supervisory role. Practice-led managers might argue that understanding the practice is also important. None the less, adding a sharpened understanding of the functions and skills of supervision seems crucial. New practitioners identify quality supervision as an essential ingredient in developing and improving practice. For the individual, the way supervision is offered and its content is important if they are to use it constructively. Lishman writes about six prerequisites for the content of supervision to meet the needs of the individual. It should:

- focus on learning
- be provided on a regular and reliable basis
- involve mutual trust and awareness of issues of authority and responsibility
- provide support and opportunities to express feelings and go 'below the surface' in the analysis of problems and situations
- address those particular issues you assess as problematic, including dealing with pain, anxiety, confusion, violence and stress
- be anti-oppressive and anti-discriminatory in its content and its process.

> (Adapted from Lishman, 1998, p. 98)

The aspirations for supervision that writers describe are understandable and laudable. However, you may feel that the gap between aspiration and reality remains too wide to support staff effectively. The following quotation from a supervisor in a home for older people reflects how difficult it can be to balance competing demands in practice.

> As the registered manager I have supervisory responsibility for all 14 members of the team. But we have six vacancies at the moment, and to keep up with the needs of all our residents, I have had to compromise on supervision. I can't remember the last time I had anything more than the

briefest of chats with staff members that was not consumed by the practical agenda of keeping this place afloat, and doing the best we can for residents. In circumstances like these any thoughts I might previously have had around supervision as an opportunity to address the professional development needs of my staff have been lost. I have had to concentrate solely on the day-to-day practical management. I feel incredibly guilty about all this as the agency we work for has a policy for supervision that I can't deliver, and I worry that the impact on the team will mean that we will lose more staff.

(Manager consultations)

It is to be hoped that this rather bleak example is uncommon. Also, supervision can become less frequent above the organisational level of frontline manager. If this is the case, who supervises the supervisors? How are issues of professional development addressed for frontline managers and senior officers in the absence of regular, planned, competent supervision? The present emphasis on quality assurance and performance management may also mean that managerial aspects of supervision are afforded greater priority than education, support and mediation. Sawdon and Sawdon (1995) suggest that the best model for the supervision of managers and frontline staff is 'a whole greater than the sum of its parts' (p. 3), by which they mean, among other things:

- Supervision needs to be central and not marginal to the work of the agency.
- All the functions of supervision (managing, educating, supporting, mediating) are balanced in practice.
- The function of supervision in the agency is understood in relation to the main tasks.
- The content of the interaction between supervisor and supervised does not include just control and monitoring but also support, empowerment and learning.
- Supervision draws from the substantial literature on the way adults learn and on supervision processes.
- Supervisors should have skills training in order to be able to offer an effective supervisory process; for instance, the uses of language, behaviours, knowledge of the use of authority/power, problem-solving strategies.

(Adapted from Sawdon and Sawdon, 1995, pp. 3–19)

There is no lack of material to draw from, including training materials (Morrison, 1999), to improve supervisory practice in care agencies. The challenging part for agencies and managers is to make these things happen in practice. For supervision to be an action that furthers departmental work, as well as a relationship that enables professional development, other aspects of the working environment must be shaped in ways that allow proper time for professional development. Supervision policies with lines of accountability for carrying them out are essential.

Key points

- Supervision has a pivotal role in the planning of professional development.

- There are many helpful models for managers to use.

- Training for supervisors, a supervision policy and time set aside for supervisory sessions need to be routine practice.

12.6 Appraisal

Appraisal provides the opportunity for managers to take stock of each worker's professional development. Where there is trust in the manager and a motivated staff team, and everyone accepts the process of appraisal as fair, there is an opportunity to recognise formally both the strengths and the skills gaps within a staff group. It can identify both achievements and areas for development in a non-judgemental and non-threatening way. Thus appraisal is an active opportunity for a manager to look to the future, and identify and plan potential development, rather than a reactive mechanism for finding fault or attributing blame.

Everard and Morris suggest that managers should see recruitment, appraisal and training as connected issues, rather than isolated events, linked into a coherent approach to professional development:

> Appraisal is, or should be, an opportunity for the individual to meet with his or her manager in order to take stock of their individual and joint achievements. As a result of the discussion, there should be agreement on action needed to:
>
> - improve the performance of the individual
> - improve working relationships
> - develop the individual's career.
>
> (Everard and Morris, 1990, p. 79)

Nevertheless, the introduction of a staff appraisal system can provoke anxiety. This is especially likely where staff 'performance' in appraisal is related to the award of enhanced pay, or where existing tensions within a staff team are perceived to be exacerbated or even exploited by the process of appraisal. It can be especially stressful for staff who already feel insecure about their abilities or competence. A teacher/manager commented:

When the new headteacher introduced the staff appraisal I can tell you I was scared. I now know I had no reason to feel that way, as the system has helped me a great deal. Then I just thought the 'new broom' wants to 'sweep clean' and saw the appraisal system as a mechanism for either turning me into a headteacher's 'yes woman', or else to get me out altogether! I've never been the most confident person at work, and at the outset the prospect of being appraised, and possibly found to be less than fully competent, scared me to death.

(Manager consultations)

The introduction of staff appraisal, and its subsequent use, has to be handled with great sensitivity and, just as importantly, needs to be fully explained to staff and take their views into account as much as possible. While this is true for both unionised and non-unionised workforces, the involvement of union representatives can help to ensure that the process is seen and accepted by everyone as equitable. It is a mistake, though, to imagine that once a system of staff appraisal has been successfully launched no further action is needed to ensure future success. For example, a health visitor said:

The appraisal system worked OK for the first two years, but then they [management] made the mistake of assuming that nothing more needed to be done. In fact, so many new staff had been recruited by that time that most people didn't have a clue what appraisal was all about. And it was then that things started to go wrong.

(Manager consultations)

Consensus about the operation of any system of staff appraisal should not be assumed just because it has worked well in the past. Changes to the work group brought about by turnover of posts and other internal and external organisational developments all need to be taken into account. Some of the complexities are described in Example 12.3.

EXAMPLE 12.3 Sybil House

Sybil House is a residential home for older people offering residential accommodation for up to 40 residents. It is run by a local charity established as an almshouse in 1513. The present building, completed in 1999, provides a high-quality environment for residents and last year won a national architectural award for residential buildings.

The management committee of the Sybil House Trust introduced a staff appraisal system for the first time earlier this year, after representations from the local authority with which the home is registered. An academic commissioned from the local university's management school drew up an appraisal policy. The registered manager, Maria, is responsible for appraising all 31 staff. The chair of the management committee will appraise her.

A special meeting of the management committee will then be called to consider the appraisal reports, especially where these recommend that posts are regraded, additional training requirements have been identified, or other serious issues are raised. Maria has completed 29 of the 30 appraisal reports, and now only has to meet with Irima, the unit nurse, in order to complete the task. The chair of the management committee is pressing Maria not to let the appraisal process go on too long.

Maria says:

> I have been dreading Irima's appraisal. She is the longest-serving member of staff at Sybil House, having been an employee of the trust for over 20 years. I have always found her to be a difficult person to manage, and there have been several occasions over the last two years where I have had to threaten to take disciplinary action in order to get her to participate in team meetings or come to supervision sessions. Irima always waits till the very last moment, but then backs down.
>
> I feel that Irima sees herself as 'different' to all other members of staff as the only nurse we employ. She can be very manipulative in order to get her own way. I know she continually undermines my authority with the rest of the staff. Irima can be very assertive and I must admit that this has often intimidated me into letting her do things in her own way. Despite all this, Irima is an excellent nurse, and very well respected by all our residents. She has also run the annual unit garden party for many years, and last year raised over £1600 for unit funds. I am concerned that appraisal with Irima will inevitably result in more confrontation, and am nervous as to how the management committee will respond to this.

Irima's view is:

> I am not looking forward to my appraisal meeting as I suspect this will be just another occasion for Maria to pick on me. She has made it clear from her attitude to me over the last 18 months that she wants me out! I think that Maria has found it very difficult to step into the manager's role, having previously been a care assistant in the unit. She now wants to 'lord it' over the rest of us. Whenever possible, I avoid contact with her in order to get on with my work.

(Source: manager consultations)

Has Maria been set an impossible task? Responsibility for so many appraisals may be a heavy burden in addition to what is already a demanding job. It is not clear what preparation Maria has had for this responsibility: she is under pressure to get the task completed but it is not evident what support is available to her. She is being asked to introduce a new system to staff who are unfamiliar with it.

However well or badly the appraisal system was introduced to the staff, Irima evidently does not trust the process or see it as working to advantage her professional development. While her response may be extreme, other workers, who are already appraised, possibly share some of her reservations, and have just 'gone through the motions' of appraisal. It is arguably easier to appraise staff who have expected it from the day of appointment.

Even then, unless appraisal is delivered sensitively, as described above, on the basis of professional respect and trust, and a developmental rather than just a monitoring process, the accuracy of the appraisal as a baseline for future staff development can be undermined.

Key points

- Appraisal is another useful opportunity to identify staff learning needs.

- Appraisal can arouse anxieties in staff members and needs to be managed sensitively.

12.7   Poor performance

Maria's situation also illustrates the difficulty for managers of handling poor performance, especially when the staff member is competent in some areas of the work. Evidence of poor performance may not be easy to find, especially when issues have been left to drift. For example, the poor relationship between Maria and Irima seems to have lingered on unexpressed. As suggested already, the existence of appraisal mechanisms helps managers both to know what problems and concerns staff have, and to be consistent about what is expected and how work is to be done. They can also identify when performance is less than what is expected and plan ways of improving things. Stewart and Stewart (1985, p. 168) suggest that managing worker underperformance falls into three categories:

1   identifying the problem
2   understanding the causes
3   trying to improve matters.

This is an area where, in the interests of service users and the organisation, a particularly active approach is needed. The early identification of difficulties before a costly incident happens is important. A robust complaints procedure and regular service user consultations provide helpful information for the manager. Stewart and Stewart suggest that managers also need to be alert to such indicators as a decline in the quality and quantity of work, absenteeism and withdrawal from work, conflict or poor relationships with other staff. An early intervention may avoid the energy spent and the stress of dealing with the aftermath of a serious disciplinary incident.

An appraisal system and clear job expectations to refer to, which are in place for everyone, give a baseline from which to draw attention to poor performance that will not mean 'picking on the individual', as Irima suggests.

It is also worth exploring the causes of the staff member's actions, in a way that offers support and feedback. They may need to develop skills for a particular part of the job or they may be demotivated through lack of challenge. They may be under too much pressure, or have personal or health problems. Selection and induction may not have gone well, and the job may not be what they expected. Working conditions and team pressures can also be a cause.

The managers consulted for this chapter said they preferred to act openly and promptly when tackling problems of performance. This gave a message to the whole team about expectations and created a climate of honesty. They used the opportunity to identify specific ways of addressing difficulties, such as changing the person's shifts, reallocating work, arranging training, or putting them in touch with agency support networks. Most difficulties can be managed if manager and staff are motivated to change. One manager acknowledged that, for her, motivating staff who were discouraged and disillusioned was hard work and a team approach and the use of peer support were helpful.

Key points

- Appraisal can identify poor performance.

- Poor performance needs to be identified, understood and improved.

- Tackling the issues sooner rather than later is best practice.

12.8 Delegation

An underlying issue in poor performance can be feeling a lack of responsibility for, or ownership of, the task. One way of encouraging individuals and teams is to share tasks and to delegate, so that everyone has the opportunity to develop the abilities that enable them to progress in their careers.

Holroyde, writing back in 1970, saw the benefit of delegating.

People must be able to get on with their work and achieve the results expected of them. They need the authority to execute decisions. Those who are near the work face know what decisions need to be made, and if

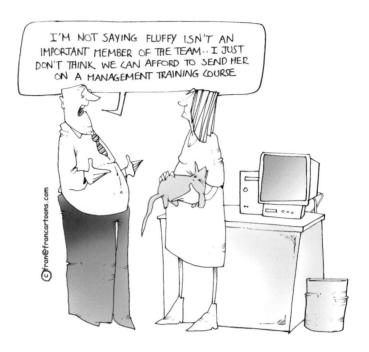

I'M NOT SAYING FLUFFY ISN'T AN IMPORTANT MEMBER OF THE TEAM.. I JUST DON'T THINK WE CAN AFFORD TO SEND HER ON A MANAGEMENT TRAINING COURSE

allowed, will get on and make them. They don't always want to be running upstairs for a decision; people enjoy and are stimulated by responsibility.

(Holroyde, 1970, p. 9)

As said in Chapter 1 about new managers, few organisations could function if managers did not delegate responsibility when appropriate. However, some managers are reluctant to delegate, often because they need to retain control, or fear that their staff will 'get it wrong' or 'steal their thunder'. There are certainly areas where managers should not delegate their authority – for example, handling disciplinary issues – but there are other circumstances in which delegation can increase efficiency through the promotion of professional development, as Example 12.4 shows.

EXAMPLE 12.4 Helping Hands

Helping Hands is a small charity in a town in South Wales that offers an interpretation and welfare service to deaf and hearing-impaired people. The charity has close links with the local church and provides services throughout the area on behalf of the council. There are two staff: Megan, a qualified social worker and interpreter, and Eirwyn, an unqualified worker, recruited after a long period of unemployment. Eirwyn has been with the charity for about two years. Megan is teaching him sign language and, although he is doing well, his communication skills are not yet at the same level as hers.

Megan says:

> One of the most important things we do for the local deaf community is to provide interpretation at events like weddings, driving tests, court appearances. This is important for two reasons. First, if we get things wrong it can have serious consequences, as well as being deeply embarrassing for the charity. On a driving test, if you tell a driver to turn left when the examiner has said turn right, this could result in them failing! Second, if we were regularly to make that sort of mistake word would get round the deaf community very quickly. If our service users did not feel that they could trust the precision and accuracy of our interpretation, then their overall confidence in our service would plummet.

> I have worked very hard over nine years to gain the trust of the local deaf community, but know how easily this could be lost. As the hearing child of two deaf parents I was signing before I was talking. I love signing, and for many years have taught and examined people learning to sign. Eirwyn is gifted with people and his appointment has really helped me to broaden the scope of what we can do. However, while he is doing very well with learning to sign, he is by no means proficient, and I have concerns that if I delegate responsibilities to him that might result in the kind of difficulties I have just described. Eirwyn has a special bond with David, who has asked him to interpret on his forthcoming Public Service Vehicle driving test. Eirwyn has asked me if this is OK, but I know he would find it difficult if I were to say no.

Eirwyn says:

> I know that Megan is concerned that I might mess up the interpretation on David's test, yet while I am anxious too, I really want to do it. I think Megan finds it difficult to remember that she does not work here on her own any more, and to let me do something means her letting go of some control. She is always so busy that it makes me feel guilty that I sometimes have little to do. Despite all this, Megan has been incredibly supportive of me over the past two years, and I respect her enormously. I just hope I can live up to her standards.

(Source: manager consultations)

Megan clearly has mixed feelings about delegating. On the one hand, she is glad of help; on the other, she fears the loss of control and worries that her own work will be undermined. However, if she gave the service user's voice more weight, she would be less hesitant. Delegating responsibility to less experienced staff carries with it the possibility of mistakes occurring, and the overall quality and sophistication of work being less.

Nevertheless, without the opportunity to learn through experience, even if it means making mistakes, it is difficult to see how new staff can acquire the skills they need to progress to senior positions. Eirwyn has been working hard to build skills and clearly wants to try them out. A period of joint work or staged handovers might help in this case. Perhaps Megan, Eirwyn and the service user might rehearse the test situation together. Once Megan sees that Eirwyn's work is competent, she can delegate with less anxiety.

However, perhaps Holroyde's introductory comments are too positive, and not all staff like the prospect of additional responsibilities and authority, as he suggests. If so, it is important to stress that delegating responsibility to staff does not mean they will not be supported and guided by more senior people. The provision of the appropriate level of support to staff with delegated responsibilities is a highly skilled managerial activity and, without the right balance, the professional development of these staff members may be undermined.

Key points

- The ability to delegate when appropriate is a valuable managerial skill.

- Delegation means supporting staff to learn new skills.

12.9 Disciplinary issues

Managers often describe disciplinary matters as complex and hard to get right. While this can be true, the disciplinary process can show up potential areas for individual and general professional development. It can also highlight issues of procedure and culture in the organisation that need to change. An ex-colleague, interviewed for this chapter, who had recently taken managerial responsibility for a complex and potentially very sensitive disciplinary investigation in a large teaching hospital, said:

> At first, there seemed to be nothing but pain for everyone involved in the disciplinary procedure. No one was winning and everyone seemed to be losing. But at the end of it all we know what we need to do to put things right. For some individual staff that means we have a much better idea of what we need to do to enhance their professional development, and it would have been a great shame if the pain of the process had prevented us from seeing, and taking advantage of, that opportunity.
>
> (Manager consultations)

In Example 12.5 a manager is faced with a complaint about a member of staff.

EXAMPLE 12.5 Broomhill Family Centre

Background

Broomhill is a local authority registered family centre run by a national charity. It provides day care services for children under seven and their families. Most of the children who attend have been assessed as being 'children in need', as defined by the Children Act 1989. Estrella, aged four, has been visiting Broomhill two days a week for the last five months. She has learning difficulties and it is suspected that when she was first referred to the centre her mother's partner had sexually abused her. He has since left the family home, and his current whereabouts are unknown.

A package of care has been set up to support Estrella and her mother, Rena, which includes her continuing placement at Broomhill. Rena works an early shift that starts at 8 am. Her next-door neighbour, Pete, is a cleaner at Broomhill. Rena has an arrangement with Pete who takes Estrella to Broomhill, picking her up from home at 7.45, and keeps an eye on her at the unit until the care staff arrive at 8.30. This arrangement has worked well so far.

Early Tuesday afternoon

Rena asks to see Carole, the manager of Broomhill. She alleges that Pete slapped Estrella earlier while waiting for the care staff to arrive. Rena has already reported the incident to the police and confronted Pete at his flat. Pete categorically denies slapping Estrella on this or any other occasion. After this conversation with Rena, Carole has learned that the police do not envisage taking matters further, unless they find clear evidence to back up the allegation. Later in the afternoon, Carole discusses the allegation with her senior manager, Sharon, who advises her that as she had received a formal complaint from a service user, a disciplinary investigation must be put into immediate effect, and that Carole should take the lead in this.

Wednesday morning

Rena has telephoned to say that she is withdrawing Estrella from Broomhill, and is furious that the police have decided to take no action against Pete. She has contacted her local councillor who, as a member of the local authority social services committee, has asked the director of social services what she intends doing about a member of staff who is abusing children, and who works in a unit registered by her department. Rena has also contacted the local press, who are very interested in getting a statement from someone at the unit.

Three weeks later

Pete was suspended from work on full pay pending the outcome of the disciplinary investigation. He has just returned to work after being cleared of any wrongdoing. However, he did say during an interview with Carole that 'kids like that sometimes need a slap'. Pete's duties at Broomhill continue to bring him into contact with children, although he has agreed that in future he will not make any informal arrangements to bring children into the unit, or supervise them before the arrival of the care staff. Pete says he feels devastated by the allegations made against him and that, despite being cleared of any wrongdoing, no one trusts him now.

(Source: manager consultations)

This is a complex but not an unusual situation. Carole must take Rena's complaint seriously, but she has no evidence of what happened. There were no witnesses, and Estrella's age and situation may limit her communication abilities. Carole is under enormous pressure from her manager, a councillor, the press and the service users. Pete is also distressed by what has happened.

It might have been better for an independent person to conduct the disciplinary investigation. Without a clear measure of independence, some of the individuals involved may possibly have thought Carole had a vested interest in dismissing the allegations against Pete. Also, after this experience, it is debatable how Pete will respond to suggestions from Carole for his professional development.

The difficulty of acting well in these situations is illustrated by the libel case brought against Newcastle Council in August 2002. The complainants were nursery workers accused of abusing children in their care. They were finally exonerated and compensated, but the process took nine years from when the allegations were made. A feature of the case was that, although the two workers were initially cleared by the courts, the council initiated its own internal review, which concluded that the workers had indeed abused children. The libel action was brought to contest the review findings and the libel judge who found in the workers' favour said that the allegations in the internal review report had no basis.

As *Community Care* (2002c, p. 18) comments, the case 'left no winners'. The parents of the children involved were left 'uncertain as to what, if anything, happened'. The two workers 'have endured a nightmare'. There are certainly lessons to be learned about review processes. This does not altogether help a frontline manager such as Carole, who is involved at the beginning of events. What it does clarify is the necessity to act with as much information as possible. It also suggests that the early involvement of someone with an independent view is essential. This could be a team of workers from another area who are accountable to an independent body. At the very least, the person initially involved might be another line manager, who could look at whether guidelines and procedures have been followed, so that what happens both protects the service user and allows for workers to be confident about how allegations against them are handled. Pete should also have had an independent adviser from the beginning to safeguard his interests.

> ### Key points
>
> - Disciplinary procedures cannot be avoided, especially when allegations of misconduct are made.
>
> - The lessons learned from such cases offer opportunities to promote professional development.

12.10   Conclusion

In this chapter I have argued that professional development is best understood as a system which, when it works well, reconciles the developmental needs of each worker with those of the team and organisation. Managers, responsible for the professional development of others, are required to balance individual, team and organisational needs so as to optimise outcomes across all these dimensions. This is by no means easy and the potential for tensions between individual needs and motivations, the needs of the agency and the views of the service users is always present.

Professional development is a complex responsibility for all managers across the spectrum of health, education and social care work. Possibly the most important managerial tool underpinning professional development is supervision: the quality of the supervisory relationship will directly influence the manager's understanding of the professional development needs of their staff. Supervision sessions provide the opportunity to discuss the work from the service user's point of view, plan responses, identify the worker's training needs and match these with training and development opportunities that arise.

Provided the manager takes account of all the needs identified in individual supervision sessions and is seen to be clearly considering the needs of all staff for professional development, supervision is an invaluable opportunity for professional development to both happen and be planned. This is particularly so if the manager is practice-led, relating the workers' training needs to the expressed needs of the agency's service users.

While supervision may have a special importance in this respect, it has to be viewed in the context of other managerial opportunities, induction, appraisal, delegation, the conduct of disciplinary issues and delegation of responsibility. These activities can operate to further promote professional development in parallel with supervision. Even exit interviews may hold opportunities to inform professional development and the employee's judgements about future work if the manager uses them positively and creatively.

Finally, professional development is basic and essential to the growth, improvement, accountability and learning of individuals and organisations. Kydd suggests:

> professional development, either individual or organizational, begins from a process of reflection on where things are, where we would like to get to and how we can get there.
>
> (Kydd, 1997, p. 2)

In this sense, without continuing professional development organisations would be incapable of evolving in step with the requirements and needs of the users of modern services.

Appendix 1: The consultation process

As part of the consultation process used to develop the course material, course team members met groups of workers and service users across Scotland, England, Wales and Northern Ireland. This Appendix briefly outlines the consultation process and puts in context the quotations from managers, practitioners and service users throughout this book and its companion volume, *Managing Care in Context*.

Adult service-user consultations

The user consultation strategy for adults' services involved (among other, less structured meetings) four workshops with groups of people who had experience of using mental health, disability, learning disability and older people's services. A facilitator with direct experience of care services was identified for each workshop and participants were contacted by facilitators through informal networks. Some of the people already knew each other, while others met for the first time at the workshops. Everyone had experience of several services, including health, voluntary sector, community-based and residential settings.

Some of the people had experienced compulsory services, and several in the mental health group had been 'sectioned' under the Mental Health Act 1983. The names of some participants and all the projects, centres, wards and professionals have been changed. Other participants were happy for their real names to be used. It was clear that, although services are split along similar lines to those chosen for the consultations, people do not fit into neat service delivery boxes. For example, Lou, a woman in the learning disability group, also had a visual impairment. Judith, from the older people group, had a physical disability and had cared for her elderly mother. People have diverse experience of services, so we identify their quotations by name alone in this book. For example, to identify Judith as belonging to a 'physical disability' service-user group would deny the range of her experience and contribution. By using names only we are highlighting the commonalities of experience and emphasising people rather than service categories.

The consultation groups had the following remit.

To consider a set range of questions from their specialist viewpoint as users of services for a specific group of people. Views on their experiences of involvement (or lack of it) in consultation and planning services are particularly useful.

For adult groups, Jeanette Henderson (a course team member) met facilitators and talked through the consultation process to ensure that participants as well as the course team would find the experience useful and relevant. Group members were sent the course outline and information about the course materials that were likely to be developed. Each member was paid a fee for taking part and travel expenses. After the workshops a representative or facilitator from each group was invited to a meeting at The Open University to discuss the content and the process of the consultations. A report was produced for each group, outlining the themes discussed and containing a selection of quotations illustrating the group's views, and an overall report summarising the sessions was circulated.

Young people, children and family consultations

The views of parents and young people are drawn from several consultations co-ordinated by Janet Seden (a course team member). In one, a Homestart staff member interviewed six families with children under five years old who were receiving services from Homestart (a voluntary befriending agency, accessed by referral from commissioning agencies). These families had experienced a crisis in their family life that led them to ask for help. The agencies they experienced include social services, health, education, housing and benefits. Their experiences of the statutory agencies are mixed, ranging from helpful (sensitive responses) to incompetent (initial telephone calls not returned). They were unanimous in valuing responsive, respectful encounters with professionals and they highly valued the peer support of the befriending agency.

In another consultation, Maya Joshi and Rukshana Owen (with Janice Whyne at the Family Service Unit) interviewed five young women who attended a group for teenagers who had experienced sexual abuse. The therapeutic group had now ended and been evaluated. These young women had also experienced a range of other interventions in their lives, and it was thought they could tell the researchers their opinions of the services and professionals they knew about. The researchers prepared questions about the following areas:

- benefits received from services
- the positive and negative aspects of the experience
- their feelings about the services they received and any improvements they could suggest.

The researchers needed to adjust the language of the questionnaire and make space for the respondents' own areas of concern as the research progressed, and they found that making space for free narrative was a useful way to work. The consultations were face-to-face interviews, which were then transcribed. In all of them the respondents had a rich experience of recent meetings with a range of professionals from several agencies, so their valuable views and insights are both genuinely felt and grounded in direct personal experience. These consultations are mainly drawn on in the companion book, *Managing Care in Context*. When referred to in this book, the source is 'service user consultations' or 'children's consultations'.

Regional and individual manager consultations

Regional consultations were held in Leeds, Edinburgh and Belfast. The regional sessions were with groups of people working in or using social care services. Participants were identified and contacted by regional academics in the School of Health and Social Welfare.

Two workshops were held with groups of managers and practitioners in the north-east of England. The first consisted of managers and practitioners from a local authority that had moved to integrated health and social care adult teams. The second workshop was for groups of senior managers, frontline managers and practitioners from adults' and children's services in one local authority.

At workshops with managers a set of questions were discussed that focused on expectations – what senior managers and staff expect of frontline managers, and what managers think is expected of them – and experiences – what senior managers and staff consider they get from frontline managers.

A total of 26 semi-structured interviews were held with individual managers in the Midlands and the north-east of England. Additional material from managers was gathered with the help of the BBC in preparing audio and video cassettes for the students of the course. Material from these interviews and workshops is used throughout this book and is referred to as 'manager consultations'.

Finally, three managers were asked to keep written diaries of their work for several weeks, and one manager kept an audio diary over several months. These are drawn on in both course books.

Some managers and service users continued their involvement with the course's development by becoming critical readers of the course materials.

Appendix 2: Understanding budget reports and accounts

Gary Spolander and Roger Gomm

Introduction

In this Appendix we explore budgets by looking at some examples. The aim is to enable readers who are not so familiar with budget reports and accounts to see some of the issues and complexities that frontline managers meet in practice.

Decisions about finance are at the heart of most organisations. Managers decide in the present about the future, and planning has to be based on predictions about what spending will be necessary. Government agendas, available funding and the demands on services fluctuate. Risk, complexity and uncertainty are inherent factors in all decision making in health and care services and need to be considered in all planning. Knowledge of past events may provide valuable pointers to the future, thus reliable information about the past may be important in providing a basis for planning.

Budgeting

At the start of a financial year (usually 1 April in the UK) the finances for a unit are allocated. This allocation is usually expected to provide the budget for the next 12 months (although some agencies may reset their budgets more frequently, for example quarterly).

Budgets are time-consuming to prepare and review but they are essential to effectively allocate and control resources for the following reasons.

- Budgeting allows the organisation's financial objectives to be stated clearly.
- Key actions are specified.
- Responsibilities for those actions are allocated to managers.
- The budgeting process encapsulates the organisation's activities.
- Financial problems can be identified quickly and dealt with.
- Budgeting and allocating target expectations, resources and responsibilities can be motivating when they are handled well.

What is a budget?

A budget is a plan for income and expenditure. Once a budget has been set it monitors and controls whether what happens is as planned. The first example is typical of one that the Child and Adolescent Mental Health Services (CAMHS) might use (see Table A2.1).

Table A2.1   **Budget report for CAMHS to end of February 2001**

	Annual budget	Budget this month	Expend this month	Budget YTD	Expend YTD	Variance
*Payroll costs**						
Manager	32 200	2 683	2 683	29 517	29 517	0
Support staff:						
Anne T	19 528	1 627	1 627	17 897	17 897	0
Harry B	19 528	1 627	0	17 897	14 643	3 254
Lynn P	19 528	1 627	0	17 897	9 762	8 135
Admin support	19 528	1 627	2 426	17 897	24 696	−6 799
Social workers:						
Joan R	24 495	2 041	2 041	22 451	22 451	0
Liz P	24 495	2 041	2 041	22 451	20 410	2 041
Psychologist:						
Sheila G	32 200	2 683	2 683	29 513	29 513	0
Nurses:						
Tom Y	27 600	2 300	2 300	25 300	25 300	0
Rachel U	21 850	1 821	1 820	20 020	20 020	0
Agency staff	21 850	1 821	5 321	20 020	58 531	−38 511
Occupational therapists:						
Colin R	26 450	2 204	2 204	24 244	24 244	0
Tessa W	26 450	2 204	0	24 244	22 040	2 204
Total	315 702	26 306	25 146	289 348	319 024	−29 676

	Annual budget	Budget this month	Expend this month	Budget YTD	Expend YTD	Variance
Non-pay*						
Advertising publicity	5 000	417	785	4 576	9 863	−5 287
Computers	12 000	1 000	0	11 000	10 200	800
Course fees	6 000	500	0	5 500	6 000	−500
Office equipment	2 500	208	269	2 288	2 459	−171
Heating	12 000	1 000	1 600	11 000	11 020	−20
Postage	1 000	83	109	913	1 022	−109
Stationery	1 300	108	500	1 188	1 499	−311
Telephones	18 000	1 500	6 321	16 500	21 330	−4 830
Rent	28 500	2 375	2 375	26 125	26 125	0
Travel expenses	20 000	1 667	9 000	18 326	32 000	−13 674
Training	8 500	708	100	7 788	5 000	2 788
Miscellaneous	1 000	83	32	913	863	50
Total	115 800	9 649	21 091	106 117	127 381	−21 264
Care packages*						
Care packages agreed	250 000	20 833	26 599	229 713	229 755	−42
Total	250 000	20 833	26 599	229 713	229 755	−42
Grand total	681 502	56 788	72 836	625 178	676 160	−50 982

In Table A2.1 the budget for the year is shown in the *annual budget* column.

The *budget this month* is produced by dividing the *annual budget* into 12 parts for each of the 12 months of the financial year, and is treated as if it were paid into the account monthly. It is usually 12 equal instalments, although some agencies may set different targets for different months, because of known variations.

Expend this month shows what was spent in the month concerned. The bills are recorded as being paid from the *budget this month* column. Good accounting practice is to record the monthly expenditure within the month the expense occurred, but when bills are quarterly, or when staff are late putting in their claims, it is often impossible to assign the expenditures to the correct months.

Budget YTD is the budget year to date. It is the budget for the year to the end of that budget period and is updated each month. Since the example is for February, *budget YTD* is eleven-twelfths of the annual budget.

Expend YTD is the expenditure in the financial year to the date of the budget report.

The *variance* column shows the difference between *budget YTD* and *expend YTD*. If a budget line is overspent the amount of the variance is sometimes shown in brackets. A minus sign indicates an overspend; a positive number indicates an underspend. If the expenditure is on budget the variance is zero.

The individual budget lines

These are listed under the asterisked headings in Table A2.1 and show the areas of expenditure in detail.

Payroll costs details staff salaries or amounts paid to agency staff to cover vacancies. The staff salaries include an extra 15% to cover the employer's costs of National Insurance, contribution to employees' pensions and other employment costs. These 'on costs' are substantial. When a team covers a vacancy, they save more than the salary for that post because on costs are saved too.

Non-pay expenditure covers all other expenses. Within the non-pay budget there are fixed and variable operating costs. Fixed costs, such as rent, cannot be altered during the year and may take a long time to change, whatever the activity level of the organisation. Variable operating costs increase as activity levels increase: the more meals-on-wheels that are delivered, the more food is purchased. On the CAMHS budget, *telephones* is a mixture of fixed costs (line rental) and variable costs (the costs of calls).

In any large organisation there are costs that cannot be allocated precisely to a particular service. For example, a local authority department may share premises, making it difficult to accurately apportion lighting, heating or shared reception services as part of the costs of providing care packages. In this case such overheads are usually apportioned between departments on the basis of a formula set at a high level in the organisation and are therefore unlikely to be under a frontline manager's direct control. Overheads are usually fixed costs. No overheads are shown on the CAMHS budget, although there are other fixed costs such as rent.

Check that you can answer the following questions by looking at Table A2.1. The answers are at the end of this Appendix.

1   What is the total annual budget?
2   What has the expenditure been so far this year?
3   What predictions can you make about overspend or underspend for the whole year?
4   Which areas are overspent?
5   Which budget lines are in budget?
6   Which budget lines are underspent?

Budget management

The manager of the budget in Table A2.1 has an immediate problem: 11 months into the financial year, the annual expenditure is heading towards an overspend of between £50,982 and £67,494. This suggests very lax budget management during the earlier 11 months. It is too late to do much in the three weeks remaining, but some reductions in the expenditure for March may be possible.

Assuming budget lines in March as in February, freezing non-essential (variable) spending in March on the following items would make a saving, as follows.

Office equipment	= £208
Computers	= £917[1]
Training	= £600[2]
Miscellaneous	= £ 83
Total	**= £1808**

[1]£1000 – £83: 'computers' includes an annual software licensing fee of £1000, which has already been paid but has been allocated in 12 fixed instalments of £83 to each month and cannot be saved.

[2]£708 – £108: £108 is already committed for training in March, thus not carrying out further training in March saves £600.

The manager could also take the following action.

Maintain the current vacancies on:

Tessa W's post	= £2204
Harry B's post	= £1627
Lynne P's post	= £1627
Freeze recruitment advertising	= £ 417
Total	**= £5875**

Before such cuts are made, the manager considers whether they would undermine the agency's ability to deliver its core services. Would making the cuts pose risks and hardship for clients? Would there be health and safety implications? Does making cuts on one budget line create costs on another? Costs for agency staff are likely to arise from unplanned savings on permanent staff expenditure.

Other possibilities for short-term savings could be investigated but these will do as an illustration. These savings add up to £7683, giving a March expenditure of £48,641 (£56,324 – £7683), if all the other budget lines can be kept within budget. Making these savings would produce an annual overspend of around £43,299, which is better than £67,494 but still considerable. However, that assumes all other items can be kept within the monthly budget, which seems unlikely.

Agency staff, telephone and travel expenses are all overspent for the year. Expenditure on these items in February may include some peak loading, and the amounts in March may not be so high. However, if, for example, travel expenses cost £2909 a month over 11 months (expend YTD divided by 11), March travel expenses are unlikely to be on budget at £1667. These budget lines should have been corrected months earlier, either by reducing expenditure or by getting authorisation for a budget increase.

Some managers only manage expenditure. Others, particularly in the independent sector, manage both income and expenditure. This means that there are additional rows on their budget sheets for income, as shown in Table A2.2. For the income rows a minus variance expresses a shortfall against planned income. This agency was planning for a small excess of income over expenditure (£370), has kept its expenditure just under budget, but has not managed to generate all the planned income. The result is an income deficit of £6975 over 11 months and a deficit of income over expenditure of £6299. If the agency continues in the same way in March, this deficit will rise further. It will be difficult for the manager to cut expenditure or raise extra income to balance the books before the end of the financial year.

Table A2.2 **Budget report for Avalon Family Centre to end of February 2001**

Expenditure	Annual budget	Budget this month	Expend this month	Budget YTD	Expend YTD	Variance
Payroll costs	87 600	7 300	7 304	80 300	80 304	−4
Non-payroll costs	24 000	2 000	1 300	22 000	21 320	680
Total	111 600	9 300	8 604	102 300	101 624	676

Income	Annual budget	Budget this month	Income this month	Budget YTD	Income YTD	Variance
Service agreement: social services	55 000	4 583	4 583	50 417	50 417	0
Service agreement: primary care trust	32 500	2 708	2 708	29 792	29 792	0
Grant: BBC Children in Need	12 500	1 042	1 042	11 458	11 458	0
Fundraising	10 000	833	0	9 167	3 000	−6 167
Donations	650	54	25	596	378	−218
Bank interest	1 320	110	62	1 210	620	−590
Total	111 970	9 330	8 420	102 640	95 665	−6 975
Balance of income and expenditure	370	30	−184	340	−5 959	−6 299

Table A2.2 oversimplifies the accounts of many independent agencies in that it shows the budget for the whole agency. This agency will probably have to keep and balance separate income and expenditure accounts for each of its major income streams (social services, primary care trust and BBC Children in Need). This is because it will not be authorised to spend social services monies on activities that should be funded by the primary care trust or the BBC.

In the language of accountancy, these funds are for 'designated expenditure' and income cannot be 'vired' (transferred) between these accounts. If an agency underspends on one account, it cannot use the spare to compensate for an overspend on another. Such underspends may be claimed back at the end of the year by the funding source. Independent agencies that provide services also have to keep VAT accounts, although this is not discussed here.

Both examples show that budgets cannot be managed easily in retrospect. It is no good allowing overspends to build up during the earlier months of the year and then trying to cut back expenditure to compensate later, or continuing to overspend in the hope that income will increase. Budgets need to be managed month by month at least. This process has to start in the previous financial year.

Budget planning

Even after making the cuts suggested above, the budget manager for Table A2.1 will end the year with an overspend of approximately £43,299, that is, over 6.3%. Managers who work in the statutory services are usually better placed than those in the independent sector. They may be criticised for overspending but somehow their overspends are lost in the overall local authority budget and are not carried forward at departmental level to the next year. In the independent sector an overspend in one year is usually carried forward as an agency debt into the next year. For a manager in the statutory services, a 6.3% overspend in one year may lead to an instruction to cut the budget by 6.3% for the coming year. For a manager in the independent sector, a 6.3% overspend in one year may require a 12.6% cut in the following year: 6.3% to pay off the debt and 6.3% to prevent further overspend.

An agency may collapse if there are insufficient reserves to pay creditors. Managers in the independent sector have to consider reserves. Most independent agencies try to maintain a reserve in the bank or in investments equal to least three months' operating costs to tide them over difficult periods. It is illegal to operate when reserves have fallen below the level which would meet the costs of outstanding debts, including salaries and staff redundancy payments. Reserves generate income, which can be added to the income side of the accounts, and some independent sector managers have considerable investment management responsibilities. Conversely, reducing the reserves reduces the income they generate.

In either sector, instead of reducing expenditure a manager might look to ways of increasing income. In the statutory sector, income is usually guaranteed for the year, barring financial crises within the authority as a whole. In the independent sector, income may come from fees, charges, donations and grants secured during the year. As shown in Table A2.2, the agency may start the financial year with only a speculative income prediction.

There are two ways of looking at the CAMHS budget (Table A2.1) and the overspend. One is to view it as the result of poor financial management during the year. The other is to think of the budget against which the overspend was judged as unrealistic. This is also poor financial management, and it occurred when the annual budget was set.

Frontline managers' responsibility for budget setting varies. Some are handed budgets, expected to manage them, however unrealistic this is, and left to take the blame for any overspends, shortfalls in service delivery, or shortfalls against income generation targets. Where frontline managers are involved in budget setting, they have an opportunity to create a budget that is realistic and manageable, representing the optimum allocation of resources for activities needed to meet their agency's objectives.

The best starting point for setting next year's budget is usually the current year's budget, partly because many financial commitments, such as payroll costs, are long-term and cannot be altered easily. The current budget also tells the manager how much it cost to do what was done before. This provides useful data for considering whether resources were used efficiently, whether the sums allocated to budget rows were realistic, and what changes should be made for the next year.

When setting the next financial year's budget it is tempting to consider only current overspends and how to reduce them. This is a mistake for two reasons. First, overspends exceed the amount budgeted for particular items. Second, overspends may occur for reasons which are of high priority in meeting the agency's objectives. Correspondingly, a budget line on or under budget does not mean that amount of expenditure was necessary. Savings on these budget lines might be reinvested in something more important. It is good practice to review the entire budget.

Setting a budget means asking two kinds of question. One kind is about restrictions. Managers can only budget to spend the income they are likely to receive. How they spend it is limited by prior financial commitments. Moreover, the next year's budget has to accommodate additional expenditure which cannot be avoided: for example, nationally negotiated pay rises, salary increments, increased fuel prices. Often, standard percentage increases in funding are made to meet such increased costs: for example, a 2% increase for local authority budgets or service agreements. However, the impact of such increased costs may be greater than the standard sum awarded to the agency.

There are sometimes planned reductions in expenditure: for example, central government might set local authorities a target to reduce the 'unit costs' of home care by 3% per year for the next three years. A unit cost is the cost of providing some standard unit of service, for example, one hour of home care. So reducing unit costs by 3% means providing 3% more home care for the same expenditure.

The other kind of question concerns aspirations: what managers want to achieve. Here the key question is not financial but 'What are our highest priorities for the service?' When that question has been answered the manager can ask, 'What are the most cost-effective ways of meeting these priorities?' and 'Is the current pattern of expenditure meeting the priorities and in the most economical way?' Although the agency may be committed to employing the same level of staff next year, does what they actually do meet the agency's key objectives?

Setting a budget should mean reviewing every budget line in relation to the agency's key objectives. On the CAMHS budget in Table A2.1, it means asking whether the vacancies need to be filled, and investigating what the staff actually do and achieve. It could mean analysing why so many hours of agency staffing were contracted; analysing the travel patterns of staff to see whether all their journeys were worthwhile; or looking at telephone usage. The care packages also need investigation. It is common for services to continue long after they are necessary. A more active approach to case review and case closure might free up resources to be reinvested in expenditure on clients with the greatest need. Budgeting is about using resources to the best effect.

Answers

1   £681,502

2   £676,160

3   The budget for the year is £681,502. In 11 months the agency has spent £676,160, leaving only £5342 for spending in March. The budget for March is £56,324 (£681,502 – £625,178). If CAMHS spent that, the total annual expenditure would be £732,484, giving an overspend of £50,982. If the agency spent in March, as in February, £72,836, the annual spend would be £748,996 with an overspend of £67,494.

4   Admin support, agency staff, advertising/publicity, course fees, office equipment, heating, postage, stationery, telephone, travel expenses, care packages.

5   Manager, Anne T, Joan R, Sheila G, Tom Y, Rachel U, Colin R, rent.

6   Harry B, Lynn P, Liz P, Tessa W, computers, training, miscellaneous.

References

Adams, S. (1996) *The Dilbert Principle*, London, Boxtree. **[Ch. 7]**

Adams, J., Hayes, J. and Hopson, B. (1976) *Transitions – Understanding and Managing Personal Change*, Oxford, Martin Robertson. **[Ch. 4]**

Ainscow, M., Hopkins, D., Southworth, G. and West, M. (1994) *Creating the Conditions for School Improvement: A Handbook of Staff Development Activities*, London, David Fulton. **[Ch. 12]**

Aldgate, J. and Dimmock, B. (2003) 'Managing to care', in Henderson, J. and Atkinson, D., pp. 3–25 (K303 Set Book). **[Ch. 1]**

Aldridge, S. (1995) 'Implementing an information strategy at local level', in Sheaff, R. and Peel, V. (eds) *Managing Health Service Information Systems: An Introduction*, Buckingham, Open University Press. **[Ch. 8]**

Alimo-Metcalfe, B. and Alban-Metcalfe, R. (2000) 'Heaven can wait', *Health Service Journal*, 12 October, pp. 26–9. **[Ch. 3]**

Allen, M. (2000) 'An underrated service', *Community Care*, 14–20 December, p. 22. **[Ch. 7]**

Antman, E., Lau, J., Kupeltruck, B., Mosteller, F. and Chalmers, I. (1992) 'A comparison of the results of meta-analyses of randomized controlled trials and recommendations of clinical experts', *Journal of the American Medical Association*, Vol. 268, pp. 240–8. **[Ch. 5]**

Argyris, C. and Schön, D. (1996) *Organizational Learning II: Theory, Method and Practice*, Reading, MA, and Wokingham, Addison-Wesley. **[Chs 1, 4]**

Armstrong, P. (1995) 'Accountancy and HRM', in Storey, J. (ed.) *Human Resource Management, A Critical Text*, London, Routledge. **[Ch. 7]**

Arnold, J., Cooper, C. L. and Robertson, I. T. (1998) *Work Psychology: Understanding Human Behaviour in the Workplace* (3rd edn), London, Financial Times and Pitman. **[Ch. 11]**

Arredondo, P. (1996) *Successful Diversity Management Initiatives: A Blueprint for Planning and Implementation*, London, Sage. **[Ch. 3]**

Ashworth, M. and Baker, A. H. (2000) 'Time and space: carers' views about respite care', *Health and Social Care in the Community*, January, Vol. 8, No. 1, pp. 50–6. **[Ch. 5]**

Atrill, P. and McLaney, E. (1997) *Accounting and Finance for Non-specialists* (2nd edn), London, Prentice Hall. **[Ch. 7]**

Audit Commission (1984) *Improving Economy, Efficiency and Effectiveness*, London, Audit Commission. **[Ch. 7]**

Audit Commission (1999a) *Best Assured: The Role of the Audit Commission in Best Value*, HMSO and Audit Commission website. www.audit-commission.gov.uk [accessed September 2001] **[Ch. 8]**

Audit Commission (1999b) *Best Value and Audit Commission Performance Indicators 1999/2000*, London, Department of the Environment, Transport and the Regions. **[Ch. 8]**

Ayre, P. (2003) 'Child protection and the media: lessons from the last three decades', in Reynolds *et al.*, pp. 315–23 (K303 Reader). **[Chs 9, 10]**

Balloch, S. and Taylor, M. (2001) 'Introduction', in Balloch, S. and Taylor, M. (eds) *Partnership Working: Policy and Practice*, pp. 1–16, Bristol, The Policy Press. **[Ch. 6]**

Banks, P. (2002) *Partnerships under Pressure: A Commentary on Progress in Partnership-working between the NHS and Local Government*, London, The King's Fund. **[Ch. 6]**

Barker, R. W. (1996) 'Child protection, public services and the chimera of market force efficiency', *Children & Society*, Vol. 10, pp. 28–39. **[Ch. 9]**

Barrett, S. (2002) *The Role of the Organisation and Managers in Promoting Wellbeing and Happiness in the Workplace*, Unpublished paper for the K303 course team. **[Ch. 11]**

Bass, B. M. (1985) *Leadership and Performance beyond Expectations*, New York, Free Press. **[Ch. 3]**

Bates, J. (2003) 'An evaluation of the use of information technology in child care services and its implications for the education and training of social workers', in Reynolds *et al.*, pp. 324–33 (K303 Reader). **[Ch. 8]**

Bebbington, A. and Miles, J. (1989) 'The background of children who enter local authority care', *British Journal of Social Work*, Vol. 19, No. 5, pp. 349–68. **[Ch. 9]**

Beedell, C. (1970) *Residential Life with Children*, London, Routledge & Kegan Paul. **[Ch. 2]**

Bennis, W. and Nanus, B. (1985) *Leaders: The Strategies for Taking Charge*, London, Harper & Row. **[Ch. 3]**

Beresford, P. (2001) 'Experience must inform the evidence', *Community Care*, 9–15 August, p. 15. **[Ch. 5]**

Bhavnani, R. and Coyle, A. (2000) 'Black and ethnic minority women managers in the UK – continuity or change?', in Davidson, M. J. and Burke, R. J. (eds) *Women in Management: Current Research Issues Volume II*, pp. 223–5, London, Sage. **[Ch. 3]**

Biggs, S. (1997) 'Inter-professional collaboration: problems and prospects', in Øvretveit, J., Mathias, P. and Thompson, T. (eds) *Inter-professional Working for Health and Social Care*, Basingstoke, Macmillan. **[Ch. 6]**

Bilson, A. and Ross, S. (1999) *Social Work, Management and Practice: Systems Principles* (2nd edn), London, Jessica Kingsley. **[Chs 2, 4, 11]**

Bion, W. (1968, 1980) *Experiences in Groups*, London, Tavistock. **[Ch. 1]**

Birkett, D. (2001) 'Remember Jade and Kieron?', *The Guardian 2*, 13 December, pp. 6–7. **[Ch. 9]**

Blanchard, K., Zigarmi, P. and Zigarmi, D. (1986) *Leadership and the One Minute Manager*, London, Collins. **[Ch. 3]**

Bosk, C. (1979) *Forgive and Remember: Managing Medical Failure*, Chicago, Chicago Press. **[Ch. 2]**

Bowlby, J. (1969, 1973, 1980) *Attachment and Loss*, Vols 1, 2 and 3, London, Hogarth. **[Ch. 11]**

Brechin, A. and Sidell, M. (2000) 'Ways of knowing', in Gomm, R. and Davies, C. (eds) *Using Evidence in Health and Social Care*, pp. 3–25, London, Sage/The Open University (K302 Reader). **[Ch. 5]**

Brechin, A., Brown, H. and Eby, M. A. (2000) *Critical Practice in Health and Social Care*, London, Sage/The Open University (K302 Set Book). **[Ch. 5]**

Bridges, W. (1988) *Transitions: Making the Most of Life's Changes*, London, Nicholas Brealey Publishing Ltd. [Ch. 4]

Bridges, R. (1991) *Managing Transition: Making the Most of Change*, London, Perseus Publishing. [Ch. 2]

Brown, A. and Clough, R. (eds) (1989) *Groups and Groupings*, London, Tavistock/Routledge. [Ch. 11]

Brown, H. and Stein, J. (1998) 'Implementing adult protection policies in Kent and East Sussex', *Journal of Social Policy*, Vol. 27, No. 3, pp. 371–96. [Ch. 9]

Burck, C. and Speed, B. (eds) (1995) *Gender, Power and Relationships*, London, Routledge. [Ch. 11]

Burns, J. M. (1978) *Leadership*, London, Harper & Row. [Ch. 3]

Burton, J. (1989) 'Institutional change and group action: the significance and influence of groups in developing new residential services', in Brown and Clough, pp. 59–79. [Ch. 10]

Burton, J. (1993) *The Handbook of Residential Care*, London, Routledge. [Chs 1, 3]

Burton, J. (1998) *Managing Residential Care*, London, Routledge. [Chs 1, 3, 10]

Care Council for Wales (2002) *Social Care Induction Framework*, Cardiff, Care Council for Wales.
www.ccwales.org.uk/english/side/publications [accessed December 2002] [Ch. 2]

Carnall, C. A. (1999) *Managing Change in Organizations* (3rd edn), London, Financial Times/Prentice Hall. [Ch. 2]

Causer, G. and Exworthy, M. (1999) 'Professionals as managers across the public sector', in Exworthy, M. and Halford, S. (eds) *Professionals and the New Managerialism in the Public Sector*, Buckingham, Open University Press. [Ch. 1]

Charlesworth, J. (2002) *Redefining Roles through Partnership Working*, Unpublished discussion paper, Milton Keynes, The Open University Business School. [Ch. 6]

Charmaz, K. (1995) 'The body, identity and self: adapting to impairment', *Sociological Quarterly*, Vol. 36, No. 4, pp. 657–80. [Ch. 11]

Clark, C. L. and Asquith, S. (1985) *Social Work and Social Philosophy*, London, Routledge & Kegan Paul. [Ch. 10]

Cochrane, A. (1973) *Effectiveness and Efficiency: Random Reflections on Health Services*, London, Nuffield Provincial Hospitals Trust. [Ch. 5]

Colenso, M. (1997) *High Performing Teams ... in Brief*, Oxford, Butterworth-Heinemann. [Ch. 2]

Collins, T. and Bruce, T. (1984) *Staff Support and Staff Training*, London and New York, Tavistock Publications. [Ch. 2]

Community Care (2000) Letters pages, 21 September, p. 16; 12 October, pp. 16–7. [Ch. 11]

Community Care (2001a) 'Editorial comment: Milburn out of touch' and 'Special report', 25–31 October, pp. 5 and 11–12. [Ch. 8]

Community Care (2001b) 4–10 October, p. 29. [Ch. 11]

Community Care (2002a) 'Editorial comment: assisted deception', 23–9 May, p. 5. [Ch. 8]

Community Care (2002b) Editorial, 27 June–3 July, p. 7. [Ch. 11]

Community Care (2002c) 'News analysis: Fallout from libel case prompts call for overhaul of review procedures', 8–14 August, pp. 18–19. **[Ch. 12]**

Conger, J. A. and Kanungo, R. N. (eds) (1988) *Charismatic Leadership: The Elusive Factor in Organizational Effectiveness*, San Francisco, Jossey-Bass. **[Ch. 3]**

Conway, D. (1993) 'The day of the manager', *Community Care*, 19 August, pp. 20–1. **[Ch. 1]**

Coombs, H. M. and Jenkins, D. E. (1991) *Public Sector Financial Management*, London, Chapman & Hall. **[Ch. 7]**

Corby, B. (1995) 'Inter-professional co-operation and inter-agency co-ordination', in Wilson, K. and James, A. (eds) *The Child Protection Handbook*, pp. 211–26, London, Ballière Tindall. **[Ch. 9]**

Coulshed, V. (1990) *Management in Social Work* (1st edn), Basingstoke, Macmillan. **[Chs 2, 10]**

Coulshed, V. and Mullender, A. (2001) *Management in Social Work* (2nd edn), Buckingham, Palgrave. **[Ch. 3]**

Curnock, K. and Hardiker, P. (1979) *Towards Practice Theory*, London, Routledge & Kegan Paul. **[Ch. 5]**

Daily Express (2002) '80 hours a week cost me my job', 2 February, p. 9. **[Ch. 11]**

Daniel, B., Wassell, S. and Gilligan, R. (1999) *Child Development for Child Care and Protection Workers*, London, Jessica Kingsley. **[Ch. 11]**

Darvill, G. (1992) 'Creating an informative environment', in Hearne, B., Darvill, G. and Morris, B. (eds) *On Becoming a Manager in Social Work*, pp. 106–16, Harlow, Longman. **[Ch. 8]**

Darvill, G. (2001) 'Creating a learning organisation', Unpublished draft material prepared for K303 course team, Milton Keynes, The Open University. **[Ch. 1]**

Davidson, M. J. and Burke, R. J. (eds) (2000) *Women in Management*, London, Sage. **[Ch. 11]**

Davidson, M. J. and Cooper, C. L. (1992) *Shattering the Glass Ceiling: The Woman Manager*, London, Chapman. **[Ch. 11]**

Davis, L. (1999) 'What do you need to know? Lessons from Joint Reviews for knowledge workers in social services', *Research, Policy and Planning*, Vol. 17, No. 3, pp. 1–6.
www.elsc.org.uk/bases/rrp/173davishtml [accessed February 2001] **[Ch. 5]**

Department of Health (1991) *Child Abuse: A Study of Inquiry Reports, 1980–1989*, London, The Stationery Office. **[Chs 2, 10]**

Department of Health (1995) *Child Protection: Messages from Research*, London, The Stationery Office. **[Ch. 9]**

Department of Health (1998a) *Partnership in Action (New Opportunities for Joint Working between Health and Social Services)*, London, The Stationery Office. **[Ch. 6]**

Department of Health (1998b) *Caring for Children Away from Home: Messages from Research*, London, The Stationery Office. **[Ch. 10]**

Department of Health (1999a) *The RAP Project, Referral, Assessment and Packages of Care in Adult Personal Social Services: Evaluation Report*, London, The Stationery Office.
www.doh.gov.uk/rapevaluation.htm [accessed December 2002] **[Ch. 8]**

Department of Health (1999b) *Effective Care Co-ordination in Mental Health Services: Modernising the Care Programme Approach*, London, The Stationery Office. [**Ch. 9**]

Department of Health (2000a) *The NHS Plan: Creating a 21st Century Health Service*, London, The Stationery Office. [**Ch. 7**]

Department of Health (2000b) *Towards a Common Cause – A Compact for Care: Inspection of Local Authority Social Services and Voluntary Sector Working Relationships*, London, The Stationery Office. [**Ch. 7**]

Department of Health (2000c) *No Secrets: Guidance on Developing and Implementing Multi-agency Policies and Procedures to Protect Vulnerable Adults from Abuse*, London, The Stationery Office. [**Ch. 9**]

Department of Health (2001a) *The Children Act Now*, London, The Stationery Office. [**Ch. 9**]

Department of Health (2001b) *Valuing People: A New Strategy for Learning Disability for the 21st Century: A White Paper*, Cm 5086, London, The Stationery Office. [**Chs 4, 9**]

Department of Health (2001c) *Making It Happen – The Key Areas for Action*, London, Department of Health. [**Ch. 8**]

Department of Health (2001d) *How Do We Meet These Challenges?*, London, Department of Health. [**Ch. 8**]

Department of Health (2002) *Care Homes for Older People: National Minimum Standards*, London, The Stationery Office. [**Ch. 10**]

Department of Health, Home Office and Department for Education and Employment (1999) *Working Together to Safeguard Children*, London, The Stationery Office. [**Ch. 9**]

DETR (Department of the Environment, Transport and the Regions) (1998) *Modern Local Government – In Touch with the People*, London, DETR. [**Ch. 7**]

DETR (1999) *Local Government Act 1999: Part I Best Value*, DETR Circular 10/99, London, 14 December. [**Ch. 7**]

Dixon, N. (1994) *The Organizational Learning Cycle: How We Can Learn Collectively*, Maidenhead, McGraw-Hill. [**Ch. 1**]

Dodd, V. (2001) 'Prison officers jailed for sadistic attack', *The Guardian*, 15 September, p. 16. [**Ch. 2**]

Dowie, J. N. and Elstein, A. (eds) (1998) *Professional Judgement: A Reader in Clinical Judgement Making*, Cambridge, Cambridge University Press. [**Ch. 10**]

Drake, R. (1999) *Understanding Disability*, Basingstoke, Macmillan. [**Ch. 9**]

Dylan, B. (1961) 'Bring It All Back Home', CBS. [**Ch. 7**]

Eby, M. (2000a) 'The challenges of being accountable', in Brechin, A., Brown, H. and Eby, M. A. (eds) *Critical Practice in Health and Social Care*, pp. 187–208, London, Sage/The Open University (K302 Set Book). [**Ch. 10**]

Eby, M. (2000b) 'Understanding professional development', in Brechin, A., Brown, H. and Eby, M. A. (eds) *Critical Practice in Health and Social Care*, pp. 48–69, London, Sage/The Open University (K302 Set Book). [**Ch. 12**]

Edge, J. (2001) *Who's in Control? Decision Making by People with Learning Difficulties Who Have High Support Needs*, London, Values Into Action. [**Chs 4, 8**]

Eley, R. (1989) 'Women in management in social services departments', in Hallet, C. (ed.) *Women and Social Services Departments*, London, Harvester Wheatsheaf. [**Ch. 3**]

Elkin, A. J. and Rosch, P. J. (1990) 'Promoting mental health at the workplace: the prevention side of stress management', *Occupational Medicine: State of the Art Review*, Vol. 5, No. 4, pp. 739–54. [**Ch. 11**]

European Disability Forum (1999) *Report on Violence and Discrimination Against Disabled People*, EDF 99/5, Brussels, EDF. [**Ch. 9**]

Evans, M. (2003) 'The quest for quality: reflecting on the modernising agenda', in Reynolds *et al.*, pp. 109–16 (K303 Reader). [**Ch. 3**]

Everard, B. and Morris, G. (1990) *Effective School Management*, London, Paul Chapman. [**Ch. 12**]

Exworthy, M. and Halford, S. (eds) (1999) *Professionals and New Management in the Public Sector*, Buckingham, Open University Press. [**Ch. 11**]

Fagge, N. (2002) 'Stressed workers' £321m in payouts', *Daily Express*, 2 February, p. 9. [**Ch. 11**]

Fallon, F. (1999) *Report of the Committee of Inquiry into the Personality Disorder Clinic, Ashworth Special Hospital*, London, The Stationery Office. [**Ch. 10**]

Farmer, E. and Owen, M. (1995) *Child Protection Practice: Private Risks and Public Remedies – Decision Making, Interventions and Outcomes in Child Protection Work*, London, The Stationery Office. [**Ch. 9**]

Faulkner, A. and Layzell, S. (2000) *Strategies for Living: A Report of User-led Research into People's Strategies for Living with Mental Distress*, London, Mental Health Foundation. [**Ch. 5**]

Fawcett Society (2000) *Where Are the Women?*, London, Fawcett Society. [**Ch. 8**]

Ferlie, E. and Pettigrew, A. (1996) 'Managing through networks: some issues and implications for the NHS', *British Journal of Management*, Vol. 7, pp. 81–99. [**Ch. 6**]

Fletcher, K. (2001) 'How to manage the fallout', *Community Care*, 21–7 June, p. 30. [**Ch. 10**]

Freeth, D. (2001) 'Sustaining interprofessional collaboration', *Journal of Interprofessional Care*, Vol. 15, No. 1, pp. 37–46. [**Ch. 6**]

Fuller, R. and Petch, A. (1995) *Practitioner Research: The Reflexive Social Worker*, Buckingham, Open University Press. [**Ch. 5**]

Furnivall, J. (1991) 'Peper Harow – consultancy – a consumer's view', in Silveira, W. R. (ed.) *Consultation in Residential Care*, pp. 123–46, Aberdeen, Aberdeen University Press. [**Ch. 2**]

Gallop, L. (2001) 'Facilitating services, managing resources and budgets', Unpublished draft material prepared for K303 course team, Milton Keynes, The Open University. [**Ch. 1**]

Gaster, L. and Deakin, N. (1998) 'Local government and the voluntary sector: who needs whom – why and what for', *Local Governance*, Vol. 24, No. 3, pp. 169–94. [**Ch. 6**]

Gaster, L., Deakin, N., Riseborough, M., McCabe, A., Wainwright, S. and Rogers, H. (1999) *History, Strategy or Lottery? The Realities of Local Government/Voluntary Sector Relationships*, London, The Improvement and Development Agency. **[Ch. 6]**

Gatehouse, M. (2001) *Information and Information Systems for Looked After Children*, Annual report, Loughborough, Centre for Child and Family Research. **[Ch. 8]**

Geddes, J. (2000) 'Evidence-based practice in mental health', in Trinder, L. and Reynolds, S. (eds) *Evidence-based Practice: A Critical Appraisal*, Chapter 4, pp. 66–88, Oxford, Blackwell Science. **[Ch. 5]**

Geneen, H. S. and Moscow, A. (1985) *Managing*, London, Granada. **[Ch. 7]**

Gilligan, C. (1982) *In a Different Voice*, Cambridge, MA, Harvard University Press. **[Ch. 11]**

Ginn, J. and Fisher, M. (1999) 'Gender and career progression', in Fisher, M., Balloch, S. and McLean, J. (eds) *Social Services: Working under Pressure*, pp. 129–40, Bristol, Policy Press. **[Ch. 3]**

Gladwell, M. (1999) *The Tipping Point: How Little Things Can Make a Big Difference*, London, Little, Brown. **[Ch. 5]**

Glasby, J. and Glasby, J. (1999) *Paying for Social Services*, Birmingham, PEPAR. **[Ch. 7]**

Glastonbury, B., Bradley, R. and Orme, J. (1987*) Managing People in the Personal Social Services*, London, Wiley. **[Ch. 11]**

Goffee, R. and Jones, G. (2000) 'Why should anyone be led by you?', *Harvard Business Review*, September–October, pp. 63–70. **[Ch. 3]**

Gomm, R., Needham, G. and Bullman, A. (2000) *Evaluating Research in Health and Social Care*, London, Sage/The Open University (K302 Reader). **[Ch. 5]**

Gould, N. (2003) 'Becoming a learning organisation: a social work example', in Reynolds *et al.*, pp. 334–45 (K303 Reader). **[Chs 1, 12]**

Greenleaf, R. (1996) *On Becoming a Servant-Leader*, San Francisco, Jossey-Bass. **[Ch. 3]**

Grimwood, C. and Popplestone, R. (1993) *Women, Management and Care*, Basingstoke, Macmillan. **[Chs 3, 11]**

Grint, K. (1995) *Management: A Sociological Introduction*, Cambridge, Polity Press. **[Ch. 7]**

Handy, C. (1999) *Understanding Organizations*, London, Penguin. **[Ch. 1]**

Hardiker, P. *et al.* (2001) 'A framework for conceptualising need and its application to planning and providing services', in Ward, H. and Rose, W. (eds) *Approaches to Need Assessment in Children's Services*, Chapter 3, London, Jessica Kingsley. **[Ch. 9]**

Harris, J. (1998) 'Scientific management, bureau-professionalism, new managerialism, and the labour process of state social work', *British Journal of Social Work*, Vol. 28, No. 6, pp. 822–62. **[Ch. 8]**

Harris, J. and Kelly, D. (1992) *Management Skills in Social Care: A Handbook for Social Care Managers*, Aldershot, Ashgate. **[Ch. 1]**

Hartley, J. and Allison, M. (2000) 'The role of leadership in the modernisation and improvement of public services', in Reynolds *et al.*, pp. 296–305 (K303 Reader). **[Ch. 3]**

Harvey, M. (2001) 'The hidden force: a critique of normative approaches to business leadership', *SAM Advanced Management Journal*, Vol. 66, No. 14, pp. 36–48. [**Ch. 3**]

Hatton, C., Azmi, S., Caine, A. and Emerson, E. (1998) 'Informal carers of adolescents and adults with learning difficulties from the South Asian communities: family circumstances, service support and carer stress', *British Journal of Social Work*, Vol. 28, No. 6, pp. 821–37. [**Ch. 5**]

Hawkins, P. and Shohet, R. (1989) *Supervision in the Helping Professions*, Buckingham, Open University Press. [**Ch. 11**]

Hay, J. (1993) *Working It Out At Work*, Watford, Sherwood. [**Ch. 7**]

Heath, G. (2000) *Accountability in the 'New NHS'*, Paper presented at the 4th International Research Conference: Dilemmas 2000, University of East London, September. [**Ch. 10**]

Henderson, J. and Atkinson, D. (eds) (2003) *Managing Care in Context*, London, Routledge/The Open University (K303 Set Book). [**Chs 1, 10**]

Henderson, J. and Seden, J. (2003) 'What do we want from social care managers? Aspirations and realities', in Reynolds *et al.*, pp. 85–94 (K303 Reader). [**Chs 3, 11, 12**]

Hermansson, A., Hornquist, J. and Timpka, T. (1996) 'The wellbeing of war wounded asylum applicants and quota refugees following arrival in Sweden', *Journal of Refugee Studies*, Vol. 9, No. 2, pp. 166–81. [**Ch. 9**]

Hersey, P. and Blanchard, K. H. (1988) *Management of Organizational Behavior: Utilizing Human Resources* (5th edn), Englewood Cliffs, NJ, Prentice Hall. [**Ch. 3**]

Hersey, P. and Blanchard, K. H. (1993) *Management of Organization Behavior: Utilizing Human Resources* (6th edn), Englewood Cliffs, NJ, Prentice Hall. [**Ch. 11**]

Hill, L. A. (1991) *Becoming a Manager: The Transformation from Individual Contributor to Manager*, Cambridge, MA, Harvard University Press. [**Ch. 1**]

Hinshelwood, R. D. and Skogstad, W. (2000) *Observing Organisations: Anxiety, Defence and Culture in Health Care*, London, Routledge. [**Ch. 2**]

Hirsch, S. K. and Kummerow, J. M. (1987) *Introduction to Type in Organizations* (2nd edn), Palo Alto, CA, Consulting Psychologists Press. [**Ch. 3**]

Holder, D. and Wardle, M. (1981) *Teamwork and the Development of a Unitary Approach*, London, Routledge & Kegan Paul. [**Ch. 2**]

Hollander, E. P. and Offerman, L. R. (1993) 'Power and leadership in organizations', in Rosenbach, W. R. and Taylor, R. L. (eds) *Contemporary Issues in Leadership*, pp. 62–86, Oxford, Westview. [**Ch. 3**]

Hollway, W. (2001) 'The psycho-social subject in "evidence-based practice",' *Journal of Social Work Practice*, Vol. 15, No. 1, pp. 9–22. [**Ch. 5**]

Holman, B. (2001) 'Upside-down studies', *Community Care*, 12–18 April, p. 14. [**Ch. 5**]

Holmes, T. H. and Rahe, R. H. (1967) 'The social readjustment rating scale', *Journal of Psychosomatic Research*, Vol. 11, pp. 213–8. [**Ch. 11**]

Holroyde, G. (1970) *How to Delegate*, Rugby, Mantec. [**Ch. 12**]

Home Office (1998) *Speaking Up for Justice: Report of An Interdepartmental Working Group on the Treatment of Vulnerable or Intimidated Witnesses in the Criminal Justice System*, Home Office, London. [**Ch. 9**]

Home Office (1999) *Action for Justice: Implementing the Speaking Up for Justice Report on Vulnerable or Intimidated Witnesses in the Criminal Justice System in England and Wales*, London, Home Office. **[Ch. 9]**

Home Office (1999) *The Stephen Lawrence Inquiry: Report of an Inquiry by Sir William Macpherson of Cluny*, London, The Stationery Office. **[Ch. 1]**

Home Office (2000) *Race Relations (Amendment) Act*, London, The Stationery Office. **[Ch. 1]**

Horwath, J. and Morrison, T. (eds) (1999) *Effective Staff Training in Social Care*, London, Routledge. **[Ch. 12]**

Howe, D. (1995) *Attachment Theory for Social Work Practice*, Basingstoke, Macmillan. **[Ch. 11]**

Howe, D. (ed.) (1996) *Attachment and Loss in Child and Family Social Work*, Aldershot, Avebury. **[Ch. 11]**

Hudson, B. (1998) *Primary Health Care and Social Care: Working across Organisational and Professional Boundaries*, Briefing paper, Leeds, Nuffield Institute for Health. **[Ch. 6]**

Hudson, B., Exworthy, M. and Peckham, S. (1998) *The Integration of Localised and Collaborative Purchasing: A Review of Literature and a Framework for Analysis*, Leeds, Nuffield Institute for Health. **[Ch. 6]**

Hudson, B., Hardy, B., Henwood, M. and Wistow, G. (2003) 'In pursuit of inter-agency collaboration in the public sector. What is the contribution of theory and research?', in Reynolds *et al.*, pp. 232–41 (K303 Reader). **[Ch. 6]**

Hunt, J. G. (1991) *Leadership: A New Synthesis*, San Francisco, Sage. **[Ch. 3]**

Huxham, C. (1996a) 'Advantage or inertia? Making collaboration work', in Paton, R., Clark, G., Jones, G., Lewis, J. and Quintas, P. (eds) *The New Management Reader*, pp. 238–54, London, Routledge/The Open University (B800 Reader). **[Ch. 6]**

Huxham, C. (1996b) 'Collaboration and collaborative advantage', in Huxham, C. (ed.) *Creating Collaborative Advantage*, Chapter 1, London, Sage. **[Ch. 6]**

Huxham, C. (2000) 'The challenge of collaborative governance', *Public Management*, Vol. 2, No. 3, pp. 337–57. **[Ch. 6]**

Huxham, C. and Vangen, S. (2000) 'What makes partnerships work?', in Osborne, S. (ed.) *Public–Private Partnerships*, London, Routledge. **[Ch. 6]**

Iles, V. and Sutherland, K. (2001) *Organisational Change: A Review for Health Care Managers, Professionals and Researchers*, London, National Co-ordinating Centre for NHS Service Delivery and Organisation R&D. **[Ch. 4]**

Information Commission (2002) 'Principles of data protection'. www.dataprotection.gov.uk [accessed November 2002] **[Ch. 8]**

James, A. (1994) *Managing to Care: Public Service and the Market*, London, Longmans. **[Ch. 11]**

Joint Reviews (2000) *People Need People*, London, Audit Commission/HMSO. **[Ch. 7]**

Josefowitz, N. (1987) *People Management*, London, Columbus Books. **[Ch. 1]**

Katzenbach, J. R. and Smith, D. K. (1993) *The Wisdom of Teams: Creating the High-Performance Organization*, Boston, MA, Harvard Business School Press. **[Ch. 2]**

Kerslake, A. (1998) 'Computerisation of the Looked After Children records: issues of implementation', *Children and Society*, Vol. 12, pp. 236–7. **[Ch. 8]**

Kerslake, A. (1998) 'Computerisation of the Looked After Children records: issues of implementation', *Children and Society*, Vol. 12, pp. 236–7. **[Ch. 8]**

Kirkwood, A. (1992) *The Leicestershire Inquiry 1992*, Leicester County Council. **[Ch. 3]**

Kitchener, M., Kirkpatrick, I. and Whipp, R. (2003) 'Supervising professional work under New Public Management: evidence from an "invisible trade",' in Reynolds *et al.*, pp. 220–31 (K303 Reader). **[Chs 1, 12]**

Kotter, J. P. (1990) *A Force for Change: How Leadership Differs from Management*, New York, Free Press. **[Ch. 3]**

Kotter, J. P. (1999) 'What effective general managers really do', *Harvard Business Review*, Vol. 77, No. 2, pp. 145–59. **[Ch. 1]**

Kouzes, J. M. and Posner, B. Z. (1987) *The Leadership Challenge: How to Get Extraordinary Things Done in Organizations*, San Francisco, Jossey-Bass. **[Ch. 3]**

Kubler-Ross, E. (1970) *On Death and Dying*, London, Tavistock. **[Ch. 11]**

Kydd, L. (1997) 'Introduction', in Kydd, L., Crawford, M. and Riches, C. (eds) *Professional Development for Educational Management*, p. 2, Buckingham, Open University Press. **[Ch. 12]**

La Valle, I. and Lyons, K. (1996) 'The social worker speaks: II – management of change in the personal social services', *Practice*, Vol. 8, No. 3, pp. 63–71. **[Ch. 3]**

Lago, C. and Thompson, J. (1996) *Race, Culture and Counselling*, Buckingham, Open University Press. **[Ch. 11]**

Larning, Sir H. (2003) *The Victoria Climbié Inquiry*, London, The Stationery Office.

Lawler, J. and Hearn, J. (1997) 'The managers of social work: their experiences', *British Journal of Social Work*, Vol. 27, No. 2, pp. 191–218. **[Ch. 11]**

Learning Disability Advisory Group (2001) *Fulfilling the Promises: Proposals for a Framework for Services for People with Learning Disabilities*, Cardiff, National Assembly for Wales. **[Ch. 4]**

Lendrum, S. and Syme, G. (1992) *Gift of Tears*, London, Tavistock. **[Ch. 11]**

Lewin, K. (1951) *Field Theory in Social Science*, New York, Harper. **[Ch. 4]**

Lewis, J. (2003) 'The contribution of research findings to practice change', in Reynolds *et al.*, pp. 166–73 (K303 Reader). **[Ch. 5]**

Lewis, M. (1998) *Achieving Best Value Through Quality Management*, Best Value Series, Paper number 9, Warwick, DETR. **[Ch. 7]**

Ling, T. (2000) 'Unpacking partnership: the case of health care', in Clarke, J., Gewirtz, S. and McLaughlin, E. (eds) *New Managerialism, New Welfare?*, London, Sage. **[Ch. 6]**

Lishman, J. (1998) 'Personal and professional development', in Adams, R., Dominelli, L. and Payne, M. (eds) *Social Work: Themes, Issues and Critical Debates*, pp. 89–102, Basingstoke, Macmillan. **[Ch. 12]**

Lord Clyde (1992) *Report of the Inquiry into the Removal of Children from Orkney in February 1991*, House of Commons 195, London, Her Majesty's Stationery Office. **[Ch. 2]**

Loxley, A. (1997) *Collaboration in Health and Welfare: Working with Difference*, London, Jessica Kingsley. **[Ch. 6]**

Lukes, S. (1974) *Power: A Radical View*, London, Macmillan. **[Ch. 6]**

Lupton, C., Peckham, S. and Taylor, P. (1998) *Managing Public Involvement in Healthcare Purchasing*, Buckingham, Open University Press. [Ch. 6]

Lyon, D. (2001) 'Virtual Citizens, Speed, Distance and Moral Selves', Paper to New Technologies and Social Welfare Conference, University of Nottingham, 17 December. [Ch. 8]

Mabey, C. and Salaman, G. (1995) *Strategic Human Resource Management*, Oxford, Blackwell. [Ch. 12]

Marks-Maran, D. (1993) 'Accountability', in Tschudin, V. (ed.) *Ethics: Nurses and Patients*, pp. 121–34, London, Scutari Press. [Ch. 1]

Marris, P. (1974, 1986) *Loss and Change*, London, Routledge & Kegan Paul. [Chs 2, 4, 11]

Marsh, P. and Triselotis, J. (1996) *Ready to Practise? Social Workers and Probation Officers: Their Training and First Year in Work*, Avebury, Aldershot. [Ch. 12]

Marshall, M. and Lockwood, A. (2000) 'Assertive community treatment for people with severe mental disorders (Cochrane Review)', *The Cochrane Library*, Issue 3, Oxford, Update Software. [Ch. 5]

Marshall, M., Gray, A., Lockwood, A. and Green, R. (2000) 'Case management for people with severe mental disorders (Cochrane Review)', *The Cochrane Library*, Issue 3, Oxford, Update Software. [Ch. 5]

Martin, V. and Henderson, E. (2001) *Managing in Health and Social Care*, London, Routledge/The Open University (B630 Set Book). [Chs 1, 3, 4]

Mawson, C. (1994) 'Containing anxiety in work with damaged children', in Obholzer, A. and Roberts, V. Z. (1994a), pp. 67–74. [Ch. 2]

Mayo, M. and Taylor, M. (2001) 'Partnerships and power in community regeneration', in Balloch, S. and Taylor, M. (eds) *Partnership Working: Policy and Practice*, pp. 39–56, Bristol, The Policy Press. [Ch. 6]

McCarthy, M. and Thompson, D. (1994) 'Sex and staff training', reprinted in Thompson, D. and Brown, H. (eds) (1998) *Response-Ability: Working with Men with Learning Disabilities Who Have Difficult or Abusive Sexual Behaviours*, Brighton, Pavilion Publishing. [Ch. 9]

McNally, S., Ben-Schlomo, Y. and Newman, S. (1999) 'The effects of respite care on informal carers' well-being: a systematic review', *Disability and Rehabilitation*, Vol. 21, No. 1, pp. 1–14. [Ch. 5]

Means, R. and Langan, J. (1996) 'Charging and quasi markets in community care: implications for elderly people with dementia', *Social Policy and Administration*, Vol. 30, No. 3, pp. 244–62. [Ch. 9]

Mental Health Foundation (1999) *The DIY Guide to Survivor Research: Everything You always Wanted to Know about Survivor-Led Research but Were Afraid to Ask*, London, Mental Health Foundation. [Ch. 5]

Menzies Lyth, I. (1988) *Containing Anxiety in Institutions: Selected Essays*, Vol. 1, London, Free Association Books. [Ch. 2]

Middlewood, D. (1997) 'Managing staff development', in Bush, T. (ed.) *Managing People in Education*, pp. 186–201, London, Paul Chapman. [Ch. 12]

Miller, E. V. (1993) *From Dependency to Autonomy: Studies in Organization and Change*, London, Free Association. [Ch. 2]

Miller, E. V. and Gwynne, G. V. (1972) *A Life Apart: A Pilot Study of Residential Institutions for the Physically Handicapped and the Young Chronic Sick*, London, Tavistock. [Ch. 2]

Milton Keynes Council (2000) *Milton Keynes Making Connections: A Guide to Effective Partnerships*, Draft document, Milton Keynes Council. **[Ch. 6]**

Milton Keynes Council (2001) *Best Value Review of Strategic Partnerships*, Policy and Resources Committee paper, Milton Keynes Council. **[Ch. 6]**

Miner, J. B. (1982) *Theories of Organizational Structure and Process*, Hinsdale, IL, Dryden. **[Ch. 2]**

Mintzberg, H. (1975) 'The manager's job: folklore or fact?', *Harvard Business Review*, Vol. 53, No. 4, pp. 49–61 (reprinted in Reynolds *et al.*, 2003, pp. 289–95, K303 Reader). **[Chs 1, 3, 8]**

Mintzberg, H. (1998) 'Covert leadership: notes on managing professionals', *Harvard Business Review*, November–December, pp. 140–7. **[Ch. 2]**

Moody, S. (1999) 'Protecting the vulnerable and including the marginal: volunteers and the law', *Journal of Adult Protection*, Vol. 1, Issue 2, November, pp. 64–70. **[Ch. 9]**

Morrison, A. M. (1992) *The New Leaders: Guidelines on Leadership Diversity in America*, San Francisco, Jossey-Bass. **[Ch. 3]**

Morrison, T. (1999) *Staff Supervision in Social Care*, Brighton, Pavilion. **[Ch. 12]**

Moss, P. and Petrie, P. (1996) *Time for a New Approach: A Discussion Paper*, London, Thomas Coram Research Unit. **[Ch. 9]**

Moylan, D. (1994) 'The dangers of contagion: projective identification processes in institutions', in Obholzer, A. and Roberts, V. Z. (1994a), pp. 51–9. **[Ch. 2]**

Nadler, D. A. (1983) 'Concepts for the management of organizational change', in Hackman, J. R., Lawler III, E. E. and Porter, L. W. (eds) *Perspectives on Behavior in Organizations*, pp. 551–61, New York, McGraw-Hill. **[Ch. 4]**

Nadler, D. A. and Tushman, M. L. (1988) 'What makes for magic leadership?', *Fortune*, 6 June, pp. 115–6. **[Ch. 3]**

Neate, P. (2000) 'Interview with John Hutton', *Community Care*, 9 November, p. 11. **[Ch. 1]**

Northouse, P. G. (1997) *Leadership: Theory and Practice*, Thousand Oaks, CA, Sage. **[Ch. 3]**

Obholzer, A. (1987) 'Institutional dynamics and resistance to change', *Psychoanalytic Psychotherapy*, Vol. 2, No. 3, pp. 201–6. **[Ch. 2]**

Obholzer, A. (2003) 'The unconscious at work', in Reynolds *et al.*, pp. 513–23 (K303 Reader). **[Ch. 11]**

Obholzer, A. and Roberts, V. Z. (1994a) *The Unconscious at Work: Individual and Organizational Stress in the Human Services*, London, Routledge. **[Ch. 2]**

Obholzer, A. and Roberts, V. Z. (eds) (1994b) 'The troublesome individual and the troubled institution', in Obholzer and Roberts (1994a), pp. 129–38. **[Ch. 2]**

O'Connor, C. (1993) 'Managing resistance to change', *Management Development Review*, Vol. 6, No. 4, pp. 25–9. **[Ch. 2]**

O'Neill, J. (1994) 'Managing professional development', in Bush, T. and West-Burnham, J. (eds) *The Principles of Educational Management*, pp. 199–222, London, Longman. **[Ch. 12]**

The Open University (2000) *Managing in Health and Social Care, Module 1: The Manager*, Management Education Scheme by Open Learning (MESOL) pack, Milton Keynes, The Open University. **[Ch. 1]**

The Open University (2001) *K260 Death and Dying*, Workbook 4, *Bereavement: Private Grief and Collective Responsibility*, Milton Keynes, The Open University. [**Ch. 11**]

Osler, A. and Morrison, M. (2000) *Inspecting Schools for Racial Equality: OFSTED's Strengths and Weaknesses*, London, Commission for Racial Equality. [**Ch. 8**]

Ousley, M. and Barnwell, M. (1993) 'Reviewing fostering services', *Local Government Policy Making*, Vol. 20, pp. 28–37. [**Ch. 8**]

Øvretveit, J. (1997) 'How to describe interprofessional working', in Øvretveit, J., Mathias, P. and Thompson, T. (eds) *Interprofessional Working for Health and Social Care*, Basingstoke, Macmillan. [**Ch. 6**]

Parkes, C. M. (1986) *Bereavement: Studies of Grief in Adult Life*, London, Tavistock. [**Ch. 11**]

Parkes, C. M., Stevenson-Hinde, J. and Marris P. (1991) *Attachment Across the Life Cycle*, London, Routledge. [**Ch. 11**]

Payne, M. (2000) *Teamwork in Multiprofessional Care*, Basingstoke, Macmillan. [**Chs 2, 6**]

Payne, C. and Scott, T. (1985*) Developing Supervision of Teams in Field and Residential Social Work*, London, National Institute for Social Work. [**Ch. 2**]

Peace, S. and Reynolds, J. (2003) 'Managing caring environments', in Henderson and Atkinson, pp. 133–58 (K303 Set Book). [**Ch. 10**]

Pearn, M., Roderick, C. and Mulrooney, C. (eds) (1995) *Learning Organisations in Practice*, London, McGraw-Hill. [**Ch. 12**]

Pearn, M., Roderick, C. and Mulrooney, C. (1997) *Learning Organizations in Practice*, London, McGraw-Hill. [**Ch. 1**]

Peck, E., Gulliver, P. and Towell, D. (2002) *Modernising Partnerships: An Evaluation of Somerset's Innovations in the Commissioning and Organisation of Mental Health Services*, London, Institute for Applied Health and Social Policy, King's College London. [**Ch. 6**]

Pederson, P. B. (1994) *A Handbook for Developing Multicultural Awareness*, Alexandris, VA, American Counselling Association. [**Ch. 11**]

Pedler, M., Boydell, T. and Burgoyne, J. (1991) *The Learning Company*, London, McGraw-Hill. [**Ch. 1**]

Pedler, M., Burgoyne, J. and Boydell, T. (1994) *A Manager's Guide to Self-Development*, Maidenhead, McGraw-Hill. [**Ch. 1**]

Pence, D. and Wilson, C. (1994) *Team Investigations of Child Sexual Abuse: The Uneasy Alliance*, Thousand Oaks, CA, Sage. [**Ch. 2**]

Pettigrew, A. and Whipp, R. (1991) *Managing Change for Competitive Success*, Oxford, Blackwell. [**Ch. 4**]

Pettigrew, A., Ferlie, E. and McKee, L. (1992) *Shaping Strategic Change*, London, Sage. [**Chs 4, 5**]

Philpot, T. (2002) 'Origin unknown', *Community Care*, 23–9 May, pp. 32–3. [**Ch. 8**]

Piachaud, D. (2001) 'Child poverty, opportunities and quality of life', *The Political Quarterly*, Vol. 72, No. 4, pp. 446–53. [**Ch. 9**]

Pickard, L. (2001) 'Carer break or carer-blind? Policies for informal carers in the UK', *Social Policy and Administration*, Vol. 135, No. 4, pp. 441–58. [**Ch. 5**]

Pine, B. A., Warsh, R. and Maluccio, A. N. (2003) 'Participatory management in a public child welfare agency: a key to effective change', in Reynolds *et al.*, pp. 215–28 (K303 Reader). [Ch. 11]

Pinkerton, J. (1998) 'Social work and the troubles: new opportunities for engagement', in Central Council for Education and Training in Social Work, *Social Work and Social Change in Northern Ireland*, pp. 15–29, London, CCETSW. [Ch. 11]

Pinnock, M. and Dimmock, B. (2003) 'Managing for outcomes', in Henderson, J. and Atkinson, D. M. A. (eds) *Managing Care in Context*, pp. 257–82, London, Routledge/The Open University (K303 Set Book). [Ch. 8]

Preston-Shoot, M. (2001) 'Evaluating self-determination: an adult protection case study', *Journal of Adult Protection*, Vol. 3, No. 1, February, pp. 4–15. [Ch. 9]

Pritchard, J. (ed.) (1995) *Good Practice in Supervision*, London, Jessica Kingsley. [Ch. 12]

Professional Social Work (1996) 'After West', 10 January, pp. 9–11. [Ch. 11]

Quigley, L. (2001) *Adult Protection in Professional Care Services: The Role of the Employer*, Brighton, Pavilion. [Ch. 9]

Qureshi, H. and Henwood, M. (2000) *Older People's Definitions of Quality Services*, York, Joseph Rowntree Foundation. [Ch. 5]

Rashid, S. (1996) 'Attachment viewed through a cultural lens', in Howe, D. (ed.) *Attachment and Loss in Child and Family Social Work*, Aldershot, Avebury. [Ch. 11]

Read, J. (2003) 'Mental health service users as managers', in Reynolds *et al.*, pp. 12–20 (K303 Reader). [Ch. 3]

Read, J. and Reynolds, J. (1996) *Speaking Our Minds: An Anthology of Personal Experiences of Mental Distress and Its Consequences*, Basingstoke, Macmillan. [Ch. 5]

Reder, P. and Duncan, S. (1999) *Lost Innocents: A Follow-up Study of Fatal Child Abuse*, London, Routledge. [Ch. 9]

Reynolds, S. (2000) 'The anatomy of evidence-based practice: principles and methods', in Trinder, L. and Reynolds, S. (eds) *Evidence-Based Practice: A Critical Appraisal*, Chapter 2, pp. 17–34, Oxford, Blackwell Science. [Ch. 5]

Reynolds, J., Henderson, J., Seden, J., Charlesworth, J. and Bullman, A. (eds) (2003) *The Managing Care Reader*, London, Routledge/The Open University (K303 Reader). [Chs 1, 6, 12]

Rice, A. K. (1965) *Learning for Leadership. Interpersonal and Intergroup Relations*, London, Tavistock. [Ch. 2]

Richards, M. and Payne, C. (1990) *Staff Supervision in Child Protection Work*, London, National Institute for Social Work Education. [Ch. 12]

Rickford, F. (2001) 'Make the evidence count', *Community Care*, 12–18 April, pp. 18–19. [Ch. 5]

Roberts, K. (2000) 'Lost in the system? Disabled refugees and asylum seekers in Britain', *Disability and Society*, Vol. 15, No. 6, pp. 943–8. [Ch. 9]

Rogers, E. (1995) *The Diffusion of Innovations*, New York, Free Press. [Ch. 5]

Rogers, R. (1999) *Performance Management in Local Government* (2nd edn), London, Financial Times/Pitman. [Ch. 7]

Rosen, G. (ed.) (2000) *Integrity, the Organisation and the First-Line Manager Discussion Papers*, London, National Institute for Social Work. **[Ch. 1]**

Royal Brompton Hospital (2001) *The Report of the Independent Inquiry into the Paediatric Cardiac Service at the Royal Brompton and Harefield Hospital*, London. **[Ch. 9]**

Sackett, D. L., Rosenberg, W. M. C., Gray, J. A. M., Haynes, R. B. and Richardson, W. S. (1996) 'Evidence-based medicine: what it is and what it isn't', *British Medical Journal*, Vol. 3, No. 12, pp. 71–2. **[Ch. 5]**

Sawdon, C. and Sawdon, D. (1995) 'The supervision partnership: a whole greater than the sum of the parts', in Pritchard, J. (ed.) *Good Practice in Supervision*, pp. 3–19, London, Jessica Kingsley. **[Ch. 12]**

Schön, D. A. (1991) *The Reflective Practitioner: How Professionals Think in Action*, Aldershot, Avebury. **[Ch. 5]**

Scott, D. (1990) 'Practice wisdom: the neglected source of practice research', *Social Work*, Vol. 35, No. 6, pp. 564–8. **[Ch. 5]**

Scottish Executive (2000) *The Same as You? A Review of Services for People with Learning Disabilities*, Edinburgh, The Stationery Office. **[Ch. 4]**

Seden, J. (1995) 'Child abuse', in Jacobs, M. (ed.) *The Care Guide*, pp. 70–8, London, Cassells. **[Ch. 9]**

Seden, J. (2001) 'Assessment of children in need: a literature review', *Studies Informing the Framework for the Assessment of Children in Need and Their Families*, London, The Stationery Office. **[Ch. 11]**

Seden, J. (2003) 'Managers and their organisations', in Henderson and Atkinson, pp. 105–31 (K303 Set Book). **[Ch. 11]**

Senge, P. M. (1990) *The Fifth Discipline: The Art and Practice of the Learning Organization*, London, Doubleday/Century Business. **[Chs 1, 3, 4, 5]**

Senge, P., Roberts, C., Ross, R. B., Smith, B. J. and Kleiner, A. (1994) *The Fifth Discipline Fieldbook*, London, Nicholas Brealey. **[Ch. 12]**

Shaw, C. (1998) *Remember My Messages: The Experiences and Views of 2000 Children in Public Care in the UK*, London, The Who Cares? Trust. **[Ch. 5]**

Shaw, C. (2003) 'Remember my messages: the experiences and views of 2000 children in public care in the UK', in Reynolds *et al.*, pp. 229–36 (K303 Reader). **[Ch. 11]**

Sheldon, B. and Chilvers, R. (2000) *Evidence-based Social Care: A Study of Prospects and Problems*, Lyme Regis, Russell House Publishing. **[Ch. 5]**

Shemmings, D. and Shemmings, Y. (2003) 'Supporting evidence-based practice and research-mindedness', in Seden, J. and Reynolds, J. (eds) *Managing Care in Practice*, pp. 111–36, London, Routledge/The Open University (K303 Set Book). **[Ch. 12]**

Shonk, J. H. (1992) *Team-based Organizations: Developing a Successful Team Environment*, Homewood, IL, Business One Irwin. **[Ch. 2]**

Simic, P. (1997) 'Social work, primary care and organisational and professional change', *Research Policy and Planning*, Vol. 15, No. 1, pp. 1–7. **[Ch. 4]**

Smale, G. G. (1996) *Mapping Change and Innovation*, London, National Institute for Social Work. **[Chs 4, 5]**

Smith, C. (1996) *Developing Parenting Programmes*, London, National Children's Bureau. **[Ch. 5]**

Smith, D. M. (2000) 'Women and leadership', in Northouse, P. G. (ed.) *Leadership: Theory and Practice*, pp. 204–36, London, Sage. **[Ch. 3]**

Smith, P. (ed.) (1996) *Measuring Outcomes in the Public Sector*, London, Taylor & Francis. **[Ch. 8]**

Social Services Inspectorate (NI) (1991) *An Abuse of Trust: Report of the Social Services Inspectorate Investigation into the Death of Martin Houston*, Belfast, Her Majesty's Stationery Office. **[Ch. 2]**

Social Services Inspectorate/Association of Directors of Social Services (2002) *Women ... Rising? Achieving Equality and Diversity in Leadership: An SSI/ADSS Sponsored Study of Women in Top Positions*, Bristol, Social Services Inspectorate. **[Chs 3, 11]**

Sorheim, T. A. (1998) *Ordinary Women – Extraordinary Challenges*, University of Oslo, Department of Medical Anthropology. **[Ch. 9]**

South Yorkshire Funding Advice Bureau (2000*) Information Sheets: Voluntary Sector Funding*, Sheffield, SYFAB. www.shef.ac.uk/uni/projects/oip/syfab/infoserv.html [accessed November 2002] **[Ch. 7]**

Statham, D. (2000) 'Guest editorial: partnership between health and social care', *Health and Social Care in the Community*, Vol. 8, No. 2, pp. 87–9. **[Ch. 6]**

Starratt, R. J. (1993) *The Drama of Leadership*, London, Falmer Press. **[Ch. 3]**

Stevenson, O. (1994) 'Child protection: where now for inter-professional work?', in Leathard, A. (ed.) *Going Inter-Professional: Working Together for Health and Welfare*, London, Routledge. **[Ch. 6]**

Stevenson, O. (1995) 'Case conferences in child protection', in Wilson, K. and James, A. (eds) *Child Protection Handbook*, pp. 227–40, London, Ballière Tindall. **[Ch. 9]**

Stewart, R. (1991) *Managing Today and Tomorrow*, Basingstoke, Macmillan. **[Ch. 1]**

Stewart, V. and Stewart, A. (1985) *Managing the Poor Performer*, Aldershot, Gower. **[Ch. 12]**

Stewart, G. L., Manz, C. C. and Sims, H. P. (1999) *Team Work and Group Dynamics*, New York, Wiley. **[Ch. 2]**

Stokes, J. (1994) 'Institutional chaos and personal stress', in Obholzer and Roberts (1994a), pp. 121–8. **[Ch. 2]**

Syer, J. and Connolly, C. (1996) *How Teamwork Works: The Dynamics of Effective Team Development*, Maidenhead, McGraw-Hill. **[Ch. 2]**

Tannen, D. (1995) 'Talking from 9 to 5: how women's and men's conversational styles affect who gets heard, who gets credit, and what gets done at work', in Reynolds *et al.*, pp. 77–44 (K303 Reader). **[Ch. 3]**

Taylor, M. and Vigars, C. (1993) *Management and Delivery of Social Care*, Harlow, Longman. **[Ch. 4]**

Thompson, A. (1999) 'High anxiety', *Community Care*, 1–7 April, pp. 18–9. **[Ch. 12]**

Thornton, P. (2000) *Older People Speaking Out: Developing Opportunities for Influence*, York, Joseph Rowntree Foundation. **[Ch. 5]**

Tichy, N. M. (1997) *The Leadership Engine: How Winning Companies Build Leaders at Every Level*, New York, HarperCollins. **[Ch. 3]**

Tilley, C. M. (1998) *Health Care for Women with Physical Disabilities: Literature Review and Theory, Sexuality and Disability*, Vol. 16, No. 2, pp. 87–102. **[Ch. 9]**

TOPSS England/Care*and*Health (2001) *The First Six Months – A Registered Manager's Guide to Induction and Foundation Standards in Social Care*, London, TOPSS England/Care*and*Health. **[Ch. 2]**

Trinder, L. (2000a) 'Evidence-based practice in social work and probation', in Trinder and Reynolds, Chapter 7, pp. 138–62. **[Ch. 5]**

Trinder, L. (2000b) 'Introduction: the context of evidence-based practice', in Trinder and Reynolds, Chapter 1, pp. 1–16. **[Ch. 5]**

Trinder, L. (2000c) 'A critical appraisal of evidence-based practice', in Trinder and Reynolds, Chapter 10, pp. 212–41. **[Ch. 5]**

Trinder, L. and Reynolds, S. (eds) (2000) *Evidence-Based Practice: A Critical Appraisal*, Oxford, Blackwell Science. **[Ch. 5]**

Tuckman, R. W. (1965) 'Developmental sequence in groups', *Psychological Bulletin*, Vol. 63, No. 6, pp. 384–99. **[Ch. 2]**

Utting, W. (1997) *People Like Us*, London, Department of Health and The Welsh Office. **[Ch. 9]**

Utting, D., Rose, W. and Pugh, G. (2001) *Better Results for Children and Families*, London, National Council of Voluntary Child Care Organisations. **[Ch. 8]**

Vettenburg, N. (1998) *Violence in Schools: Awareness Raising, Prevention and Penalties*, Strasbourg, Council of Europe. **[Ch. 9]**

Vince, R. (1996) *Managing Change: Reflections on Equality and Management Learning*, Bristol, Policy Press. **[Ch. 2]**

Vinkenburg, C. J., Jansen, P. G. W. and Koopman, P. L. (2000) 'Feminine leadership – a review of gender differences in managerial behaviour and effectiveness', in Davidson, M. J. and Burke, R. J. (eds) *Women in Management: Current Research Issues Volume II*, pp. 120–37, London, Sage. **[Ch. 3]**

Waine, B. and Henderson, J. (2003) 'Managers, managing and managerialism', in Henderson and Atkinson, pp. 49–74 (K303 Set Book). **[Ch. 3]**

Walker, S., Shemmings, D. and Cleaver, H. (2001) *Write Enough: Effective Recording in Children's Services* (a Department of Health funded project). www.writeenough.org.uk [accessed September 2002] **[Ch. 5]**

Walsh, J. A. (1987) 'Burnout and values in the social services profession', *Journal of Contemporary Social Work*, May, pp. 279–83. **[Ch. 11]**

Ward, A. (1993) *Working in Group Care: Social Work in Residential and Day Care Settings*, Birmingham, Venture Press. **[Ch. 2]**

Ward, H. (1995) *Looking After Children: Assessing Outcomes*, London, HMSO. **[Ch. 8]**

Ward, B. and Associates (1992) *Good Grief: Exploring Feeling, Loss and Death with Over-11s and Adults* (2nd edn), London, Barbara Ward and Associates. **[Ch. 11]**

Ward, A., McMahon, L., Cain, P. and Howard, T. (1998) 'The function of the staff meeting', in Ward, A. and McMahon, L. (eds) *Intuition Is Not Enough: Matching Learning with Practice in Therapeutic Child Care*, London, Routledge. **[Ch. 2]**

Waterhouse, R. (2000) *Lost in Care: Report of the Tribunal of Inquiry into the Abuse of Children in the Care of the Former County Councils of Gwynedd and Clwyd since 1974*, London, The Stationery Office. **[Ch. 10]**

Watson, T. J. (1994) *In Search of Management: Culture, Chaos and Control in Managerial Work*, London, Routledge. **[Ch. 1]**

Webb, S. A. (2001) 'Some considerations on the validity of evidence-based practice in social work', *British Journal of Social Work*, Vol. 31, pp. 57–79. **[Ch. 5]**

Weber, M. (1947) *The Theory of Social and Economic Organizations*, translated by Henderson, A. M. and Parsons, T., Oxford, Oxford University Press. **[Ch. 3]**

Weiss, J. A. (1981) 'Substance vs. symbol in administrative reform: the case of human services co-ordination', *Policy Analysis*, Vol. 7, Part 1, pp. 21–45. **[Ch. 9]**

West, J. (1997) 'Caring for ourselves: the impact of working with abused children', *Child Abuse Review*, Vol. 6, pp. 291–7. **[Ch. 11]**

Wiener, R. (1997) *Creative Training: Sociodrama and Teambuilding*, London, Jessica Kingsley. **[Ch. 2]**

Wigfall, V. and Moss, P. (2001) *More Than the Sum of Its Parts? A Study of a Multi-Agency Child Care Network*, London, National Children's Bureau. **[Ch. 6]**

Wilde, O. (1892) *Lady Windermere's Fan* (first published 1893), London, E. Mathews and J. Lane. **[Ch. 7]**

Winchester, R. (2001) 'Secret service', *Community Care*, 16–22 August, pp. 20–1. **[Ch. 8]**

Wistow, G. (1990) *Community Care Planning: A Review of Past Experiences and Future Imperatives*, Leeds, Nuffield Institute for Health. **[Ch. 6]**

Worden, J. W. (1991) *Grief Counselling and Grief Therapy*, London, Tavistock. **[Ch. 11]**

Wyre, R. (2000) 'The arena of safety and the aware culture', *Practitioners Guide 10*, RWA Publishing. **[Ch. 10]**

York City Council (2001) *Best Value Performance Plan 2001/2002.* www.york.gov.uk [accessed 20 March 2002]. **[Ch. 7]**

Zalzenik, A. (1993) 'Managers and leaders: are they different?', in Rosenbach, W. E. and Taylor, R. L. (eds) *Contemporary Issues in Leadership* (3rd edn), pp. 36–56, Oxford, Westview Press. **[Ch. 3]**

Web addresses

Department of Health: www.doh.gov.uk **[Ch. 5]**

The Electronic Library for Social Care: www.elsc.org.uk/ksf.htm/researchmindeness/usingthisresource/supporting resources/glossary **[Ch. 5]**

Making Research Count: www.uea.ac.uk/swk/research/mrc/welcome.htm **[Ch. 5]**

NHS Critical Appraisal Skills Programme: www.phru.org.uk/~casp/ **[Ch. 5]**

Research in Practice: www.rip.org.uk/main.html **[Ch. 5]**

Social Care Institute for Excellence: www.scie.org.uk **[Ch. 5]**

Index